Boyd, William
An Introduction to
Science   4th Ed.

DATE DUE			
APR 2 0 1989			
APR 9 1990			

AN INTRODUCTION TO
MEDICAL SCIENCE

An Elementary Text on Pathology

BY

WILLIAM BOYD 1885 —

M.D., Dipl. Psych., M.R.C.P. (Edin.), F.R.C.P. (London), F.R.C.S. (Canada),
LL.D. (Sask.), M.D. (Oslo), F.R.S. (Canada).

Professor of Pathology, University of British Columbia, Vancouver, B. C., Canada

Fourth Edition, Thoroughly Revised,
With 124 Illustrations and 3 Colored Plates

LEA & FEBIGER

PHILADELPHIA

1952

1 6 1
PRACTICAL NURSING

TO

ENID

PREFACE

ANYONE beginning a professional career which is destined to bring him or her in contact with disease, be the work that of the nurse, the laboratory technician, or the physiotherapist, is bound to be overwhelmed by the complexity and multitude of the studies which lie ahead. Anatomy, physiology, bacteriology, medicine and surgery are vast subjects in which one is apt to be submerged so deeply that one loses sight of the disease which afflicts the sick person. The present book is a general introduction to the study of disease, an airplane view of that subject, its causes and the bodily changes which accompany it. When one descends to earth again it is easier to understand the details of the country over which one has flown. With a picture of disease as a whole the nurse should be better able to see the component parts of nursing, why it is she studies anatomy, bacteriology, materia medica, and all the other subjects in the curriculum. The same is true of the laboratory technician and the physiotherapist. Such a survey must necessarily be brief, but this is no disadvantage provided that the fact is recognized. A little knowledge is a dangerous thing, but not if you know how little it is.

The first section of the book deals with the general principles of disease, the second with the diseased organs, and the third with some practical applications. Chapter 1 is intended for those who know nothing. It can be skipped by those who do not belong to this class. There is a brief summary of the structure and function of each organ, but only those facts are mentioned which are essential for understanding the changes that occur in the diseased organ, and the symptoms which these changes produce. Such a summary of course does not in any way replace the use of textbooks dealing with anatomy and physiology. When the pathological changes are understood the symptoms and also the possible complications at once become intelligible. The nurse who understands what a gastric or a typhoid ulcer really is must realize the danger of hemorrhage and perforation. It is hoped that the book will give her a sound beginning, and that it will be in deed as well as in name an introduction to medical science.

In the present revision of the book the most important changes have been those in the sections on treatment. Much of the material in the chapter entitled The Principles of Treatment has been transferred to the sections dealing with specific diseases, and at the same time altered and elaborated.

The antibiotics, the sulfonamides, and cortisone and ACTH have revolutionised our outlook on therapy. My indebtedness to Dr. R. B. Kerr, Professor of Medicine in the University of British Columbia, for assistance in this work is profound. Indeed the word assistance is quite inadequate, for Dr. Kerr has entirely rewritten many of these sections. The chapter formerly entitled The Nurse and the Laboratory has been treated in a similar way, much of the content has been transferred to the body of the book, and the title of the chapter changed to The Collection of Material for the Laboratory. For help in bringing up to date the sections dealing with laboratory tests and the collection of material for these tests I am greatly indebted to Dr. John Eden, in charge of Chemical Pathology at the Vancouver General Hospital. The former chapter on The Prevention of Disease has been omitted, the material being incorporated in the body of the book.

Some of the other principal changes may be enumerated. New sections have been added on congenital heart disease, diseases of arteries, edema, shock, fluid balance, stress, the functions of the adrenal cortex, virus pneumonia, the dust diseases of the lungs, and diseases of the male reproductive system. Much of the descriptive material on bacteria has been omitted from the chapter dealing with that subject, as it is dealt with more adequately in books devoted to bacteriology. A number of new figures and 2 new color plates have been added and some old ones have been replaced. It is hoped and believed that the present edition reflects and embodies the more important of the extraordinary advances in medical science which have been made in the last few years.

WILLIAM BOYD

VANCOUVER, CANADA.

CONTENTS

PART I. SOME GENERAL PRINCIPLES

An Introduction to Medical Science

PART I. GENERAL PRINCIPLES

Chapter

1

THE LIVING BODY

THE human body, that miracle of mechanical perfection, is composed of an infinite number of minute elements known as *cells*, which are collected to form definite structures or *tissues*, these again being grouped into *organs*. Thus certain cells with definite properties are set aside to form muscle tissue, and others with quite different properties to form nervous tissue; these and other tissues are combined to form organs such as the heart and stomach. A tissue consists of cells of the same kind. An organ is composed of tissues of different kinds.

In the earliest stage of development the cells of the embryo are not notably different from one another. Later a finished muscle-cell and a finished nerve-cell and a finished liver-cell are as far apart in visible structure as in what they do. Some of the cells will pour out cement which binds them together, as in cartilage and bone, some become fluid as water so as to flow along tubes too fine for the eye to see. Some become clear as glass, as in the cornea of the eye, some opaque as stone, some colorless, some red, some black. Some become factories of a furious chemistry, some develop into a system transmitting electrical signs. Each one of all the millions upon millions finally specializes into something helpful to the whole. This is the miracle of life and its development.

We have seen that the body is composed of cells as a house is of bricks. But it is as if a house originated from one brick, a magic brick that would set about manufacturing other bricks. These bricks, without waiting for the architect's drawings or the coming of the bricklayers, assemble themselves into walls, and become changed into windowpanes, roofing-slates, coal for heating, and water for the kitchen and the bathroom.

There is a striking contrast between the durability of our body and the transitory character of its elements. Man is composed of a soft matter which can disintegrate in a few hours, and yet he lasts longer than if made of steel. Moreover, he accommodates himself marvelously to the changing conditions of his environment. The body seems to mould itself on events. Instead of wearing out like a machine, it changes.

The cells are the fundamental units of every living body, whether it be animal or vegetable, and in the last analysis it is they that eat the food,

drink the water, and breathe the air which are necessary for the life of the body. The marvellous arrangements of structure (*anatomy*) and function (*physiology*) are simply a complex mechanism to bring to the cells this food, water, and air which are so far beyond their reach, as well as to perpetuate the species to which the organism belongs.

The most important single constituent of the body is water. Life started in the water, for the sea is the original home of all life on the globe; even vertebrate life first appeared as a marine form. It is still lived in water, not, as we fondly imagine, in the air. For the surface of the body in contact with the air is either dead (the horny layers of the skin) or is separated from the air by a layer of water (eyes, nose, and mouth). We carry the memory of the remotely ancient ocean from which we originated in the salt content of the blood plasma and the film of salt water through which we look upon the outside world.

The cells of the body are bathed in salty fluid; without that fluid they cannot live. In many diseases such as cholera this fluid is drained away from the body, the tissues become dehydrated, and they will die unless the fluid is replaced by injections of salt solution.

Hunger can be endured for days or weeks; thirst is unendurable. Lawrence, in *Seven Pillars of Wisdom*, describes death from thirst in the desert: "Not a long death—even for the very strongest a second day in summer was all—but very painful; for thirst was an active malady, a fear and panic which tore at the brain and reduced the bravest man to a stumbling babbling maniac in an hour or two; and then the sun killed him." Such thirst is maddening because the cells of the whole body are crying out for water, not merely the parched mouth. Cannon, the physiologist, paints the picture with vivid accuracy: "A flowing stream brings to the simple organisms fixed on the rocks of the stream bed the food and oxygen needed for existence, and carries away the waste. These single-celled creatures can live only in watery surroundings; if the stream dries they die or enter a dormant state. The same conditions prevail for the incalculable myriads of cells which constitute our bodies. Each cell has needs similar to those of the single cell in the flowing stream. But the body cells are shut away from any chance to obtain food, water, and oxygen from the environment or to discharge the waste materials resulting from their activity. To provide these necessities, moving streams of fluid have been developed to take from the moist surfaces of the body food, water and oxygen, which they deliver to the cells in the remotest nooks of the organism, and from the cells they bring back to the moist surfaces the useless waste to be discharged."

The body fluids are of three kinds: tissue fluid, blood, and lymph. (1) The *tissue fluid* surrounds and bathes the cells; it is immobile, a lake, not a stream (Fig. 1). (2) The *blood* is contained in the bloodvessels, and nowhere comes in direct contact with the tissues except in the spleen. It is carried to an organ in arteries. These break up into a vast network of capillaries through whose infinitely thin walls the fluid of the blood (plasma or serum) is able to pass, mixing with the tissue fluid and carrying it to the food and oxygen which the waiting cells absorb. The capillaries open into the veins, by which the impoverished blood is carried away from the

part. As the tissue fluid is being continually added to, it is obvious that there must be some means of escape. This is provided by (3) the *lymph*, which, like the blood, is contained in a set of vessels, the lymphatics. The tissue fluid laden with waste products from the living cells passes through the thin walls of the lymphatics and is carried away as lymph. This is really a round-about way of getting back into the veins, for all the lymphatics eventually form one or two main ducts which open into the large veins in the neck. The advantage of this method is that the lymph has to pass through a series of filters known as the lymphatic glands or lymph nodes in which bacteria and other injurious agents which may have gained access to the tissue fluid are strained out and usually destroyed. A small proportion of the tissue fluid passes directly back through the walls of the veins into the blood stream.

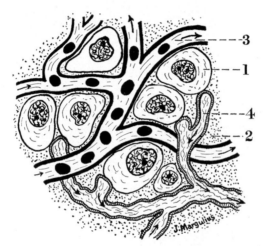

Fig. 1.—Tissue fluid bathing body cells. 1, Tissue cell; 2, tissue fluid; 3, bloodvessel; 4, lymphatic.

It is possible to estimate the rate of passage of water from the vessels into the tissue spaces by injecting some traceable substance, such as a radioactive isotope, into a vein and noting the rapidity with which it disappears from the blood. The rate of exchange shown by this method is incredibly fast, for more than 70 per cent of the water of the blood is exchanged with extravascular water every minute. The walls of the smaller bloodvessels appear to be veritable sieves with regard to water. This is the reason why the older method of using saline solution to replace lost blood was of so little use, and why it has been replaced by the use of blood plasma which remains inside the vessels.

An adequate and constant supply of tissue fluid is necessary for the health of the body cells. If this supply is insufficient or if the fluid is withdrawn too quickly a condition of *dehydration* develops, which can be recognized by the sunken appearance of the face and the wrinkled condition of the skin. This may develop very quickly, as after a night of hard drink-

ing, or in acute diseases associated with severe vomiting or profuse diarrhea. On the other hand, tissue fluid may accumulate in excessive amount, so that the part becomes water-logged, a condition known as *edema*, which can be recognized by the fact that when a finger is pressed into the swollen part a temporary pit is formed owing to the fluid being forced away into the surrounding tissues. Edema may be caused in many ways. (1) In inflammation the walls of the capillaries become unduly permeable and too much fluid passes from the blood into the tissue spaces. (2) In heart and kidney disease edema is an important symptom; its method of production will be considered in connection with these diseases. (3) Pressure on the lymphatics by a tumor will naturally be accompanied by edema.

The *circulatory system* is the mechanism by which fresh material is sent to the tissue fluid and waste material is removed from it. The fresh material is of two kinds, food and oxygen. The food is contained in the blood from the intestine, the oxygen in the blood from the lungs. As the blood has to circulate from the intestine and lungs to the tissue fluid and back again a pump is required. This pump is the heart. Contraction of the muscles helps to force the lymph through the lymphatics. When this is interfered with as the result of disease, massage may take its place. The blood from the tissues is impure. It contains waste products in the form of solid material in solution and gas (carbon dioxide) also in solution. The solid material in solution is excreted, mainly by the kidneys but also by the skin. If the kidneys go on strike the skin may be stimulated to do at least part of the work through increased perspiration. The carbon dioxide in the blood is given off in the lungs and expired; in this way the blood is purified. At the same time oxygen is breathed in and taken up by the blood, as a result of which the color of the blood becomes a much brighter red.

The tissues contain abundant reserves of water, salts, proteins, carbohydrates and fat. These reserves can be used when need arises. Unfortunately oxygen is not stored anywhere; it must be unceasingly supplied to the body by the lungs. That is why the absence of oxygen or anoxia can only be tolerated for the shortest time, and is rapidly fatal to a tissue such as heart muscle and to life itself.

An organ is like a pond completely filled with aquatic plants and fed by a small brook. The water in the pond is almost stagnant, and is polluted by waste products of the plants. The degree of stagnation and pollution depends on the volume and rapidity of the stream. This is the reason why the health of every organ suffers in the condition of prolonged heart disease known as congestive heart failure.

The impure blood from the body is carried to the heart by veins, and is then sent to the lungs to be purified (Fig. 2). The pure blood from the lungs is also carried to the heart by another set of veins. It is evident that if these two kinds of blood were allowed to mix in the heart, the whole object of the circulation would be defeated. The cavity of the heart is therefore divided by a longitudinal partition into two sides, right and left. The right side receives the impure blood from the body and sends it to the lungs. The left side receives the pure blood from the lungs and sends it throughout the body in the arteries. Like any other pump the heart is

provided with valves, so that the blood will always move in one direction. If these are diseased the blood may leak back through the valve with great disturbance to the circulation. The names and arrangment of the valves and of the various chambers of the heart will be considered in connection with diseases of that organ.

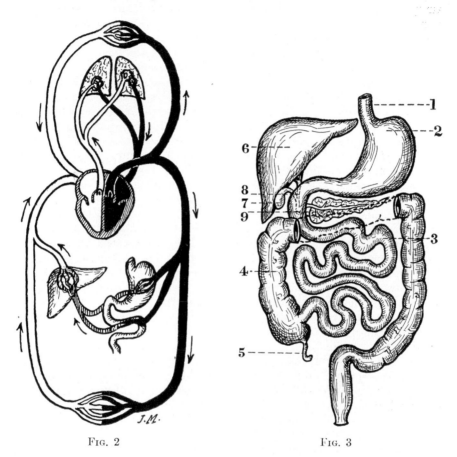

Fig. 2   Fig. 3

Fig. 2.—Diagram of the circulation. The pure arterial blood is black, the portal blood is shaded and the impure venous blood is colorless.

Fig. 3.—Alimentary canal. 1, Esophagus; 2, stomach; 3, small intestine; 4, large intestine; 5, appendix; 6, liver; 7, gallbladder; 8, bile duct; 9, pancreas.

The *respiratory system* is designed to bring air, or rather oxygen, from the outside to the cells in the innermost recesses of the body. The air is inhaled through the trachea or windpipe into the lungs, where it is brought into intimate contact with a vast network of capillaries through the thin walls of which the oxygen is able to pass. It is seized upon by the red blood corpuscles and carried by them throughout the body. When the capillaries of the tissues are reached the oxygen leaves the red blood cor-

puscles, passes through the capillary walls, enters the tissue fluid and is taken up by the cells. The energy of cells is obtained from burning food with oxygen. At the same time the tissues give off one of their waste products in the form of the gas carbon dioxide, which is taken up by the disengaged red blood corpuscles, carried back to the lungs, discharged into the air spaces of those organs, and exhaled into the outside air. Tissue respiration is therefore the real meaning and reason for the rising and falling of the chest which we commonly call respiration.

The *digestive system* is concerned with providing the food which is to be carried by the blood to the tissue fluid for the nourishment of the cells. The tissue fluid must receive its food in the simplest form, analyzed into the *building stones* of the body and the *fuel* which drives the engine. A beefsteak would be out of place in the tissue spaces; the cells would not know what to do with it. The work of preparing the food so that it may be utilized by the tissues is performed by the *alimentary canal* and by certain *digestive glands* which are derived from the alimentary canal and pour their digestive juices into it (Fig. 3). The alimentary canal consists of the *mouth*, where the food is broken up by the teeth and acted on by the saliva, the *esophagus* or gullet which is a mere passageway, the *stomach* where the food is retained for some hours and is acted on by the gastric juice, the *small intestine* where it is further digested and liquefied and from which it is absorbed, and the *large intestine* which conducts the indigestible part of the food to the exterior. The food is converted into a soluble absorbable form by digestive juices which are produced by collections of cells known as *glands*. The glands line the interior of the stomach and intestine and are also collected to form a most important digestive organ, the *pancreas*, which pours its digestive juice into the very beginning of the intestine. *Bile* from the liver also enters the bowel at the same point and assists in the digestion of fats.

The *liver* plays a much more important rôle in the utilization of foodstuffs than merely by the production of bile, which in may respects is simply a waste product. The three main constituents of food are proteins, carbohydrates, and fats. All contain carbon, hydrogen and oxygen, but proteins are also distinguished by possessing nitrogen, which has to be built into the cells to make up for the loss which occurs in the wear and tear of activity. The complex proteins of the food are broken down in the intestine into their simplest elements, the *amino-acids* or building stones of the body, still characterized by the possession of nitrogen. The amino-acids and carbohydrates are absorbed into capillaries in the wall of the small intestine and carried to the liver by the *portal vein*. In the liver the portal vein breaks up into fine capillaries which come into intimate contact with the liver cells, each of which is a little chemical factory. Some of the amino-acids pass on to the heart and are distributed to the tissues where they serve their important function of body building. The rest of the amino-acids lose their nitrogen in the liver, where it is converted into urea, a waste product which reaches the kidneys by the blood stream and is excreted in the urine. The valuable non-nitrogenous portion (carbon and hydrogen) of these amino-acids reaches the tissue cells where it is utilized in the production of energy. This process of breaking down the

protein of food into its constituents and rebuilding these into the tissues of the body is graphically portrayed by Best and Taylor (*The Living Body*) in the following passage: "The utilization of protein in the construction of body tissue may be compared to the building of a number of houses of different types from materials derived from the wrecking of other structures. Each brick and stone in the old buildings must be separated and then sorted and carted to the new sites. Some of this building material will be more suitable for one type of house, some more suitable for other types. Other materials again will not be utilizable at all, and will therefore be discarded as refuse. The new buildings, though constructed from materials taken from the old, will be quite different in structure and in general plan."

The *carbohydrates* of the food are converted in the intestine into glucose or sugar. From the intestine the glucose is absorbed into the capillaries and carried by the portal vein to the liver, where most of it is changed into a storage form known as *glycogen* and retained temporarily in the liver cells. Glucose is one of the important fuels of the body, necessary for muscular action and heat production. When fuel consumption is rapid the carbohydrate depôt, the liver, is called upon to convert some of its glycogen into readily available glucose and give it back to the blood for transportation to the muscles.

Some of the *fats* are carried to the liver by the portal vein; here they are converted into a form more readily utilized. The rest of the fat is absorbed into lymphatic vessels known as *lacteals*, and is carried by the *thoracic duct* to the great veins of the neck, where it enters the general circulation and is stored in the fat depôts of the body.

It will be seen that the journey of the blood stream from the intestine to the tissues is somewhat in the nature of a cafeteria, various additions to the tray being made on the way. Denatured amino-acids, now freed from their nitrogen and therefore no longer deserving of their name, are added by the liver; glycogen is converted into glucose when the storehouse in the liver is called upon by the tissues; oxygen is added as the blood passes through the lungs; and fat is poured into the veins at the root of the neck.

This reference to an organ being "called upon" to do something raises the very important question of how the various highly specialized parts of the body are brought to work together for the common good. What are the integrating influences which make the organs members one of another? They are of two kinds. The one is telephonic or telegraphic in type, urgent in character, demanding instantaneous response; the messengers are *nervous impulses*, electrical in nature, and they are transmitted by the nervous system. The other may be compared to a special delivery service, slower but more detailed in character; the messengers are the *hormones*, chemical instead of electrical in nature, produced by the endocrine or ductless glands, and carried by the blood stream.

The *nervous system* is singularly like a gigantic telephone system. There is a central exchange, an infinite number of wires, and receivers at the end of these wires. The exchange is the brain and spinal cord, known collectively as the *central nervous system*, whilst the wires are represented by the nerves which form the *peripheral nervous system*. Some parts of the system act like automatic telephones without any conscious control;

purely automatic messages are concerned in such functions as the beating of the heart, the contraction of dilatation of the bloodvessels, the swallowing of food, the movement of food along the intestine, the process of childbirth. The automatic messages are carried for the most part by a special set of nerves known as *autonomic* or *sympathetic*, which form the *involuntary nervous system*, although *reflex action* also plays some part in automatic responses.

The greater part of the nervous system is operated on the principle of a non-automatic telephone exchange. On the surface of the body as well as in its interior there are myriads of receivers which when stimulated transmit sensations of various kinds to the spinal cord and thence to the brain, or directly to the brain. These receivers are known as *receptors*, some of which are specialized for the reception of sensations of sight, sound, taste, etc. (the special senses), whilst others respond to stimulation by giving rise to sensations of touch, pain, heat, and cold. These varied sensations are carried to the central nervous system by *afferent* or *sensory nerves*, where they are sorted out and analyzed by the nerve cells of the brain. The sensory nerves form part of the *voluntary nervous system*, the other part of which is constituted by *efferent* or *motor nerves*. These nerves carry electrical messages from the nerve cells of the brain to the muscles, in response to which muscular contraction occurs. The actual stimulus which acts on the muscle fibers is apparently chemical in nature, for chemical substances of various kinds are liberated at the nerve endings when the nerves are stimulated.

The other means by which intercommunication between organs is established is through the agency of the chemical messengers, the hormones. These are produced by the *endocrine* or *ductless glands*. Ordinary glands such as the salivary glands and pancreas pour out their secretion into the mouth or intestine through ducts. The endocrine glands have no ducts, and so discharge their secretion directly into the bloodvessels with which they are in contact. These glands are amongst the most important structures in the body, for they control metabolism and regulate personality. Metabolism is the sum of the building up and breaking down processes of of the body. In addition to controlling metabolism they influence growth and reproduction. The effect which the ductless glands exert on the mind is equally striking, and the difference between endocrine health and disease may mean the difference between the finest mental power and imbecility. The principal endocrine glands are the pituitary at the base of the brain, the thyroid and parathyroids in the neck, the adrenals, the islets of Langerhans (pancreas), and the sex glands in the abdomen.

It would be absurd to attempt even to outline the complex functions of the endocrine organs in this place, but it may be noted that not only do they regulate the behavior of many of the tissues (*e.g.*, the parathyroids determine the amount of lime salts in the bones), but they also influence one another so as to act in harmony. They are like the instruments of a string quartet noted for its perfect ensemble, and the leader of the glandular orchestra is the pituitary, the master gland of the body. The pituitary produces hormones which influence the activity of the thyroid, the parathyroids, the adrenals, and the ovaries, as well as other organs and glands.

The endocrines are stimulated to activity not only by hormones from other endocrine glands but also by nervous stimuli. One simple example of this remarkable interrelationship must suffice. When a person is intensely activated by great rage or great fear he is impelled to immediate muscular activity either for purposes of attack or flight. The muscles are called on to contract to the utmost of their ability, and therefore require a maximum supply of carbohydrate fuel in the shape of glucose. This is lying stored in the liver in the form of glycogen. A nervous stimulus passes from the brain along the nerves to the adrenal glands, and causes them to pour out their hormone, adrenalin. This is carried by the blood to the liver, where it causes the conversion of inert glycogen into active glucose. The glucose is carried by the blood to the muscles, supplying them with the fuel necessary for intense activity.

The *excretory system* is concerned with the removal of waste products from the body. This is brought about by the coöperation of a number of organs, *i.e.*, the intestine, kidneys, skin, and lungs. The *intestine* offers the simplest example of an excretory organ. Food contains elements which are indigestible and cannot be utilized. These are passed on into the lower part of the bowel, the large intestine, from which they are discharged periodically as feces or stools. The *kidney* is a complex structure, the details of which will be considered in a later chapter, but the essential arrangement is not unlike that of the lung, except that fluid instead of gas leaves the blood. The arteries to the kidneys break up into fine capillaries, through the walls of which pass fluid from the blood together with waste substances in solution. The fluid or urine passes into tubules which open into a duct, the ureter; this carries the urine to the bladder, from which it is periodically discharged. The excretory function of the *lungs* has already been indicated. Here the waste product is carbon dioxide which passes through the capillary walls into the air spaces or alveoli of the lungs and is breathed out through the trachea. The *skin* is an excretory organ by virtue of its sweat glands which remove waste substances from the blood and pour them out on the surface in the fluid form of sweat. If the kidneys are not working properly the sweating function of the skin can be stimulated by heat, etc., and thereby relieve the kidneys of part of their load. The skin is a remarkable structure. Despite its thinness it effectively protects the delicate internal structures and fluids against the unceasing variations of external conditions. It is moist, supple, elastic and durable. Its durability is due to its being composed of several layers of cells which continually multiply. These cells die while remaining united to one another like slates on a roof, slates which are continually blown away by the wind and continually replaced by new ones. All the openings in the skin except the nostrils are closed by elastic and contractile rings known as the sphincters. Thus it is the almost perfectly fortified frontier of a closed world.

Reproduction is the most complex of the mechanisms of the body, but in its elements it is essentially simple. In the lowest forms of life, as in such a unicellular organism as the amœba, reproduction is asexual. A line of division is formed along the middle of the cell, and the cellular constituents divide into two, one set passing to one half of the cell, the

2

other set to the other half.   Finally, the line of division becomes complete
and two new individuals are formed.

In all the higher forms of life reproduction is sexual in type, and is brought
about by the union of two cells specially set aside for this purpose, the
male and female elements.   The sex cells are produced by the male and female sex glands or *gonads*, the *testicle* in the male, the *ovary* in the female.
The male sex cells are the *spermatozoa* or sperms, the female sex cells are
the *ova*.   In the human female an ovum is liberated every month from the
ovary, and passes along a duct, the *Fallopian tube*, to reach the *uterus*
or womb, from which it is soon discharged in a flow of blood known as
menstruation.   If impregnation occurs the male elements, the spermatozoa,
ejected by the *penis* into the *vagina*, pass through the uterus and enter the
Fallopian tube.   Should they chance to encounter an ovum on its way
down the tube, one spermatozoön unites with the ovum, the process of
fertilization, and a new individual is formed.   The fertilized ovum continues
on its way down the tube and enters the uterus.   This time, however, it
is not discharged, so that menstruation does not occur.   In the uterus it
develops into an *embryo*, the original single fertilized cell dividing and mul-
tiplying, the resulting cells becoming differentiated and arranged to form
the infinitely varied tissues and organs, until in the fullness of time, nine
months in the case of the human, a child is born.

Chapter

2

THE EVOLUTION OF MEDICAL SCIENCE

THE practice of medicine is an art based on a science. So also is the practice of nursing. Let us review briefly the development of this science. When we look into "the dark backward and abysm of time" we see primitive man terrified by the world around him and ascribing disease, as well as his other misfortunes, to supernatural malevolent forces, to the influence of spirits to be placated by sacrifice. It was the age of the witch doctor, the medicine man, the fetish and amulet, an age which has perhaps even yet not entirely passed away.

The old civilizations of *Egypt* and *Babylon* had their medicine, and developed a knowledge of drugs and methods of embalming. The practice of medicine in Babylon must have demanded care, for we read that if a physician treats a severe wound successfully with a bronze lancet, or opens an abscess of the eye and cures the eye, "he shall take ten shekels of silver"; but if the patient dies of his wound or loses his eye, "one shall cut off his (the physician's) hands." Such a practice would at least encourage conservative methods of treatment.

Jewish medicine developed about the same time as that of Assyria. It was remarkable for its regulations for the prevention of disease and contagion, its hygiene of menstruation and the puerperium, and the establishment of social hygiene, details of which can be read in the Book of Leviticus.

Scientific medicine was born in *Greece* in the fourth century B.C.; it died in Rome six hundred years later; it was resurrected after nearly fifteen hundred years in the Rennaissance or rebirth of learning. Hippocrates was its father, for he separated medicine from mystery and magic, relieved the gods of their responsibility for the prevention and treatment of disease, and laid that burden on the shoulders of man, its proper place. Dawson remarks with truth about Hippocrates that "probably no character in all history has through a single principle exerted so great an influence on civilization, upon the conditions of humans, as did he whom we revere as the father of modern medicine." He developed a system of thorough case-taking. His methods of physical examination are still used. He advocated clean hands and nails and boiled water for operations! He preferred the "vis medicatrix naturæ," the healing power of nature, to drugs.

With the decline of Greece, due in part to the prevalence of malaria, the candle of learning continued to burn feebly in *Rome*. Here progress was marked by practical organization rather than by originality. The outstanding contribution of Roman medicine was sanitation: clean streets, pure water, public baths, sewage disposal—all necessary to public health.

The only great figure thrown up by Roman medicine was Galen, who lived in the second century A.D. He was the real originator of experimental research methods in medicine, but he was dogmatic to a degree, and made facts fit his theories, instead of theories fitting the facts, which is the modern method. His dogmatism was fatal for a thousand years or more, because men soon lost the power of doubting, without which no progress is possible, and regarded his writings as those of an infallible medical Pope.

Galen died in 200 A.D., and in 410 A.D. the German barbarians under Alaric entered Rome. Then the dark night of the Middle Ages fell upon Europe. Medicine ceased to be a science; it again became mystery and magic. Life itself was too precarious for mental development. Even when it became relatively safe, the authority of the Church did not encourage research in medicine, for it was far more interested in the immortal soul than in the frail and mortal body. When men become slaves to authority they lose the power of independent thought, in medicine as in other things. And so the clear stream of scientific medicine was lost in the morass of the Dark Ages. In Osler's moving words: "Following the glory that was Greece and the grandeur that was Rome, desolation came upon the civilized world in which the light of learning burnt low, flickering almost to extinction." The Arabs kept the flame alight, translating many of the Greek and Roman texts, but it was not until the revival of learning and the founding of the universities that this knowledge became available to western Europe.

The *sixteenth century* saw the dawn, for in 1543 Vesalius, a young Italian anatomist, published a textbook of anatomy in which he recorded what he saw and not what authority said that he should see. Ambroise Paré, a great French military surgeon, made surgery an art. He introduced the use of ligatures, the truss in hernia, massage, artificial eyes, and other innovations. His most famous aphorism: "I dressed the wound; God healed it."

The *seventeenth century* was marked by one of the greatest advances in the whole history of medical science, the discovery of the circulation of the blood by William Harvey, an English physician, in 1628. It is difficult to picture medical thought without this vital information. The function of respiration, diseases of the heart, hemorrhage, embolism, the spread of infection, the distribution of tumor metastases by the blood stream, and a host of other phenomena would be unintelligible without the magic words of Harvey: "I began to think whether there might not be a movement, *as it were in a circle*." As usually happened in those days, the epochmaking discovery was greeted with ridicule and abuse. In reality it formed the beginning of modern medical science. The great practitioner of this century was Sydenham, who has been called the English Hippocrates. He was not interested in theories or experiment, but if you fell sick in those days with one of the infectious fevers, you would do better with Sydenham than with Harvey as your physician.

In the *eighteenth century* there was little of the stirring of spirit and uprush of new ideas which characterized the seventeenth. This was a period of consolidation, an age of criticism rather than discovery in medicine, of philosophers and philosophizing. There were many gifted clinical ob-

servers, Laennec in France, Addison, Bright and a host of others in England. The great Italian observer, Morgagni, really founded pathological anatomy, for he systematically explained the symptoms of disease by changes which he found in the diseased body. But two men of this period stand out from the others as imbued with the true spirit of research. These are John Hunter and Edward Jenner. We have seen that Paré in the sixteenth century made surgery an art. Two hundred years later Hunter, an extraordinary and turbulent personality, made it a science. He correlated surgery for the first time with physiology and pathology, and introduced a spirit of scientific enquiry which had been entirely lacking in surgical practice. So great was his influence that it is no exaggeration to say that surgery may be divided into two periods, before Hunter and after Hunter; but the surgery was still only the surgery of the surface of the body and the extremities. Jenner, by introducing vaccination against smallpox, was the founder of preventive medicine, as well as one of the greatest benefactors of mankind. Some idea of the ravages and prevalence of the disease which he did so much to eradicate may be gained from the old saying "mothers counted their children only after they had had the smallpox." In spite of rapid strides made in the eighteenth century in chemistry and physics, anatomy and physiology, there was no real advance in the actual treatment or prevention of disease over that which was available to the patient in the time of Hippocrates. Nor was there any true knowledge of the nature of the *causes* of disease.

The *nineteenth century* dawned with no indication of the stupendous and revolutionary discoveries which it had in store. As late as the end of the eighteenth century the kings and queens of England and France still "touched for the King's Evil," *i.e.*, laid their healing hands on those suffering from scrofula (tuberculous glands in the neck)! The first forty years were quiet, but in the remaining years of that century medicine advanced further than in the entire course of recorded history. It was a triumph for the application of experimental methods to medical problems. Time now has to be reckoned not in centuries but in decades.

1840–1850. In 1846 Morton demonstrated to an audience of Boston doctors that ether would abolish the pain of a surgical operation. In the following year Sir James Young Simpson of Edinburgh introduced chloroform to relieve the pain of childbirth as well as for general surgery. For the first time in the world's history it was possible for a surgeon to operate without inflicting terrible anguish on his patient.

1850–1860. Nursing is as old as the human race, but in this decade Florence Nightingale organized it, made it a profession, and one for trained gentlewomen. In the early Victorian period the level of nursing had sunk very low indeed. "The hospitals were dirty; the patients poorly cared for. Actual nursing was relegated to a degraded type of woman of low intelligence, often dissolute, still more often dishonest—the type that Dickens has portrayed as Sairey Gamp" (Haggard). How incredible a change to the modern nurse, that compound of science and sympathy! In this same decade some of the most valued medical instruments of precision were invented; the ophthalmoscope by von Helmholtz, a German professor of physics, the laryngoscope by Manuel Garcia, a Spanish teacher

of singing in London. Darwin's "Origin of Species" was published, and Virchow's "Cellular Pathology." Virchow is the father of modern pathology as we know it, for he showed for the first time that the underlying structural changes in disease are to be found, not in the organ as a whole, but in the cellular elements of which the organ is composed; what the molecule is to the chemist and the electron to the physicist, the diseased cell has been to the pathologist since Virchow.

1860–1870. The greatest discovery in the long history of medical science, namely the rôle which bacteria play in the causation of disease, was made in this and the following decades. The existence of bacteria was well known. They had been guessed at by Kircher in the seventeenth century, and seen and accurately described by the Dutchman Leeuwenhoek later in the same century. For our knowledge of the overwhelming importance of bacteria as agents of disease we are indebted to three men, a Frenchman, Louis Pasteur, an Englishman, Joseph Lister, and a German, Robert Koch. Pasteur was a chemist, not a physician, but he became interested in the problem as to why wine spoils, and he came to the conclusion that the fermentation of wine and beer was due to the action of living bacterial agents. From this he was led to the study of putrefaction, *i.e.*, the decomposition of meat and other dead organic material. This was again found to be due to the same living agents, and the process could be prevented by heating organic fluids, such as milk, to a temperature below the boiling point, the procedure now known as pasteurization. At this time the surgeon, Joseph Lister, afterwards Lord Lister, was pondering on the problem of wound infection following surgical operations, which rendered the most brilliant operation worse than useless, and gave origin to the popular gibe "the operation was successful but the patient died," when he came across Pasteur's work. At this time the mortality from operations, now frequent owing to the use of anesthetics, was appalling. At least 45 per cent of amputations resulted in death from septicemia, pyemia and gangrene. Lister had previously realized that putrefaction of dead organic material and infection of wounds were intimately related, and now he saw in one lightning flash that if putrefaction was bacterial in origin, so also was wound infection. Destruction of bacteria in infected wounds (antisepsis), and later exclusion of bacteria from the field of operation (asepsis), wrought a revolution in surgery so far-reaching, so overwhelming, that surgery as we know it today is essentially the gift of Lister to humanity. His work alone made possible the surgery of the abdomen, chest, brain and joints, as well as rendering a hundredfold more safe operations on the limbs and the practice of obstetrics.

In this same wonderful decade there is evidence of an awakening social conscience in medical matters in the founding of the International Red Cross by a Swiss, Henri Dunant, an organization designed to help sufferers in war and great natural disasters.

1870–1880. This is the decade of bacteriological advance. Pasteur and Koch are the two supreme figures. Koch, at first a German country practitioner, may be regarded as the founder of modern bacteriology, for he introduced the methods of bacteriological investigation, such as the use of pure cultures and special stains, which are employed at the present day.

In this decade a large number of infectious diseases (as opposed to wound infections) were shown to be due to specific bacteria. Pasteur also introduced the idea of ultramicroscopic filterable viruses, agents of disease so small that they could not be seen with the microscope and were able to pass through the finest filter, although ordinary bacteria were held back by such a filter.

1880–1890. The two outstanding discoveries of this period were preventive inoculation against disease, and the fact that the microscopic animal parasites known as protozoa may cause widespread epidemics. Jenner's discovery in 1798 of the value of vaccination against smallpox (now known to be a virus disease) was an isolated miracle which led to no further advances. Pasteur now introduced the principle of preventive inoculation by means of "vaccines" against bacterial and virus disease. In the war of 1914–1918 hundreds of thousands of men were saved from illness and death from typhoid fever by means of inoculation. The discovery of protozoa as agents of disease was of special importance in the case of malaria, the most widespread disabling and killing disease in the world. It was Laveran, a French Army doctor, who first discovered the malaria parasite.

1890–1900. The nineteenth century ends with a tremendous burst of activity in scientific medicine, but only three outstanding achievements can be mentioned here. These are the discovery of x-rays and radium and their application to medicine; the treatment of infectious disease by antitoxins; and the discovery of the insect transmission of disease. The use of the x-rays has revolutionized diagnosis in every region of the body, and radiations either of this type or those of radium constitute the greatest recent advance in the treatment of many forms of cancer. The first and the most successful of the antitoxins was against diphtheria, but serum treatment, especially of tetanus, pneumonia and scarlet fever, is becoming more and more important. The demonstration that infection can be carried by insects was one of the most important contributions ever made to preventive medicine. We know now that the mosquito carries malaria and yellow fever, the flea bubonic plague, the louse typhus, the tse-tse fly sleeping sickness, and so on. Haggard, in his delightful little book, "Mystery, Magic, and Medicine," sums up the effect of these discoveries as follows: "Six hundred years ago men believed that disease was due to the wrath of the gods; they prayed—and died. Three hundred years ago they believed it due to meteorological disturbances and contaminated air; they closed their windows at night and burned coal and powder in the streets—and died. Today we turn from such omniscient powers as the gods and the weather to prosaic matters such as exterminating of the mosquito, the killing of the rat and its fleas, and the delousing of the traveller—and we live free from plague, malaria and yellow fever."

As regards the *twentieth century* the most striking achievements of medical science so far may be grouped under the three headings of chemotherapy, organotherapy, and the discovery of the importance of dietary factors in the causation of disease. The great advances in what may be called social medicine lie outside the scope of this review.

The first triumph of *chemotherapy* was with respect to syphilis, and in the first decade of the new century the spotlight was directed on that disease. At that time the cause was unknown, accurate diagnosis was difficult and often impossible, and treatment was unsatisfactory and inefficient. Incredible though it may appear these three problems were solved in the space of five years. In 1905 Schaudinn discovered the cause of syphilis (Spirochæta pallida), in 1906 Wassermann introduced his famous blood test, and in 1910 Ehrlich demonstrated that arsenical preparations provide a specific treatment against the disease. Seeing that these preparations have a direct action on the spirochete of syphilis, it was hoped that other chemicals would soon be found which would have a similar action on other bacteria. No major success attended repeated efforts until 1935, when the sulfonamide group of agents, the so-called sulfa drugs, were introduced. This produced a revolution in the treatment of bacterial infections. An even more remarkable discovery was that of the dramatic effectiveness of penicillin in 1940. The sulfonamides are synthetic chemicals invented and manufactured in the chemist's laboratory. Penicillin, on the other hand, is a substance naturally produced by one of the common green molds growing in nature, called Penicillium notatum. As it prevents the growth of certain bacteria it is known as an antibiotic. Penicillin was followed by streptomycin, which acts on another group of bacteria, and later by aureomycin, terramycin and chloromycetin. All of these antibiotics have their particular use, which will be described later. Both penicillin and the sulfonamides are not antiseptic or rather bactericidal for they do not kill bacteria directly; they are bacteriostatic, that is to say they inhibit the growth of the bacteria, thus leaving them an easy prey to the defensive forces of the body. These dramatic and epoch-making therapeutic advances are due to the entry of chemistry into medicine, one of the most important features of twentieth century progress.

Organotherapy, i.e., treatment by the administration of organs or extracts of organs, has also made great advances, particularly in the field of endocrine diseases. In the days when medicine was compounded of mystery and magic primitive man ate the heart of a lion to make him brave. Now, with considerably more satisfactory results, he eats liver so that he may recover from pernicious anemia, that hitherto invariably fatal disease, or receives injections of extract of the thyroid gland for myxedema, or insulin (the extract of the pancreas first prepared by Banting) for diabetes. Hormones from the sex glands, especially those of the female, are extensively used in the practice of gynecology. The most recent and exciting of the hormones are those obtained from the cortex of the adrenal gland (cortisone), and the hormone of the pituitary (ACTH) which stimulates the production of the adrenal hormone.

Dietetics is largely a twentieth century product, although scurvy, that scourge of armies and navies, had already been conquered by fruit juice. Knowledge of vitamins and the mineral requirements of food is extremely modern. It is of importance in the prevention rather than the cure of disease, and will go far to the future physical betterment of the race.

In this lightning review of the development of medical science far, far more has been omitted than has been mentioned. Only a few men and a

few supreme achievements have been picked out. The aim has been to show the different position of the sick person now compared with that in bygone days. The healing art from the humblest beginnings has developed into the greatest benefactor of mankind, but this development of the art has been entirely due to the progress of medical science. The leaves of its tree are for the healing of the nations. This wonderful story of progress affects the nurse no less than the doctor, and it is therefore fitting that she should at least be aware of its existence.

REFERENCES

DAVIDSON, L. S. P.: The evolution of modern medicine, with special reference to medical research, Edin. Med. Jour., *38*, 113, 1931.
DAWSON, BERNARD: The History of Medicine: A Short Synopsis, London, 1931.
HAGGARD, H. W.: Mystery, Magic, and Medicine, New York, 1933.
OSLER, SIR WILLIAM: The Evolution of Modern Medicine, London, 1921.

Chapter

3

THE NATURE AND CAUSES OF DISEASE

It is singularly difficult, indeed impossible, to give a concise definition of disease. Health is a state in which the body is in complete harmony with its surroundings; disease is the opposite, a condition of discomfort or dis-ease. In other words, health is harmony, disease discord. This conception, however, refers to the *clinical* or bedside aspect, the question of symptoms. There is another aspect, that of *lesions* or structural changes in the organs. The study of lesions forms part of the science of *pathology*. Only part however, for pathology may be defined as that branch of medicine which deals with the essential nature of disease. It might be thought that these two would go hand in hand, and usually this is true. The pain of acute appendicitis corresponds with the acutely inflamed appendix, the cough of a tuberculous patient is due to the tuberculous lesion in the lung. But there may be symptoms without lesions, just as there may be lesions without symptoms. The presence of lesions distinguishes *organic disease* in which there are definite observable changes in the organs from *functional disease* in which there is some temporary disturbance of function without any corresponding organic change. The nervous system offers some of the best examples of functional disease. In this book we shall concern ourselves only with organic disease, although at the same time considering the disturbances of function which are produced by the lesions in the organ.

The causes of disease are known as the etiological factors: *etiology* is causation. The outcome of disease will vary between the extremes of complete recovery and death. This outcome is *prognosis*; it is a forecast of what may be expected to happen. *Diagnosis* is the art of determining not only the character of the lesion but also its etiology. It is often difficult, but accurate prognosis is much more difficult and calls forth the very highest powers of the physician. It is largely the result of experience and judgment.

Disease processes and the lesions which accompany them may be divided into three main groups: (1) *Inflammation* due to bacterial and other irritants, (2) *degenerative changes* due to insufficient food supply to the organs and tissues or to the action of poisons on them, and (3) *tumors*.

Bacteria.—By far the commonest cause of disease is bacteria. These properly belong to the vegetable kingdom, but certain lowly forms of animal life known as the *animal parasites* may also live in the body and produce disease. Finally there are *filterable viruses*, forms of living matter so minute that they pass through the pores of filters fine enough to hold

back bacteria, so tiny that they cannot be seen with the most powerful microscope, and are therefore said to be ultramicroscopic. This last group has attracted a great deal of attention in recent years.

Bacteria, microörganisms or germs can be divided into three main groups: (1) cocci which are round; (2) bacilli which are rod-shaped; and (3) spirilla or spirochetes which are spiral like a corkscrew. They produce disease either by their presence in the tissues or by producing toxins (poisons) which either act on the surrounding structures or are carried by the blood stream to distant organs; in both instances they cause inflammation and degeneration.

It would be useless to give in this place a list of the bacteria which may cause disease, for it would be merely a list of names with little meaning. Many of these are considered in Chapter 6 (Some Bacterial Infections), and others in connection with the organs which they are most prone to attack.

Ischemia.—Loss of blood supply to a part is called ischemia. This is a local loss of blood, in contrast to anemia which is a general condition of bloodlessness affecting the entire body. As the food and oxygen are carried by the blood it is evident that if the supply of blood is diminished by narrowing of the lumen of an artery, the part of the body deprived of its blood supply will suffer and become diseased. An example of this is seen in arteriosclerosis (hardening of the arteries) of the vessels supplying the leg; the tissues of the foot will finally die, a condition known as *gangrene*. An even more important example of ischemia is blockage of the coronary arteries to the heart muscle either by arteriosclerosis or thrombosis, resulting either in sudden death or in permanent damage to the heart.

Overwork or Overstrain.—Overwork or overstrain is an occasional cause of disease. It is best seen in the heart, which may be permanently damaged by the chronic strain thrown upon it by prolonged high blood-pressure.

The concept of *stress*, although an old one, has reasserted itself through the work of Selye. This will be discussed in connection with the endocrine glands. Here it may be said that stress of various kinds, both physical and mental, may upset the normal hormonal balance, especially that between the pituitary and adrenal, with resultant disturbance of health. This far-reaching concept has aroused widespread interest. Health indeed may be regarded as the result of success in the ceaseless struggle between man and his environment, and much of this struggle is with stress. The outcome of the struggle depends largely on the adrenal cortex, itself controlled by the pituitary. When the stress is continued over too long a period, the adrenals become exhausted.

Trauma.—Trauma or injury may damage a part to such an extent that the tissues may be killed. Trauma may take the form of a blow, a wound, or a sprain to a joint. Lesser degrees of trauma cause inflammation.

Temperature and Radiation.—Excessive heat or cold, and radiation in the form of x-rays or radium, may damage or kill the tissues, with resulting burns, frost-bite, or radiation necrosis. It must be borne in mind that radiation, so valuable for destroying cancer cells, can also destroy normal tissue more certainly and extensively than any other known agent. What is powerful for good is also potent for evil.

Poisons.—Poisons provide another example of this truth. Many of our most useful drugs, such as strychnine, arsenic, and digitalis, are stimulants in small doses but poisons in large amount. The same is, of course, true of alcohol.

Heredity.—Heredity is a factor in the causation of disease the importance of which is recognized by life insurance companies. If one has the misfortune to inherit poor materials from one's ancestors the machine constructed from those materials can never be first class, and the "causes of disease" may wreck that machine, whereas they might have little effect on one of high grade. In most diseases, certainly in all bacterial infections, there are two factors to be considered, an extrinsic or external factor, such as the bacillus of tuberculosis, and an intrinsic or internal factor, which we may call the constitution of the patient, the body's power of defense, etc. It is a question of the seed and the soil. If the soil is suitable, even a minute quantity of seed will grow abundantly and bring forth a rich harvest of disease. Some people get every infection that is going around, whilst others never seem to be ill. Much of this is a question of heredity.

Constitution.—The constitution comprises those features of the mind and body that a man derives from heredity and upbringing. It is the sum total of his being. There can be little doubt that nutrition is a factor of great importance, especially in the early formative years of life. Every day and every hour the cells of the body are taking up elements from the food, including vitamins, and if these are deficient in quantity or quality the constitution as a whole cannot fail to suffer. It has been said, with what truth I am unable to tell, that if all the diseases now described in the textbooks could be removed by the wave of a wand, doctors would still be left with 80 per cent of their patients. Their ill-health would be due not so much to any known disease as to the failure of the constitution to adapt itself to the life led. A good constitution is not to be confused with a good physique; it is something more and something more valuable. Those who have it seem able to do whatever they wish without impairing it in any way. When it is poor, small causes may impair health or even endanger life. The athlete with the most perfect physique may be attacked by every infection which he encounters, and may early develop arteriosclerosis and other degenerative conditions. Constitution can be divided into the hypersthenic, the hyposthenic and the normal. The hypersthenic individual is bubbling over with energy; he is the man of action. The hyposthenic may be the very reverse of this, but it is this group which supplies the great thinkers. It is obvious that a doctor must distinguish between these groups if he is going to give advice of value as to the way of life which a patient should follow.

It is sometimes said that the nature of disease is changing, that we hear much more about people dying of heart failure and cancer than used to be the case. This does not mean that these diseases have become actually more common, although more people do die from them. Long ago Addison, in the *Vision of Myrza*, drew a picture of the great masses of mankind walking over the bridge of life which spans the dark river of death. In the bridge there were many hidden trapdoors through which the unwary travellers dropped into the flood below. Their numbers became ever fewer

as they approached the far side, but none succeeded in completing the journey. The trapdoors represent diseases. At the near end of the bridge there are many trapdoors—infantile mortality, typhoid, malaria, small-pox—which have been so securely closed by medical science that they seldom open now. But at the far end there is a small number of wide trap-doors—cancer, heart failure, apoplexy—and great numbers must fall through these into the dark flood of oblivion.

DEFICIENCY DISEASES

The idea that disease may be due to something lacking rather than to some positive hostile factor such as bacteria, injury, or poison, is a comparatively new one, but enormously important and far-reaching. It has, of course, always been recognized that starvation will affect the health of the body and will eventually result in death. But there may be an insufficient supply of some particular element in the food, such as proteins, carbohydrates and fats. Even more important as a cause of disease is an inadequate supply of minerals and of the essential food factors known as vitamins. Even though actual disease may not be present, *perfect* health is impossible if there are deficiencies in the food. This is particularly true of the growing period of life.

With every year that passes the importance of nutritional deficiencies is becoming more apparent. It is the quality rather than the quantity of the food that is essential. During starvation the demands of the body are so much lowered that true deficiency disease may not become apparent. But if the food is abundant, particularly in carbohydrates, but deficient in minerals or vitamins, the health of the cells is impaired and evidence of disease becomes manifest.

The most obvious method of production of nutritional deficiency is lack in certain elements in the diet. But the same result may be brought about in a number of other ways. If a patient suffers from persistent vomiting he cannot assimilate his food, no matter how excellent it may be. Such conditions as gastric ulcer and diabetes may necessitate the long-continued use of diets which may be deficient in particular food elements. Widespread disease of the intestine, commonly associated with diarrhea, may interfere so seriously with the absorption of food that deficiency must result. Even when satisfactory absorption has occurred, such an important digestive organ as the liver may be unable to deal with the food elements owing to cirrhosis, etc., and once again symptoms of deficiency may appear. This list, which could be extended considerably, will indicate how readily a condition of dietary deficiency may arise.

Resistance to infection appears to depend to some extent on the food supply, and particularly on the proteins, for it is from proteins that antibodies to bacteria are manufactured. It is for this reason that a state of chronic starvation is associated with a greatly lowered resistance to such infections as tuberculosis. A tragic demonstration of this fact is provided by the high incidence of tuberculosis and other serious infections amongst the peoples of Europe impoverished by a great war.

The earlier work on food deficiency, particularly vitamin deficiency, was concerned with what may be termed full-blown diseases such as scurvy, rickets and beri-beri. It is now realized that minor manifestations of deficiency are much more common, though they have been overlooked in the past. In certain localities, where for geographic or economic reasons there is a grave lack of such essential foods as milk and fresh vegetables, a large proportion of the population may exhibit symptoms and signs of deficiency disease, though they may be quite unconscious of that fact.

The minerals and vitamins have been called the *"protective elements"* of the diet, and they are really more important than proteins, carbohydrates and fats, which are energy foods necessary for running the engine. Without the protective foods a child cannot enjoy buoyant as compared with merely satisfactory health.

Mineral Deficiency

The three important minerals are calcium, iron, and iodine. *Calcium* is necessary both for the formation and the continued health of bone. If it is deficient in the diet during early childhood there is danger that *rickets* may develop; the bones which are deficient in calcium are soft and easily bent, so that bow-legs and other deformities develop. In adult life calcium deficiency may also lead to softening of the bones or *osteomalacia* (the same thing in Greek). *Iron* is absolutely necessary for the health of the red blood corpuscles, and when it is deficient in the diet *anemia* or bloodlessness inevitably develops. As will be seen when diseases of the blood are studied, anemias are now divided into iron-deficiency anemias and other forms of anemia. It is of interest to note that the most important member of the latter group, pernicious anemia, is also a deficiency disease. *Iodine* is essential to the proper functioning of the thyroid gland, and when it is deficient one form of *goiter* develops. Although minerals are so essential for the health of the body, the actual amounts needed are extraordinarily minute. For instance, the amount of iodine needed to prevent the development of goiter is only 10 to 20 mg. *a year*.

In addition to the three minerals which have been described there is a host of others which cannot even be mentioned, although an exception may be made in the case of potassium and phosphorus.

There is a curious relationship between mineral metabolism and the ductless glands, which will be discussed in more detail when diseases of those organs are considered. Iodine metabolism is regulated by the thyroid gland, and as we have just seen, lack of iodine will cause disease of the thyroid, just as disease of the gland will cause disturbed iodine metabolism. The parathyroid glands bear the same relation to calcium metabolism, and more recently it has been discovered that the adrenals govern the metabolism of sodium chloride.

Vitamin Deficiency

An adequate supply of protein, carbohydrate, fat and mineral salts is not sufficient for the needs of the living body. Certain "accessory food

factors" are also necessary for life. These are therefore called vitamins. They are formed or synthetized by plants, not by animals. Man's supply therefore comes directly from plants, or from animals (including fish) which have eaten the plants and stored up the vitamins. They need only be present in minute amounts, but their absence (avitaminosis) leads to profound pathological changes. Some of these deficiency diseases such as rickets and scurvy have been known for centuries. Although it was not recognized that they were due to a simple deficiency in diet, empirical methods of treatment were successfully employed. The old explorers recognized the value of fresh fruit in the prevention of scurvy, and cod-liver oil has been used in the treatment of rickets for more than a hundred years.

The original list of four vitamins (A, B, C, D) has been extended to thirteen, and the end is not in sight. Moreover vitamin B, a complex, has been separated into a number of distinct chemicals. With such complexity, the alphabetical system of names has broken down, and the chemical names have come into general use. An exception to this rule are vitamins A and D, which are not manufactured chemically, but are sold as concentrates from fish-liver oils. Originally all the vitamins were obtained from animal or vegetable sources, but now they are produced synthetically in the chemical laboratory. The mystery which used to shroud the nature of the vitamins has therefore largely disappeared.

Vitamin A.—This is a fat-soluble vitamin, so that it is found in butter, cream, egg yolk, fish-liver oils, as well as in yellow and green vegetables such as carrots, spinach, peas and beans. The plants do not really contain vitamin A, but a yellow pigment called carotene which is converted by the liver into the vitamin. The vitamin A content of milk and butter depends on the carotene content of the plants the animal eats. Even the vitamin in fish-liver oil comes from marine plants (plankton). Minute invertebrates feed on the plants; they are devoured later by small fish; these in turn serve as food to large fish in whose livers the vitamin is stored.

Lack of vitamin A in the diet leads to degeneration of the epithelium lining mucous membranes in the respiratory and digestive tracts as well as in certain glands such as the lachrymal and salivary. Such mucous surfaces are especially susceptible to infection. In children, in whom the deficiency is most likely to develop, drying of the cornea, known as *xerophthalmia* (*xeros*, dry) may occur, due to lack of secretion of the lachrymal glands. This may lead to ulceration of the cornea and subsequent blindness. Bronchopneumonia in children may be caused by the changes in the mucous membrane of the bronchial tree. A peculiar symptom is night blindness, or inability to see in a dim light. This due to deficiency in visual purple of the retina, a substance necessary for vision in poor light.

Under ordinary conditions of life vitamin A deficiency is seldom seen in Europe and North America, although quite common in India, China and other countries where the diet is often of low quality. Where war brings restrictions in diet, however, night blindness and xerophthalmia may become common, the former being particularly dangerous during blackouts. Governments have recognized this to such an extent that they have added vitamin A to bread when necessary.

The Vitamin B Complex.—One of the earliest discoveries regarding vitamins was that beri-beri, a disease of the Orient, was due to eating "polished" rice, *i.e.*, rice from which the outer covering and the germ had been removed in the milling process. The vitamin responsible was called vitamin B. It is now known that what was thought to be a single vitamin is really a complex, from which a number of components have been separated. The three best known of these are thiamin, niacin, and riboflavin. The chief sources of the vitamin B complex are yeast and cereals, particularly wheat-germ.

Thiamin (formerly vitamin B_1) is the antiberi-beri factor. The principal features of *beri-beri* are peripheral neuritis (marked by weakness of the limbs), widespread edema, and myocardial weakness. When rice is polished the skin and the germ which contain the vitamin are removed, so that in rice-eating countries such as China beri-beri is a common disease. Thiamin is now added to enriched white flour, to restore what is lost from the whole wheat in milling.

Riboflavin (formerly vitamin B_2) is also desirable for the enrichment of bread, but the supply is still small. Mild symptoms of its absence (ariboflavinosis) are not uncommon among the undernourished and those women who subsist on absurdly inadequate diets with the object of improving their figure. Severe manifestations are seen principally in the southern states of America and in Newfoundland. There may be fissured lesions at the corners of the mouth (cheilosis) and erosions around the eyes and the sides of the nose. The tongue may acquire a characteristic magenta color. The most serious disturbances are those involving the eye. In persons whose occupation exposes them to bright light, including workers with the microscope, there may be eye strain and redness of the conjunctiva and the lower lids. In advanced cases there is invasion of the cornea by capillaries. In the past these ocular symptoms were never attributed to the real cause, namely, vitamin deficiency. The principal source of riboflavin is milk.

Niacin (formerly nicotinic acid) is the pellagra-preventing vitamin. *Pellagra* is a disease common in Italy and the southern United States, but not confined to these regions. It is characterized by reddening and scaling of the skin on the exposed parts of the body, as well as gastrointestinal, nervous and mental disorders. The tongue may become smooth and fiery red. Although a deficiency disease, it is also in some way connected with eating diseased maize.

Other constituents of the former B complex are pyridoxin and pantothenic acid. Not enough is known about their physiological action to justify discussion here.

Vitamin C (Ascorbic Acid).—This is the antiscorbutic vitamin, which prevents scurvy or scorbutus. It occurs in fruits and fresh vegetables rather than in fats. It is particularly abundant in tomato, orange, lemon, and grapefruit. It is destroyed by heat and drying, so that preserved foods and fruits are lacking in it. In vitamin C deficiency the level of ascorbic acid is low in the urine and very low in the blood. By estimation of this level deficiency of the vitamin can be readily detected.

When ascorbic acid is lacking the cement substance, which holds together the endothelial cells lining the capillaries, becomes deficient. The vessels thus develop leaks through which bleeding occurs into the tissues.

Scurvy or scorbutus is the great manifestation of vitamin C deficiency. It used to be a common disease amongst sailors, soldiers, arctic explorers, and others deprived of fresh fruit and vegetables. The old Elizabethan seaman, Captain Hawkins, called it "the plague of the sea and the spoil of mariners," adding that "the sea is natural for fishes and the land for men." That was all changed by Captain Cook's discovery that limes and lime juice would prevent the disease, and now even that is not necessary, for the vitamin can be put up as tablets of ascorbic acid.

Hemorrhage occurs owing to lack of cement substance in the capillaries. The gums are soft, spongy, bleed readily and are heavily invaded by bacteria, whilst the teeth fall out, so that the condition of the mouth becomes foul and very distressing. The skin presents numerous small hemorrhages (petechiæ). There is hemorrhage into the joints and the internal organs. If the condition is not relieved it will end fatally.

Infants who are artificially fed may develop infantile scurvy (*Barlow's disease*), of which the chief symptom is extreme tenderness of the legs due to hemorrhage under the periosteum of the tibia. The disease should never occur, as it can so readily be prevented by including tomato or orange juice in the feedings.

Vitamin D.—Much of the romance of the vitamins centers around this member of the group. Several factors are concerned in the action of this vitamin, and the unraveling of these might easily have taken half a century, but the whole problem was cleared up in little more than half a dozen years by workers in many widely separate countries.

Vitamin D is the antirachitic vitamin; it prevents rickets or rachitis. It does this by controlling calcium metabolism. It is a fat-soluble vitamin, so, as might be expected, it is found in milk, butter, egg yolk, and other fats, but by far the most abundant supply is in cod-liver oil.

One of the most remarkable discoveries was that the vitamin is formed by the action of ultra-violet light on certain waxy compounds known as sterols, particularly ergosterol, found in yeast, and cholesterol, present in the skin. When the skin is exposed to abundant sunlight, a sufficient amount of the vitamin is formed from the cholesterol. In darkened gloomy climates, however, and in the slums of cities, there is not enough light to form the vitamin. It is prepared commercially by irradiating yeast, which is rich in ergosterol, by the mercury vapor lamp, and is then called *viosterol*. The vitamin has been synthetized in the laboratory; it is a yellow crystalline substance, which has been named calciferol because of its influence on calcification.

Without a sufficient sypply of vitamin D the proper calcification of bone in the child cannot take place, and rickets is the result. It is also required for the formation of normal teeth in the growing child. Marked deficiency of the vitamin is rare in adults, but when present it may produce *osteomalacia* or softening of the bones. This disease is more likely to be seen in such countries as India and China, where the diet is deficient, and commonest in women who are little exposed to sunlight in these countries.

3

Rickets or rachitis is a disease of young children. The bones are not properly formed, owing to insufficient deposition both of calcium and phosphorus. The bones are therefore soft and bend easily, so that deformities (bow-legs, etc.) result. These are described in more detail in connection with diseases of bones (page 282). The disease occurs usually in bottle-fed babies, and in young children brought up in the slums of smoky cities in northern latitudes. It is unknown in the tropics. As we have seen, it may be due to one of two factors. or often to a combination of the two: (1) insufficient vitamin D in the diet; (2) insufficient sunlight (ultra-violet) which could produce the vitamin by activating the cholesterol in the skin.

The disease is easily arrested by the administration of cod-liver or halibut-liver oil or viosterol, or by exposing the child to ultra-violet radiation from sunlight or the mercury vapor lamp or carbon arc.

Vitamin E.—This vitamin is necessary for normal reproduction, so it has been called the antisterility vitamin. The chief sources are the germ of of various cereals and green vegetable foods. Wheat germ oil contains a large amount of the vitamin. Knowledge as to its action is limited to animals. Deficiency in female rats causes the embryo to die early, and in males spermatozoa are not produced because of degenerative changes in the testes.

Vitamin K.—The story of vitamin K is quite as remarkable as that of vitamin D. In 1930 a Danish observer, Dam, noticed that chicks fed on a deficient diet developed hemorrhage and that this was prevented when they were given alfalfa. There was evidently some factor in the alfalfa which was necessary for the coagulation of the blood and without which hemorrhage would occur. Soon this factor was extracted and crystallized. It was called Koagulationsvitamin, being German for the vitamin which promotes coagulation; this became shortened to vitamin K.

The prothrombin of the blood (page 40) must be at a normal level if the coagulation of blood which is necessary to stop hemorrhage is to occur in a normal way. It was soon found that animals deficient in vitamin K were also deficient in prothrombin, so it became apparent that vitamin K is necessary for the formation of prothrombin. The mere presence of a sufficient amount of vitamin K in the food is not enough; it has to be absorbed before it can be used for the manufacture of prothrombin.

The next discovery was that the vitamin is not absorbed unless bile is present in the intestine. It had long been known that operations on jaundiced patients were apt to be followed by hemorrhage, often fatal, at the site of operation. In jaundice the bile is unable to reach the intestine. Now it was clear that the reason for the bleeding tendency in jaundice was lack of vitamin K, that lack being due to failure in absorption, which in turn was due to absence of bile in the bowel. The prothrombin in the blood was found to be very low in cases of jaundice, as was to be expected.

This was a discovery of great practical importance, because now it is possible to raise the prothrombin in the blood of jaundiced patients before operation. This is done by administering bile, or rather bile salts, combined with vitamin K. The vitamin is absorbed, the prothrombin rises to normal, and the operation can be performed without danger of hemorrhage.

Another condition in which the prothrombin is low is hemorrhagic disease of the newborn. Shortly after birth the baby may show a tendency to bleeding, and if there has been any birth injury to the head there may be fatal intracranial hemorrhage. This is due to vitamin K deficiency in the baby, and can readily be prevented by administering the vitamin to the mother before delivery.

The various vitamins are necessary for perfect health. Deficiency in any one of them may lead to disease. It is important, however, to remember the following facts, which are apt to be overlooked in view of the flood of articles on vitamins in the press and periodicals, not to mention the persuasive pamphlets from the pharmaceutical houses: (1) Under modern conditions outspoken deficiency disease is uncommon except in a few less favored localities, in Oriental countries, or as the result of war, although minor degrees are far from rare. (2) An average mixed diet including fresh fruit and green vegetables contains an ample supply of vitamins. (3) While pure vitamin deficiency can be produced in the experimental animal, in human cases an inadequate diet is likely to be lacking in more than one vitamin, so that the clinical picture will tend to be a mixed one. (4) More than $100,000,000 are spent by the United States public in buying vitamins. (5) It is better and infinitely cheaper to get your vitamins from the grocery store, where they have been manufactured by Nature than from the drug store where they have been manufactured by man. While this is true for healthy persons, it may not be true for those suffering from avitaminosis. When the condition is of long duration it may be necessary to administer artificially prepared vitamins for a correspondingly long period before the needs of the tissues are fully satisfied and the normal balance of vitamins is restored. Finally, it must be borne in mind that vitamins, although essential to life, are no substitute for food. They provide no energies, calories or body-building materials, and are merely accessory to diet.

HOW THE DOCTOR MAKES A DIAGNOSIS

The detection of disease is as elaborate and sometimes as difficult a matter as the detection of crime. The methods employed fall into two main groups, the clinical and the laboratory.

Clinical Methods.—The *clinical* group can be subdivided into symptoms and physical signs. *Symptoms* include the complaints of the patient, either voluntary or elicited by careful cross-examination. It is often possible to make a correct diagnosis from the symptoms alone. Thus the agonizing pain over the heart in coronary thrombosis, or the digestive distress and pain relieved by taking food so characteristic of ulcer of the stomach, may tell the doctor in clear and unmistakable language the disease from which the patient is suffering. In the majority of diseases there is a close relationship between the symptoms of the patient and the lesions which the pathologist may be able to demonstrate. Thus if the air spaces of the lung are filled with inflammatory material in pneumonia it is only natural that the patient should be severely short of breath. This close relationship of lesions to symptoms is one of the chief reasons why a

knowledge of pathology is of value to the doctor. One of the peculiar effects of cortisone is that it may break this relationship without having actually altered the lesions and therefore without having benefitted the patient, no matter how much better he may feel. Unfortunately the number of symptoms of which a patient can complain are limited, and pain, shortness of breath, fever, and loss of strength can be caused by many very different diseases. On this account the doctor has to turn to physical signs for further help.

Physical signs are elicited by physical examination of the patient. By listening to the heart a murmur may be heard, palpation of the kidney may show it to be enlarged, pressure over the appendix may elicit tenderness even though the patient has complained of no pain. These signs are of the greatest help in diagnosis.

Simple visual inspection of the patient may tell the doctor or the nurse all that needs to be known. The patient with pneumonia can be recognized by reason of the rapid respiration, cough, and flushed feverish appearance. In chronic heart failure there is shortness of breath (dyspnea), swelling of the legs, and the bluish tinge of cyanosis. In an acute heart attack, such as that of coronary thrombosis, the face is clammy and ashen in color, the expression that of deep anxiety, and there is a strange immobility as if the patient feared to move a muscle. In nephritis the face and eyelids are swollen and the skin presents a typical pallor. Acute intestinal obstruction can be suspected from the sunken appearance of the eyes due to extreme loss of fluid (dehydration), the leaden skin, and the board-like rigidity of the abdomen. The wasted and emaciated appearance (cachexia) of the cancer patient is only too readily recognized.

What may be called the *scopes* can be included in a discussion of physical signs. They are instruments which enable the doctor at the bedside to see what would otherwise remain hidden from him. They consist of a tiny electric light bulb at the end of a metal tube. When this is introduced into one of the hollow organs of the body, the walls of the organ can be studied by means of an ingenious system of mirrors. The *laryngoscope* reveals the interior of the larynx, the *bronchoscope* the interior of the bronchial tree, the *gastroscope* the interior of the stomach, the *sigmoidoscope* the interior of the colon (sigmoid), the *cystoscope* the interior of the bladder, and so on. In the case of the *ophthalmoscope* a beam of light is directed into the eye, the interior of which is illuminated and can be studied.

Laboratory Methods.—These comprise tests which cannot be done at the bedside but require the use of laboratory apparatus such as the microscope, the test tube, and the x-ray machine. They do not provide the doctor with a ready-made diagnosis; they merely give him additional information which, taken in conjunction with the clinical evidence (history of the illness, symptoms and signs), enable him to arrive at a correct conclusion. Laboratory methods are numerous and complex. Only a few of the more important will be mentioned here.

Urinalysis is the commonest of all laboratory tests. Examination of the urine serves not only to indicate the condition of the kidneys, but may also reveal disease of the bladder and urethra. Other diseases not connected

with the urinary tract may be detected by urinalysis, *e.g.*, the presence of sugar in the urine in diabetes.

Examination of *stomach contents* and *feces* gives valuable information as to the presence of disease in the stomach and intestine.

A *blood count* shows the number and the condition both of the red blood cells and leucocytes. The red cells are diminished in various forms of anemia. The number of the leucocytes is increased in acute infections (appendicitis, pneumonia), and in the blood disease leukemia.

Blood chemistry is becoming of ever increasing importance. Thus the blood sugar is increased in diabetes; the urea and non-protein nitrogen are increased in Bright's disease, the phosphorus is lowered in rickets, etc.

The *cerebrospinal fluid* shows changes in many diseases of the nervous system. Thus the diagnosis of acute meningitis is made by finding large numbers of leucocytes in this fluid, together with the bacteria causing the infection. The fluid, which is obtained by means of lumbar puncture, is a mirror in which is reflected disease of the brain and spinal cord.

Bacteriological examination is of the greatest importance in the diagnosis of many of the infectious diseases such as diphtheria, pneumonia, and tuberculosis. A blood culture may show the presence of streptococci, etc., in the circulating blood.

Serology, which is a branch of bacteriology, consists in the examination of the blood serum for substances which indicate the presence of bacterial infection. The two commonest of such tests are the Widal test for typhoid fever and the Wassermann test for syphilis. It must be understood that these are not tests for the bacteria, but for substances produced by the body in response to the infection.

Tissue diagnosis is the microscopic examination of pieces of tissue. When such a piece is removed during life for the purpose of diagnosis the procedure is called a *biopsy*, in contrast to the examination of tissues at autopsy. It is usually done to determine whether or not a tumor is malignant.

The *electrocardiogram* is an electrical record of the contractions of the heart. All contracting muscles produce an electric current, and such a current is produced by the contractions of the auricles and ventricles. The current is made to write a permanent tracing (electrocardiogram) which is of one pattern when the heart muscle is healthy, but of a different pattern when the muscle is diseased. These finger prints of the heart's action are of great value to the heart specialist.

Basal metabolism or the *basal metabolic rate* (B.M.R.) is the heat production of the body. It is determined from the amount of carbon dioxide eliminated or the amount of oxygen consumed over a given period of time. The two important conditions which raise the basal metabolic rate are fever and overactivity of the thyroid gland (hyperthyroidism, exophthalmic goiter). The chief value of the test is to estimate the functional activity of the thyroid in cases of goiter.

X-ray examination is used in medical diagnosis because the rays have the power of passing through solid objects and affecting a photographic film on the other side of that object. But their use is limited by the fact that they can only show differences in density. An opaque object like a bullet will stand out clearly; large solid organs can be seen on the film,

but the outlines of hollow structures, such as the stomach, intestine, gallbladder, bronchi, etc., are indistinguishable. It is these outlines, however, which are most likely to be altered in disease.

This serious limitation to the usefulness of x-ray examination has been largely overcome by the ingenuity of the radiologist. He has found it possible to introduce into the cavities of the body substances such as barium and iodine which are opaque to x-rays and thus provide the contrast necessary for the making of a picture. The method has its greatest use in examination of the gastrointestinal tract, which when filled with a barium meal becomes opaque to the rays, so that an exact outline of the stomach or intestine appears on the film. An ulcer stands out on the edge of the stomach as a crater, whilst a tumor shows as a dent (filling defect) which the barium cannot fill out. A *cholecystogram* is a picture of the outline of the gallbladder; an opaque substance is administered which is excreted by the liver in the bile and thus enters the gallbladder where it becomes sufficiently concentrated to throw a shadow on the film. Similarly in *urography* an opaque substance is injected into the ureters through the bladder and thus shows an outline of the renal pelvis. Or similar material (uroselectan) can be injected intravenously; this is excreted by the kidneys, and the outline of the renal pelvis again becomes visible. *Lipiodol* is an oil containing iodine which can be injected into the bronchi or the spinal canal, so that an outline of these spaces is seen. A *ventriculogram* is a picture of the ventricles of the brain obtained by injecting air into these cavities through an opening made in the skull. As air is less dense than the surrounding brain, an outline of the ventricles is obtained.

In all of these cases a photograph is made on a film by the rays which have passed through the body. An equally valuable method of examination is by means of the *fluoroscope*. This is a sensitive screen on which a faint outline of opaque structures becomes visible when x-rays pass through the body. The value of the fluoroscope is that it shows movement; an aneurysm of the aorta can be seen to pulsate, the movements of the diaphragm can be studied, the ability of the stomach to empty itself is noted, and the peristaltic movements of the intestine can be observed. The fluoroscopic screen shows the observer what is happening in the body from moment to moment, but the x-ray film gives a permanent record of any structural changes which may be present.

Chapter

4

DISTURBANCES OF THE BLOOD FLOW

THROUGH every organ and tissue of the body the life blood flows cease-lessly night and day. Health is dependent on the maintenance of that flow which is governed partly by the heart, the pump of the circulation, partly by the intact conditions of the bloodvessels. Heart disease will be considered in a later chapter. In this place we shall concern ourselves with three topics: (1) The intactness of the vessel walls and the possibility of hemorrhage; (2) clotting of blood circulating in the vessels, a process known as thrombosis; (3) narrowing of the lumen of the vessel with the production of ischemia.

HEMORRHAGE

When a vessel is ruptured blood will naturally escape into the surround-ing tissue or on to a free surface. The hemorrhage may be large and form a tumor-like swelling known as a *hematoma*. Or the hemorrhages may be as small as a pin's head and are then called *petechiæ*. The effect depends on the size and the site of the hemorrhage. If it occurs into a muscle it does little damage, but if it takes place into the brain or on to a free surface such as the interior of the stomach where it cannot be arrested it may cause death. *Rupture of a vessel* may be produced in several ways: (1) The commonest cause is *trauma* in the shape of a wound or bruise. (2) A *de-structive process* in the neighborhood of a large vessel may finally perforate the wall and give rise to profuse hemorrhage; this may happen in ulcer of the stomach or in a tuberculous cavity in the lung. (3) The wall of the vessel may be weakened by a degenerative condition such as *arteriosclerosis*, and finally give way under the pressure of the blood; this is what happens in apoplexy or cerebral hemorrhage.

But the remarkable thing about hemorrhage is not that it should occcur, but that it should ever stop. If a hole is made in a pipe through which water is passing, the water will flow out until the pipe is empty. It is true that if we fill the pipe with a glue-like material too thick to pass through a small hole none will escape, but such a material would never be able to flow through the small arteries and the minute capillaries. The problem to be solved in the case of hemorrhage is how a fluid thin enough to pass through the finest channels ceases after a short time to flow through a comparatively large opening in the vessel wall.

The *arrest of hemorrhage* is brought about by the coagulation or clotting of the blood. As long as the blood is inside the vessel it does not clot, but when it escapes into the surrounding tissue or on to the surface of the

skin it at once begins to coagulate, and soon the clot thus formed is able to plug the hole in the vessel unless that hole be too large. The clotting of blood is due to the interaction of two substances in the plasma called *fibrinogen* and *thrombin*. The thrombin is formed by the interaction of *prothrombin* with *calcium salts*. Prothrombin has recently become a substance of great importance; it appears to be formed from vitamin K, and when a person suffers from vitamin K deficiency his blood prothrombin is low and the blood has lost the power of clotting. What prevents this mechanism from making the blood clot in the vessels of a normal person is the presence of *heparin (antithrombin)*, which prevents the prothrombin and calcium from uniting to form thrombin. Heparin is present in extremely minute quantities in the blood. It was first obtained from the liver, hence its

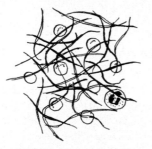

FIG. 4.—Network of fibrin containing red blood cells and one leucocyte in its meshes.

name (*hepar*, liver), but is also present in large amount in the lung and intestine, from which it can be extracted. When blood is shed the blood platelets disintegrate and liberate *thromboplastin*; this neutralizes the heparin, and when it is eliminated the whole complex machinery of clotting is set in motion. The clot is formed of interlacing threads of *fibrin* (Fig. 4), and these threads seal over the opening in the vessel in much the same way as the threads of a spider's web might do. This plug is greatly reinforced by the *blood platelets*, tiny particles which float in the plasma and which form a sticky mass which effectually seals up the hole in the vessel wall. In course of time this emergency plug is converted into fibrous or scar tissue, just as an inflammatory exudate becomes changed into scar tissue, and the opening is closed safely and permanently.

When a surgeon ties a catgut ligature round a bleeding vessel during the course of an operation, he does not intend it to remain in place permanently. In the course of a few weeks the ligature will be absorbed, but its place will be taken by a firm, permanent clot. In studying inflammation we shall see that healing will not take place properly as long as infection is present. The same is true of the formation of the permanent clot. In an infected wound there is always the danger that the temporary plugs may become weakened by the action of bacteria, and that severe hemorrhage may occur a week or two after the operation. This is called *secondary hemorrhage*.

Occasionally, though fortunately rarely, it happens that the mechanism for the temporary arrest of hemorrhage is defective, so that the blood continues to flow out. This is most marked in the hereditary disease called *hemophilia*, sufferers from which are known as bleeders, and may die of hemorrhage from a trivial wound, cut, or tooth extraction. It appears that the essential defect is a lack in the globulin fraction of the plasma. When this is added to hemophilic blood it causes coagulation to occur, and when it is injected into the patient clotting time is reduced. The prothrombin seems not to be utilized properly in the hemophiliac. Hemophilia is a striking example of sex-linked heredity; only the males of a

family suffer from the disease, and only the females transmit it. Everyone is familiar with the fateful part which hemophilia has played in the misfortunes of the house of the Romanoffs and in the matter of the Spanish succession. Excessive bleeding may also occur to a lesser degree in patients suffering from jaundice and in a number of blood diseases.

THROMBOSIS

Clotting of the blood should occur when the blood escapes from the vessel but not when it is flowing through the lumen of the vessel. Should this occur the process is called *thrombosis* and the clot within the vessel is known as a *thrombus*. This consists mainly of platelets, which adhere to the vessel wall on account of their stickiness and gradually form a mass which may finally close the lumen of the vessel and stop the flow of blood through it.

The *causes* of thrombosis are injury to or inflammation of the vessel wall and slowing of the blood stream. As all of these factors are commoner in veins than in arteries it is natural that thrombosis should usually occur in veins. The normal vessel has an exquisitely smooth lining known as the endothelium. When this is destroyed by injury or inflammation the platelets adhere to the rough spot and gradually build up a thrombus from the blood as it flows past. The slower the flow the more likely are the platelets to fall out of the stream and adhere to the vessel wall, so that thrombosis is associated with varicose (dilated and tortuous) veins, failing heart, etc. A very important form of thrombosis is that which follows abdominal operations, particularly on the pelvic organs. Closely related to this is the thrombosis which may occur in the puerperium, the period following childbirth.

The principal *sites* of thrombosis are the veins and the heart. Thrombosis may occur in the arteries, particularly the coronary arteries, the cerebral arteries, and the arteries to the leg in old persons. In all of these cases there is preliminary narrowing of the lumen by arteriosclerosis. The veins of the leg are frequently affected because of the tendency for postoperative and puerperal thrombosis to involve these veins. Thrombosis of the veins of the leg is also common in chronic heart failure owing to the sluggish circulation, particularly when a patient is confined to bed for some time. A number of cases of thrombosis in the legs followed by fatal pulmonary embolism occurred in London air raid shelters in elderly persons who sat all night in deck chairs, the wooden supports of which pressed continuously on the thighs. The leg is swollen owing to interference with the return of blood and the thrombosed vein may be felt as a hard tender cord. In the heart a common site of thrombus formation is an inflamed valve, on which the platelets are deposited as the blood flows past, until they form a large thrombus which in this situation is known as a vegetation. Even more common is thrombus formation in one of the auricles, particularly in the part called the auricular appendix, which is a kind of cul-de-sac in which the blood is apt to stagnate.

Thrombosis may be a serious complication in surgical operations, particularly in operations on large bloodvessels such as arteries. This can now be controlled by the use of heparin, which prevents the platelets from sticking together and to the vessel wall, so that a thrombus is not formed. Heparin has also been used to prevent thrombosis in the veins of the leg after an operation. The substance Dicumarol resembles heparin in prolonging the coagulation time, and it has the advantage that the action is much more prolonged and that it can be taken by mouth instead of being injected intravenously.

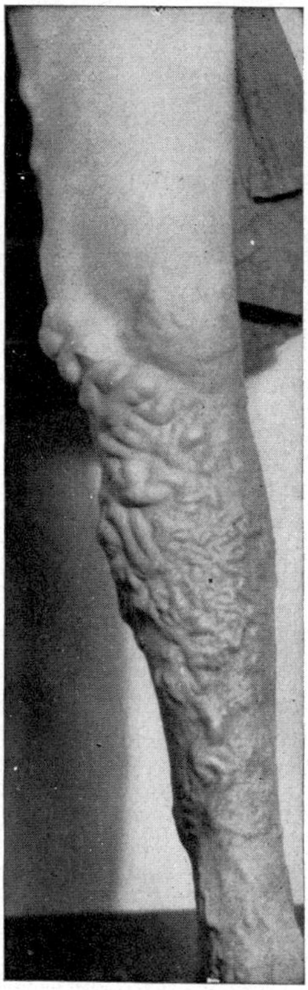

The *subsequent history* of a thrombus varies: (1) The thrombus may become converted into fibrous tissue with permanent closure of the vessel. (2) It may contract so as partially to reopen the lumen and allow the blood to flow through it again. (3) Finally, the thrombus may become detached from the vessel wall and enter the blood stream as a floating body known as an *embolus*, a catastrophic occurrence, as we shall see in the next section. This detachment of the thrombus is particularly likely to occur when there is sepsis at the site of thrombosis, as the infection causes the thrombus to break down and become loosened. Another factor is rough handling of the part. It is evident that a thrombosed leg has to be treated with the greatest care and anything in the nature of massage must be avoided.

Fig. 5.—Varicose veins. (Boyd's Surgical Pathology; courtesy of W. B. Saunders Company.)

The opportunity may be taken now to say something about two conditions in which thrombosis is common and often serious, namely, varicose veins and piles. The two really belong to the same group, for piles or hemorrhoids are merely varicose veins at the lower end of the intestinal canal.

Varicose Veins.—A varicose vein is one that is dilated and tortuous (Fig. 5). The dilatation may be extreme in degree, so that the valves which normally guard veins and prevent a backflow because of gravity become incompetent and cease to function. As a result of this the stagnation and accumulation of blood in the vein becomes increasingly great. The common site of varicose veins is in the superficial veins of the leg just under the skin. Bluish knuckles of veins can be seen pushing the skin in front of them. These are liable to injury, with resulting *hemorrhage* into

the surrounding tissue. Thrombosis is liable to occur due partly to the slow flow in the dilated vessels, partly to the frequency of injury to the vessel wall. The circulation in varicose veins is gravely interfered with, the legs become swollen, and *varicose ulcers* are formed in the lower part of the leg. These ulcers used to be extremely chronic and difficult to treat, but the outlook has been completely changed by modern methods of treating the varicose veins.

The *causes* of varicose veins are obscure. Heredity undoubtedly plays a part and the condition may run in a family for generations. The active factor is increase of pressure in the vein. This may be due to prolonged standing, muscular straining (in the case of piles) or the pressure of a tumor in the pelvis, a pregnant uterus, or even a continually loaded rectum.

The *treatment* of varicose veins is directed to the relief of the congestion, the accumulation of stagnant blood, in the dilated vessels. This may be accomplished by the application of a uniform support to the leg in the form of an elastic bandage or stocking; this should extend to the groin rather than to the knee which is the common practice. If this fails to relieve the condition the veins may be obliterated by the injection of irritating solutions (sodium morrhuate, etc.) which injure the vessel walls, leading to thrombosis and finally fibrosis. The varicosity only affects the superficial veins, and as these communicate with the deep veins of the leg by small collateral channels, the circulation is reëstablished through the leg veins. For the same reason there is no danger of emboli passing from the superficial veins into the general circulation.

Hemorrhoids or Piles.—Hemorrhoids or piles is a condition in which the veins at the lower end of the rectum become varicose and enlarged. *Internal hemorrhoids* are those covered by the mucous membrane of the lower end of the rectum; they may "come down" through the anal opening and appear on the surface, although they can be replaced by pressure. *External* hemorrhoids are covered by the skin in the neighborhood of the anus.

The *causes* are those of varicose veins, *i.e.*, heredity and increased pressure in the vein. The commonest cause of increased pressure is chronic constipation accompanied by undue muscular straining while the bowel is being emptied. A condition which must always be borne in mind, especially in a man over middle age, is cancer of the rectum, which may produce piles by causing pressure on the veins coming from the lower end of the bowel. In this case the piles are merely a symptom of a much more serious condition.

The possible *effects* which may render the condition serious are hemorrhage, phlebitis, and thrombosis. *Hemorrhage* when the bowels are moved is usually small in amount, but may be continued over a long period, so that a grave degree of anemia may be produced without the patient suspecting its cause. *Phlebitis* or inflammation of the dilated veins together with inflammation of the surrounding tissue is commonly referred to as an "attack of the piles." Its danger is that it may lead to the formation of an infected thrombus, which readily becomes converted into an embolus.

The *treatment* of hemorrhoids is partly indirect, partly direct. By indirect treatment we mean keeping the bowels loose by means of bland

bosis or embolism of the cerebral arteries. The most important sites of infarction are the heart, lung, brain, spleen, kidney, and intestine.

Before leaving the general subject, reference must be made to *pulmonary embolism* and *infarction*. As the blood from the veins passes to the right side of the heart, and as the pulmonary artery to the lungs arises from that side, it is evident that emboli from the veins will lodge in the lungs. The effect on the patient depends entirely on the size of the embolus. If it is small it will not be arrested until it reaches a correspondingly small arterial branch, and the area of the infarct produced will be equally small. The patient will experience a sharp pain in the chest, and may cough up a little blood during the next few days, after which recovery will be complete. Tragically different is the course of events when the embolus is large enough to block the main pulmonary artery or one of its principal branches. The blood is suddenly cut off from an entire lung or even from both lungs, the shock is so great that the heart rapidly fails, and the patient dies in the course of a few minutes. The full tragedy of this accident is evident in those cases where the embolism occurs about a week after an abdominal operation or after childbirth when the patient is convalescing splendidly, but after sitting up in bed suddenly feels faint, drops back on the pillow panting for breath, and is dead in the course of a few minutes. Often, however, embolism is a complication of medical rather than surgical cases, and it is particularly likely to complicate heart failure.

In all these cases the patient is confined to bed, and the condition (failing heart, childbirth, an abdominal operation, immobility) tends to interfere with the flow of blood from the veins of the leg to the heart. It is in these veins that thrombosis occurs, the thrombus becomes dislodged by some sudden movement, and pulmonary embolism is the result. Nursing precautions can be of real value in preventing the stagnation of circulation which leads to thrombosis. Voluntary movements of the legs, frequent change of position, and elevation of the foot of the bed all contribute to this end. Circulation is assisted by stimulating the respiration, and this may be done most conveniently by getting the patient to breathe into a rubber bag, the carbon dioxide which he is thus forced to inhale being the most powerful of known respiratory stimulants. In order to counteract the tendency to thrombosis which is associated with prolonged rest in bed after pelvic operations and childbirth it is becoming the fashion to make the patient get up, if only for a short time, at a much earlier date.

ISCHEMIA—ITS CAUSES AND EFFECTS

Ischemia is a condition in which the blood supply to a part is diminished or stopped. It is a local rather than a general bloodlessness. As the blood is carried to the part by an artery, it is evident that ischemia will be caused by anything which narrows or closes the lumen of an artery, provided that the collateral circulation is not sufficiently abundant to compensate fully for the primary loss of blood supply.

The closure of the artery may be sudden or slow, and the effect will vary accordingly. We have already studied the effect of *sudden closure* of an artery whether by the formation of a thrombus or by the lodgment of

an embolus. If the collateral circulation is inadequate the result will be an infarct. *Slow closure* is due to the degenerative disease of arteries known as *arteriosclerosis* or *atheroma*, commonly called hardening of the arteries (Fig. 8). The exact cause of this condition is not known but it is a degenerative condition of advancing years, just as is graying of the hair. The bloodvessels begin to feel the effect of the sharp tooth of time. Occasionally, however, it may begin before the age of thirty, and a person of advanced years may be singularly free from the disease so that the saying that "a man is as old as his arteries" is profoundly true. The essential change is a nodular thickening of the inner coat of the artery, as a result of which the lumen slowly becomes narrowed, until finally a mere chink may be left through which the blood can only trickle with difficulty. The smooth endothelium lining the vessel in time becomes lost over the nodules of

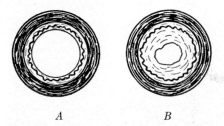

A   *B*

FIG. 8.—Arteriosclerosis. *A*, Normal artery; *B*, arteriosclerotic artery showing great thickening of inner coat (pale part) and narrowing of lumen.

atheroma, so that the inner surface is now roughened, and as the platelets tend to stick to the rough surface a thrombus may form which suddenly completes the closure of the already narrowed vessel. This is what happens in *coronary artery thrombosis*, one of the commonest causes of sudden death in persons over fifty years of age. The coronary arteries are the vessels which supply blood to the heart muscle, the most essential muscle in the body, and if that supply is suddenly cut off the heart will stop beating.

For some reason at present not understood arteriosclerosis is not a general process affecting all the arteries in the body, but a selective process which picks out an artery here and there. The three principal sufferers are the heart, kidneys, and brain, to which must be added the arteries of the leg. Not all of these are attacked in the same person so that one person may have symptoms pointing to injury to the heart, another to the kidneys, and a third to the brain. It is probable that a hereditary or inherited weakness plays a part in the selection, for several members of one family may die of coronary thrombosis about the same age.

The effect of ischemia is gradual death of the specialized cells of the part, *i.e.*, nerve cells in the brain, heart muscle cells, etc., and their replacement by scar tissue, so that the organ loses the power to do its proper work. In the brain there is failure of memory and of the power of accurate thinking, and there may be actual softening of the part of the brain affected due to degenerative processes.

Necrosis is the name applied to the death of cells whether caused by the cutting off of the blood supply or for any other reason such as the toxins produced by bacteria, or physical and chemical injurious agents like marked heat and cold, chemical poisions, etc. When a cell dies it undergoes degeneration. The nucleus breaks up and eventually disappears, and the outline of the cytoplasm becomes very indistinct. In an infarct the general outline of structure can still be recognized, such as the tubules and glomeruli of the kidney. In the case of some bacterial infections such as tuberculosis and syphilis the outlines are wiped out. This process is known as caseation, because the gross appearance of the material is cheesy or caseous. The microscopic structure of the organ is now unrecognizable. The difference between the necrosis of an infarct and caseation is the difference between the site of ancient Pompeii in which the outline of the streets can still be recognized compared with that of the destruction at Hiroshima.

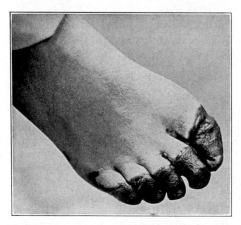

FIG. 9.—Gangrene of the toes. (Bell, Textbook of Pathology.)

Closure of the arteries in the leg and rarely in the arm may lead to death of the parts farthest from the heart, the toes or fingers, as in them the circulation is likely to be most sluggish. Here another change becomes evident, for bacteria invade the dead tissue through the skin and cause decomposition and putrefaction of the dead tissue, a process known as *gangrene* (Fig. 9). The gangrenous part undergoes a series of color changes, becoming first green and finally black. The gangrene tends to spread slowly up the limb as the narrowing of the arteries becomes more extreme and widespread. Diabetes often leads to the occurrence of marked atheroma in the arteries of the leg, so that *diabetic gangrene* is a common complication in elderly patients.

Principles of Treatment.—When a patient shows evidence of marked interference with the circulation in the leg, the nursing becomes a question of preventing the onset of gangrene. Any injury, however trivial, may start the process in the devitalized tissues. Special care must be taken in cutting the nails lest the toe be injured, and of course a hot-water bottle that is too

hot is a particular source of danger. Bandages must not be tight, and the limb must be kept warm to encourage any circulation which may still remain in the collateral vessels. The most modern method of stimulating the collateral circulation is by means of an appliance which produces what has been called "passive vascular exercise," and the appliance is known as the Pavex machine, pavex being the first letters of passive vascular exercise. The idea is to make the remaining healthy arteries contract and relax until they are sufficiently vigorous to carry the additional burden of circulation. A large hollow "glass boot" is fitted around the leg as far as the knee and hermetically sealed. Air is then pumped into and sucked out of the glass chamber many times a minute, so that the vessels of the leg are alternately compressed and dilated, and in this way are passively exercised. By this means threatened gangrene may be averted and amputation of a foot often rendered unnecessary.

EDEMA

Edema or dropsy is an abnormal collection of fluid in the tissue spaces. This accumulation may be local or general. The fluid can be moved from one place to another, so that when the edematous part is pressed on, a pit is left; this is known clinically as "pitting on pressure." The accumulation of fluid is most marked and most readily recognized in the subcutaneous tissue of the skin. An edematous tissue has a pale watery appearance. Subcutaneous tissue may come to resemble jelly. In the lung where edema of the alveolar spaces is very common, the affected part may feel solid, but fluid pours from the cut surface.

Causes of Edema.—There are three main causes of general edema. The *first* of these is increased permeability of the capillary wall. All edema fluid comes from the blood and passes into the tissues. It is evident that if the permeability of the smallest blood vessels is increased, fluid will pass from the blood into the tissues. It must be remembered that this passage of fluid through the wall of the small vessels is a normal one, for it is the process by which nourishment is carried to a part and reaches the individual tissues. The most important cause of increased permeability of capillaries is inflammation. This is the explanation of the large amount of edema fluid which collects during the inflammatory process, and is mainly responsible for the swelling of inflammation. The *second* cause is a decrease of the osmotic pressure of the plasma proteins. These proteins exert an osmotic influence on the fluid in the blood which holds it in the vessels and prevents it from escaping. It is evident that in the event of a reduction in the amount of proteins there will be a corresponding loss of this "pool" which normally keeps the fluid from escaping. If proteins such as albumin are lost in the urine in such a condition as Bright's disease a development of edema may be expected. The *third* cause is an increase in the pressure in the small veins and capillaries. This has nothing to do with high blood pressure, but is the result of chronic heart failure in which the blood is prevented from reaching the heart readily and accumulates in the veins. As a result of this the fluid tends to pass from the inside of the vessel to the tissues outside.

4

From what has been said it will be apparent that there are three principal types of edema encountered by the physician. These are inflammatory edema, renal edema, and cardiac edema. Inflammatory edema will be localized. Renal edema is general, but appears first in the face and the lower eyelids, giving a puffy appearance. Cardiac edema is also general, but usually makes its first appearance in the dependent parts of the body, particularly the ankles and feet. The *fourth* cause of edema, local rather than general, is lymphatic obstruction. If the lymphatics are obstructed by inflammation or by the pressure of a tumor, the lymph within the lumen will pass outward and accumulate in the tissues. A striking example of lymphatic edema is sometimes seen after extensive operations for the removal of cancer of the breast or radiation to the part for the treatment of that disease. The subsequent swelling of the arm is not due to a recurrence of the cancer, but to an accumulation of lymph fluid which is unable to escape from the tissues.

The subject of edema is very involved and the accumulation of tissue fluid is dependent upon many complex disturbances of chemical processes. A detailed account of the subject would be out of place here.

SHOCK

In a state of health not all the capillaries of an organ are open at the same time, for some parts of the organ are working and some are resting. If all the capillaries and venules in the body were filled with blood at the same time, the entire supply would be contained in these vessels. The heart would have insufficient blood to contract on, the stimulus to work would be lost, and the heart would fail. This is essentially the state of shock, where there is an enormous dilatation of the capillary bed in which the blood collects, and the effect on the heart is disastrous.

Shock may be produced in a variety of ways. Very severe injury or prolonged surgical operations may cause so severe a nervous disturbance that the capillaries are allowed to dilate to a dangerous degree. The blood disappears into the vast capillary bed as if sucked up by a sponge, so that the patient may be said to bleed into his own capillaries. Great loss of fluid from the body, either loss of blood itself as in severe hemorrhage or loss of fluid from the stomach as in continuous vomiting or from the bowel as in continuous diarrhea, may deplete the blood volume so much that the heart has not sufficient to work upon, even though the capillaries are not unduly dilated. Many other pathological conditions may lead to shock.

The appearance of a person in shock is characteristic. He lies quite still, his face is pale and gray, drawn and anxious, and the skin is cold and clammy. The temperature is subnormal, the pulse feeble, the respirations shallow and sighing, and the blood pressure alarmingly low. Shock is usually a temporary condition, a step towards death which the patient can retrace, but sometimes the step is final and return impossible.

It is obvious that the most important point in the *treatment* of shock is to refill the empty vessels and give the heart fluid to work on. Saline solution is of no value, because it pours through the permeable walls of the vessels

into the interstitial tissue as fast as it is administered. Blood plasma when given intravenously remains in the vessels, because its large protein molecules cannot pass through the walls of the capillaries, and the protein in turn holds back the fluid by virtue of the osmotic pressure which it exerts.

WATER BALANCE

The discussion of shock has introduced the idea of the fluid both inside and outside the vessels, an all-important subject known as water balance. Water, which comprises about 70 per cent of the weight of the body, is present in the vessels (in the form of plasma), in the interstitial tissue, and in the cells. These may be regarded as three compartments between which a continual exchange of fluid is going on. Water lost from one compartment can be supplied from another compartment. Thus loss of plasma is made up by fluid from the interstitial compartment. There is 12 times as much water in the cells as in the blood, and 4 times as much in the interstitial tissue. Water balance is the remarkably constant balance between the fluid in the vessels and the fluid in the tissues, both cellular and interstitial. It is in the cells themselves that the correct content of water is so important. The balance will be influenced both by the intake and output of water.

Dissolved in the water there are salts known as electrolytes, by reason of their being dissociated into their constituent elements by the passage of an electric current through the solution. These have an important effect on the amount of water because of the osmotic pressure which they produce; this pressure exerts a pull on the water. The salt content in the cellular compartment is quite different from that of the interstitial and vascular compartments. Potassium is the chief constituent in the cellular compartment, whilst sodium and chlorine are present in the other two compartments. The chief function of the sodium and chlorine, combined as sodium chloride, is, by means of its osmotic pressure, to maintain the delicate water balance which is controlled by the kidneys. The renal glomeruli excrete water and sodium chloride, but these are reabsorbed by the renal tubules in the right quantities to maintain the correct balance.

Under normal conditions more water is taken in than is needed, and the excess is excreted in the urine by the kidneys. If the intake is insufficient, the output due to evaporation from the skin and the lungs and the excretion in urine and feces results in a negative water balance and a state of *dehydration*. Death occurs when the loss reaches 15 per cent of the body weight. As this percentage is reached twice as quickly in an infant as in an adult, it is evident that the water in the tissues will be exhausted at twice the rate of an adult and that the infant will die in half the time. Dehydration is therefore a much more acute problem in infants and young children than in adults.

From what has been said it is obvious that fluid balance depends not only on water but also on salt. If both water and salt are lost, as in vomiting and diarrhea or even in profuse and continued sweating as in the tropics or in men working at blast furnaces, salt must be replenished as well as

water. One of the hormones of the adrenal cortex controls the excretion of sodium chloride by the kidneys. If this hormone is insufficient there will be excessive loss of salt in the urine, the salt content of the plasma will fall, water is not retained in the tissues, and dehydration will result. This is seen in marked degree in Addison's disease, which is due to destruction of the adrenal cortex.

Disturbance in the water (and salt) balance may occur in a number of diseases, some of which will be discussed in this book. Important examples are shock, acute intestinal obstruction, renal failure and Addison's disease.

Chapter

5

INFLAMMATION, IMMUNITY, AND ALLERGY

INFLAMMATION

OF all the forms of disease which the doctor or nurse are called upon to minister to, inflammation is the commonest, the most important, and the most amenable to treatment. Every disease whose name ends in *itis* is a form of inflammation, so that appendicitis is inflammation of the appendix, tonsillitis, is inflammation of the tonsil, and so on. Some important examples of inflammation, such as pneumonia and pleurisy, were given their names long ago, so that they do not follow the usual rule regarding nomenclature.

Inflammation is the *local reaction of the body to an irritant.* Now there are many kinds of irritants, but they can all be placed in one or other of three great classes, physical, chemical, and bacterial. The simplest example of a *physical irritant* is a *foreign body*, that is to say some solid substance introduced into the tissues from outside, like a splinter in the finger. The foreign body injures and irritates the tissues, and the attempt which the body makes to remove the irritant is the process of inflammation. Sometimes the attempt is crowned with success, sometimes it is a miserable failure, and occasionally a truce is established between the invader and the defense forces of the body. For inflammation is like life: it is a continuous struggle between two opposite forces, the one friendly, the other hostile. *Trauma* or injury may cause inflammation even though no bacteria are present, as every footballer knows who has wrenched his knee. When tissue is traumatized a substance known as histamine is liberated, and this causes the local changes of inflammation. Other physical irritants which may produce intense inflammation are great *heat* (burns) and *cold* (frostbite), *light* (sunburn), *roentgen rays* and *radium.* It is true that here there is no question of expelling the irritant, but the changes in the tissues are similar to those produced by a foreign body. Examples of *chemical irritants* are strong acids and alkalis, and poisons of every description.

The *bacterial irritants* are by far the most important, because bacteria are universally present, and are continually gaining access to the tissues. They are destroyed by the process of inflammation, but the fight is usually so short and so localized that the patient is not aware of its existence; it is only when it becomes more severe that symptoms develop which demand medical attention. The great majority of acute infections are caused by staphylococci (which are always present in the skin) and streptococci (which are similarly present in the throat), but pneumococci cause the

inflammation of pneumonia, meningococci the inflammation of meningitis, and so on.

The *symptoms* of inflammation have been known since the beginning of medical history; they are *heat, redness, swelling,* and *pain.* The infected finger or the finger containing a sliver is hot, red, swollen, and painful. The meaning of these symptoms has only become apparent in recent times, and in order to understand them we must ask what we mean by saying that inflammation is the local reaction to an irritant, or an attempt to remove the irritant from the body.

The main defense of the body against bacteria, which we shall take as the standard type of irritant, is the leucocytes of the blood. These blood cells have the power of engulfing the bacteria and finally digesting them, an operation known as *phagocytosis* (*phago* ,to eat; *cytos*, cell). Bacteria damage the tissues not merely by their physical presence in enormous numbers, but by the poisons or toxins which they produce. Antagonizing substances called *antitoxins* are produced in the blood which neutralize the bacterial toxins. It is evident, then, that the most important defense forces against bacterial infection lie in the blood. But unfortunately the invaders against which these forces are to operate are not in the blood stream but in the tissues outside the bloodvessels. Something has to be done to bring the defenders out to meet the invaders, and it is this something that is largely responsible for the heat, redness, swelling, and pain which constitute the clinical picture of inflammation.

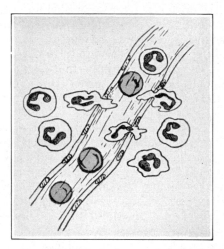

FIG. 10.—Leucocytes passing through vessel wall and collecting outside. No emigration of red cells. (Best and Taylor, The Human Body; courtesy of Henry Holt & Co.)

There are two great phases of the inflammatory process: (1) the vascular or bloodvessel changes, and (2) the formation of the inflammatory exudate. It will be evident in what follows that these two cannot be sharply separated from one another, but it is of help to keep them in mind. In the inflamed finger or appendix we can only guess what is going on, although microscopic examination of the tissue will show us the state of affairs at the particular moment the tissue is removed. But the whole process can be watched under the microscope in the living animal if we use a transparent tissue such as the web of a frog's foot. When an irritant such as a drop of weak acid is applied to the frog's foot the small bloodvessels and capillaries are seen to dilate, so that very much more blood comes to the part, bringing with it great numbers of leucocytes. An increased blood supply means that

the part becomes red and hot, and this is the basis for the heat and redness of the inflamed finger.   If we continue to look down the microscope it will be seen that the blood flow becomes slower in the dilated vessels, and that the leucocytes collect along the walls of the vessels to which they become adherent.   The vessel wall becomes looser in texture, and through this loosened wall the leucocytes, which are of jelly-like consistency, can be seen to make their way, much as a soap bubble might pass through a closed door by flowing though the keyhole (Fig. 10).   In this way great numbers of leucocytes accumulate in the tissues immediately outside the vessels, where they have the desired opportunity of attacking the bacterial irritant. (Fig. 11).

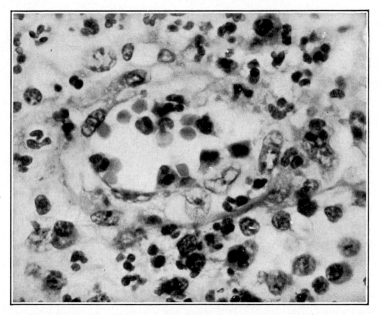

Fig. 11.—Inflammation; separation of elements of vessel wall; emigration of leucocytes.
× 800. (Boyd, Textbook of Pathology.)

Still further assisting the local accumulation of leucocytes is the fact that the bone-marrow, which is the storehouse and factory of the leucocytes, pours out vast numbers into the blood, so that the total number of leucocytes is greatly increased.   This increase is known as *leucocytosis*, and is an indication that inflammation is going on in some part of the body.   A blood examination (leucocyte count) is therefore an invaluable test for determining whether a pain in the right side of the abdomen is due to appendicitis or a pain in the chest is due to pneumonia.   The normal leucocyte count is about 6000 (6000 leucocytes in each cubic millimeter of blood), but in severe inflammation the count may be 30,000 or even higher.

Let us now consider more in detail the elements of the blood which pass through the vessel walls whose permeability has become so greatly in-

creased. The white cells of the blood are of various kinds, but the two important ones in acute inflammation are the polymorphonuclear leucocytes and monocytes. The *polymorphonuclears* are the first to collect outside the vessels; they are the first line of defense. Later they are followed by the *monocytes*, which perform a very different function. Finally there is the fluid part of the blood, the *plasma*. This also passes through the permeable vessel walls and collects in the tissues around the irritant. The plasma which passes out is changed in character and is called serum or inflammatory lymph. The various leucocytes and the serum together form what is known as the *inflammatory exudate*. It is this exudate which is responsible for the swelling that is such a striking clinical feature of inflammation. The swelling causes tension and pressure on the nerves of

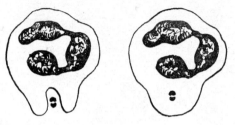

Fig. 12.—Phagocytosis by polymorphonuclear leucocyte.

the part, and this is the cause of the pain, the fourth and most important of the symptoms. It is obvious that the more dense the tissue, the more severe will be the pain, so that the pain will be worse in inflammation of bone (mastoid disease, toothache, etc.) than in inflammation of a loose structure such as the skin. The throbbing of an inflamed finger is caused by the increase of pressure in the dense tissues each time the heart beat forces more blood into the part.

Now that the defense forces have passed from the inside of the vessels to the outside it is time to enquire what part the various elements of the inflammatory exudate play in disposing of the irritant, which we shall presume to be invading bacteria. The first line of defense, the polymorphonuclear leucocytes, approach the bacteria, and when they meet them they throw out arms of protoplasm (the jelly of which they are composed), arms which surround the germ with a deadly embrace, and draw it into the interior of the leucocyte, where it is slowly digested (Fig. 12). The process is known as *phagocytosis* or swallowing by a cell, just as the esophagus is the structure which swallows food. Inflammation is essentially a fight between the defenders and invaders of the body, and the result depends largely on the shock troops, the polymorphonuclears. But the fight is not entirely one-sided. The bacteria discharge their poisonous toxins, which kill great numbers not only of the polymorphonuclears but also of the tissue cells. The battlefield therefore becomes strewn with the dead bodies of cells. At this stage if the defense forces are in the ascendant the monocytes begin to arrive. They also are actively phagocytic and on that account, and also because of their large size, they are called *macrophages* (*macro*, large;

phago, devour). These macrophages are the scavengers of the body, for they remove the débris of the battle by the simple process of engulfing the dead cells. In more chronic inflammations, such as tuberculosis, they also devour the bacteria.

In addition to the polymorphonuclears and the macrophages other cells may play an important part in the inflammatory process. The chief of these are the lymphocyte, the plasma cell, and the eosinophil. The *lymphocyte* is a small round cell which is present in enormous numbers in the lymphoid tissue and lymph nodes of the body. It may put in an appearance in the acute stage of inflammation, but is more characteristic of the later stages. For many years its function was completely unknown, but it is now believed to be an important source of the immune bodies which are so essential for the neutralization of bacterial toxins and for damaging the bacteria themselves. The *plasma cell* is probably derived from the lymphocyte. It is somewhat larger, and is characterized by the fact that its nucleus is at one side of the cell rather than in the center. It also is concerned with the production of immune bodies. The *eosinophil* is similar to the polymorphonuclear lymphocyte, but contains granules which stain intensely with the red stain eosin. Its function is not certain, but it appears in large numbers in those types of inflammation in which allergy plays a part. It is of interest to note that the eosinophils of the blood disappear almost entirely when cortisone is administered.

So far the conflict has been prehistoric in type, a hand-to-hand encounter. But more subtle methods are also employed by both sides, suggestive rather of modern warfare. Reference has already been made to the toxins of the bacteria. Against these the phagocytes are of no avail, but the value of the serum in the inflammatory exudate now becomes apparent. The serum contains antibacterial and antitoxic substances, which increase steadily in amount as the infection progresses, and which are, of course, present not only in the circulating blood but also in the serum which pours through the vessel walls into the inflammatory exudate. The antitoxins neutralize and destroy the toxins of the bacteria, and the antibacterial substances paralyze the bacteria so that they readily fall prey to the phagocytic leucocytes. Antitoxins can be prepared by injecting an animal repeatedly with small doses of toxin until the animal becomes immunized. When the serum of such an immunized animal is injected into a patient suffering from a bacterial infection, the antitoxins which it contains destroy not only any toxins which may be in the patient's blood, but also those which are being produced in the tissues. One of the best examples of this method of treatment is afforded by diphtheria antitoxin.

When the serum is poured out on the surface of a serous membrane such as the pleura or peritoneum, it tends to clot with the formation of *fibrin*. This takes the form of fine interlacing threads (Fig. 13), and a surface covered with fibrin becomes sticky so that it tends to adhere to a neighboring surface. In this way *adhesions* are formed between adjacent coils of bowel, between the pleura covering the lung and that lining the chest wall, etc. These adhesions usually disappear when the inflammation subsides, but sometimes they persist and may cause serious subsequent trouble in the abdominal cavity.

Varieties of Inflammation.—Inflammation has been divided into a number of varieties, although the essence of the process is always the same. The principal types are acute inflammation, chronic inflammation, and granulomatous inflammation. In *acute inflammation* the process is of rapid onset and of comparatively short duration. The characteristic cell is the polymorphonuclear leucocyte. *Chronic inflammation* is a more long-drawn-out process, and is sometimes described as a low type grade of inflammation. The characteristic cells are the lymphocyte and plasma cell. *Granulomatous inflammation* is really a subvariety of chronic inflammation. Whereas acute inflammation is characterized by the formation of an exudate from the bloodvessels into the tissues, granulomatous inflammation is characterized by a proliferation of cells at the site of inflammation. It is spoken of as proliferative or productive in type. The result is that a mass of new tissue is formed which is called a *granuloma*, because of a somewhat fancied resemblance to the microscopic picture of granulation tissue which will be described in connection with the healing of inflammatory lesions. The best known examples of infective granulomas, as they are called, are tuberculosis and syphilis.

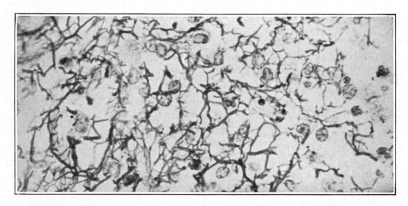

Fig. 13.—Exudate consisting mainly of fibrin. × 600. (Boyd, Textbook of Pathology.)

Results of Inflammation.—The outcome of the conflict depends on two factors, the virulence or destructive power of the bacteria and the resistance of the patient. In most cases the former is weak and the latter is strong. When a needle infected with germs is run into the finger of a healthy person a mild degree of inflammation ensues, but there is every chance that the defenders will overpower the invaders before the latter have time to multiply, and the resulting heat, redness, swelling, and pain may be so trivial as hardly to attract the notice of the patient. Sometimes, however, the bacteria are of such overpowering virulence, as in the case of a pathologist who receives a prick in the finger when performing an autopsy on a patient who has died of streptococcal septicemia, that they paralyze the leucocytes with their toxins, invade the blood stream, set up *septicemia* (blood poisoning), and spread throughout the body with fatal results. This is particularly likely to happen with streptococcal infections.

More frequently the infection is kept within bounds or localized, although there may be extensive damage to the tissues. Infections caused by staphylococci generally remain localized. A digestive ferment is liberated from the bodies of the dead polymorphonuclear leucocytes, and this ferment digests and liquefies the tissue cells which have been killed by the bacterial toxins. *Pus* or matter is a thick yellow fluid consisting of liquefied tissue and the fluid of the inflammatory exudate, and containing polymorphonuclear leucocytes, known here as pus cells, and living and dead bacteria. Inflammation accompanied by the formation of pus is called *suppuration*, and the bacteria responsible are known as *pyogenic* or pus-producing (*pyon*, pus). A cavity is produced in the tissues as the result of the destruction, and this cavity is called an abscess, and is filled with pus (Fig. 14). The cavity is surrounded by a wide barrier of leucocytes which prevent the infecting bacteria from spreading further into the tissues. If the abscess extends and reaches the surface it is said to point; finally it bursts, and pus is discharged on the surface. This may be regarded as a method which the body has of ridding itself of infection and the bursting of the abscess is likely to be followed by healing.

If the abscess is some distance from the surface, the track leading from the abscess to the surface is called a *sinus* (Fig. 15). A sinus may remain open for a considerable time. If the abscess should discharge onto both skin and a mucous surface the track is known as a *fistula* (Fig. 15). Thus if an abscess of the appendix should open on to the skin a fistula is formed between the skin surface and the interior of the bowel.

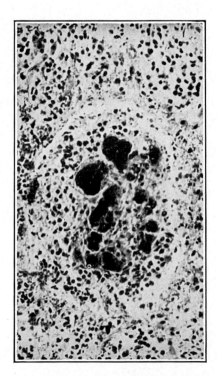

Fig. 14.—Abscess of kidney showing dark masses of bacteria and destruction of tissue. × 275. (Boyd, Textbook of Pathology.)

An *ulcer* is a superficial lesion caused by destruction of the skin or of a mucous membrane (*e.g.*, ulcer of the stomach) (Fig. 16). The cause of the destruction may be a focus of inflammation a short distance below the surface leading to disintegration of the overlying skin or mucous membrane. Or it may be in the nature of a shallow wound which subsequently becomes infected. A *boil* is an abscess of the root of a hair due to bacteria which have penetrated from the skin, often owing to friction, so that it is commonest on

the buttocks and the back of the neck. The root of the hair is a dense
fibrous structure, so that an inflammatory swelling within it causes much
tension and pain until softening occurs and the hard "core" of the boil is
liquefied and extruded. Spontaneous softening may fail to occur owing
to lack of the liquefying ferments of the polymorphonuclears, but the local
application of heat will cause an outpouring of leucocytes and greatly
hasten the process. A *carbuncle* is a group of boils which are connected by
underground channels. It is a much more serious lesion, with extensive
destruction of tissue and great absorption of septic material.

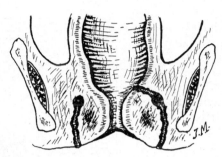

Fig. 15.—Sinus (left) opening on to skin. Fistula (right) connecting rectum and
skin surface.

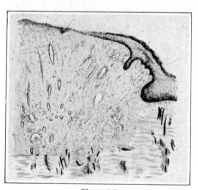

Fig. 16

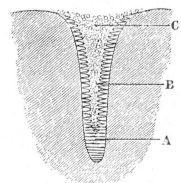

Fig. 17

Fig. 16.—Ulcer of skin, showing epithelium to the right and raw surface to the left.

Fig. 17.—A healing wound. *A*, Wound closed by connective-tissue cells; *B*, gap filled
by exudate; *C*, discharging surface of wound. (Bowlby and Andrewes' Surgical Pathology; courtesy of J. and A. Churchill, Ltd.)

Healing or Repair.—In the living body destruction of tissue is followed
by healing or repair. The process is the same whether destruction has
been due to inflammation or to a wound, surgical or otherwise. The
first requisite for healing is complete destruction of bacteria. Neither an
inflammatory lesion nor a wound can heal if it is infected. The next step
is removal of dead fragments of tissue by macrophages. When this has

been done, healing can commence. In the case of a surgical incision where the edges can be brought together the *fibroblasts* or connective tissue cells in the sides of the wound proliferate and bridge across the narrow gap (Fig. 17). At the same time they form fibers of connective tissue which sew together the edges of the wound much more securely than can the surgeon; the sewing is completed in about five days. The thin connective tissue fibers are then converted into strong, dense scar tissue, a process which takes about three weeks.

When the edges of a wound cannot be united or when healing of an abscess takes place, young vascular connective tissue fills up the cavity from below. This gives the surface of the wound or cavity a granular appearance, so that it is known as a granulating surface and the new connective tissue is called *granulation tissue*. The granulating surface is slowly covered by epithelium which grows in from the edges. At first this is a very thin blue

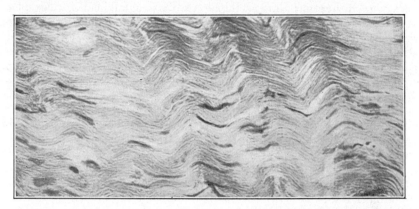

Fig. 18.—Scar tissue. Bundles of collagen fibers, between which are flattened fibroblasts. × 400. (Boyd, Textbook of Pathology.)

layer, like ice forming on a pond in the fall of the year, but after a few weeks it becomes thick and white. At the same time the underlying granulation tissue is becoming converted into dense *scar* tissue (Fig. 18). This has an unfortunate tendency to contract as it gets older, and marked deformities may result in this way. The adhesions of fibrin to which reference has already been made also become converted into scar tissue, and if these adhesions are between loops of bowel, the subsequent contraction may lead to kinking of the bowel and serious intestinal obstruction.

It will be noted that although the word repair has been used, the repair is but a makeshift. The human machine has no replacement parts. If the greater part of a kidney is destroyed by inflammation, it is not replaced by new kidney tissue but only by scar tissue. This is useful for plugging a hole but it has no other use. With advancing years many tissues wear out, but they can only be replaced by scar tissue, a poor substitute. Any house runs down in the wear and tear of seventy years' continuous occupancy by the same tenant. Unfortunately with the human body, as with

the automobile, the older the model is the more repairs are required, and the harder it is to make them.

The process of *healing* is a complex one. Suffice it to say here that newly formed connective tissue grows in from the walls and fills up the abscess cavity, and this is followed by an ingrowth of the skin epithelium which covers the new connective tissue. The process is exactly the same as the *healing of a wound* (Fig. 17).

In this discussion of inflammation we have taken for convenience the example of a finger infected with staphylococci or streptococci. But it will be realized that inflammation may occur in any organ and that it may be caused by many different bacteria. Pyogenic bacteria cause acute inflammation with suppuration and the production of pus. Other bacteria produce a slow or chronic form of inflammation without the formation of pus. Tuberculosis, syphilis, and other important diseases are examples of chronic inflammation, but in these cases the defense forces are the cells of the tissues rather than those of the blood. Here again healing takes place by the formation of scar tissue, so that a former tuberculous lesion in the lung or the glands of the neck can be recognized by the scar which it leaves.

Principles of Treatment.—In the treatment of any infectious disease the doctor may adopt one or both of two methods; he may assist the healing powers of Nature, what the old writers used to call *vis medicatrix naturæ*, or he may directly attack the infecting bacteria. *Rest* to the inflamed part is the most important of all therapeutic measures. Exercise not only acts as an additional irritant, but serves to disperse the bacteria through the tissues and thus increase the area of inflammation. It tends to break down the barrier which the leucocytes try to build up around the bacteria. Thus the inflamed finger is tied up, the inflamed arm is placed in a sling, the inflamed eye is shaded so that it cannot be used, and purgatives are avoided like poison in the treatment of the inflamed appendix.

The second principle is *free drainage*. The quickest way to get an abscess to heal is to open it and let out the pus. This not only allows the infecting bacteria to escape, but also relieves the tension in the inflamed area, and thus encourages the further flow of healing substances from the bloodvessels in addition to relieving the pain. But if pus has not yet formed and a barrier of leucocytes has been built around the bacteria, the knife may do more harm than good, for it may open up fresh channels for spread of the infection.

Heat in the form of fomentations, poultices, etc., is one of the oldest and most efficient methods of treating inflammation. The warmth sends messages up the sensory nerves of the part to the spinal cord; these pass down the nerves to the bloodvessels and cause the latter to dilate, so that additional blood is brought to the part, thus adding to the supply of leucocytes and antitoxins. *Cold* in the form of an ice-bag or cold compresses will relieve the pain by causing the vessels to contract and thus diminish the swelling of the tissues which is responsible for the pain, but it will not increase the local resistance.

In addition to local applications of heat, treatment by means of *hyperthermy* or the artificial production of *fever* has recently come into vogue. A rise in temperature used to be regarded as a sign of disease which had

to be actively combated and forced back to normal. Fever is now known to be a defense mechanism necessary to the protection of the body, although an excessively high temperature is extremely harmful to the brain, heart, and other vital organs. Fever acts beneficially in the following ways: (1) It prevents the growth of certain bacteria and tends to destroy them; (2) it favors phagocytosis and the movement of leucocytes; (3) it stimulates the formation of immune bodies which have an antibacterial action. Various methods can be used for raising the temperature of the body, such as hot baths, radiant heat from lamps, the injection of proteins into the blood stream, the use of a fever-producing agent such as the malaria parasite which can be readily controlled by means of quinine, and high-frequency (short-wave) electrical energy. The most favored method at the present day is the *hypertherm*, an air-conditioned chamber which contains the entire body except the head and neck. The principal infections for which fever therapy has been used are gonorrhea, syphilis, and chronic infective arthritis. By far the best results have been obtained in gonorrhea. The gonococcus is killed outside the body by a temperature of 106° F. for five hours. When the patient is subjected to this temperature for six to eight hours remarkable results have been obtained. It is probable that other bacterial infections will also be found to yield to fever therapy. This form of treatment cannot be used in old age, or in advanced disease of the heart or kidneys. The patient, moreover, must be kept under constant supervision during the period of hyperthermia.

Direct attack on the infecting bacteria may be made by chemotherapy or by immune serum. *Chemotherapy* or treatment of infections by chemical agents is no new invention. Malaria has been controlled for very many years by means of quinine, and in 1910 arsenic in the form of salvarsan, neoarsphenamine, etc. was found to be a specific against the spirochete of syphilis. But an enormous and epoch-making advance was made in 1935 with the introduction of the sulfonamide (abbreviated to sulfa) group of drugs. The first of these was sulfanilamide, which attacks in particular hemolytic streptococci, meningococci, Bacillus coli and other important disease-producing bacteria. This was followed by sulfapyridine, which has a special action on pneumococci, sulfathiazole which is used against the staphylococcus, sulfaguanidine, and others. Just as the medical world was recovering from its astonishment at the remarkable results achieved by the sulfonamides, an even more resounding victory was heralded by the announcement of a new therapeutic miracle, penicillin, which is not a drug supplied by the chemical laboratory, but a product of the common mold, Penicillium notatum. The extreme importance of the new agent lies in the fact that it is potent against organisms which resist the action of the sulfonamides, that it is effective in the presence of pus and is therefore of the greatest value in suppurating wounds, whilst the reverse is true of the sulfonamides, and that it is without the toxic effects which may mar the action of the sulfonamides and sometimes may prove fatal. The method of action and the results achieved is discussed more fully in the chapter on The Treatment of Disease.

Immune sera are of greater value against toxins than against the bacteria which manufacture the toxins. Diphtheria antitoxin is by far the most

potent. Sera prepared against the pneumococcus and meningococcus are of considerable use.

IMMUNITY

Inflammation is a protective phenomenon, one of the means by which the body defends itself against infection. In our discussion much stress has been laid on phagocytosis, which is so easily recognized under the microscope. But there are other and more subtle means by which the body can defend itself, means which are not necessarily associated with the inflammatory process. Bacteria may invade the body and die or be killed before they can gain a foothold and set up inflammation. This is the most perfect type of defense, and the person in whom this occurs is said to be *immune* to the infecting agent.

Immunity to infection depends largely upon properties of the blood serum, although the tissue cells also play a part. The blood of all persons contains a substance called *complement*, which under suitable conditions has the power of destroying bacteria. The amount of complement may be lowered by long-continued infection, starvation, etc., and in such a person the power of resistance is correspondingly diminished. But in order that the complement may unite with and destroy the invading bacteria, there must be a link or connecting substance which brings the two together. This all-important link is known as an *immune body* or antibody, because upon its presence and amount depends the degree of immunity which the person possesses against infection. The antibodies are *specific* with regard to the various bacteria, *i.e.*, there is an antibody against the staphylococcus, one against the streptococcus, one against the typhoid bacillus, and so on. There are antibodies against bacteria (antibacterial immune bodies) and antibodies against toxins (antitoxins).

A person may have antibodies normally in his blood, so that he has a *natural immunity* against a particular infection. Such an individual will pass through an epidemic without acquiring the disease. There is also *acquired immunity*, which is the result of an infection from which the patient has recovered, the tissue cells producing the specific antibody in response to the stimulus of the infecting organisms. Thus a person who has had typhoid fever is immune against a second attack for a number of years.

The fact that immunity can be acquired is utilized by medical science in two very different ways; these ways are summed up by the words vaccines and antitoxins. A *vaccine* is an emulsion of bacteria which have been killed, usually by heat. Although they have now lost their power to produce disease, they still retain the power to stimulate the tissues to the production of antibodies, which will enable the patient to resist this particular infection should he be exposed to it subsequently. Two of the best examples of the prophylactic or preventative use of vaccines are vaccination against smallpox and inoculation against typhoid fever.

The principle of *antitoxin* treatment is entirely different. Here an animal is used to make the antitoxin, and the blood serum of the animal is then injected into the patient, so that the antitoxin may neutralize the toxins in the patient's blood. The words antitoxin and serum are often used

interchangeably. In the preparation of an antitoxin repeated injections of toxin are given to a large animal, such as a horse, in doses at first small but gradually increasing in size. More and more antitoxin is produced by the animal, which thus becomes immune (active immunity), and this immunity is then transferred to the patient (passive immunity). One of the best examples of immunity production by means of antitoxin is the case of diphtheria. From what has been said it is evident that vaccines are of special use in the *prevention* of infectious disease and antitoxins in its *treatment.*

There are two other antibodies which deserve mention, for they play an important part in the defense mechanism; these are opsonins and agglutinins. An *opsonin* in Greek is a sauce or appetizer. Leucocytes washed free from blood serum will not phagocytose bacteria, but when a trace of serum is added they will commence to do so. The serum evidently contains something which makes the bacteria appetizing to the leucocyte, and this something is opsonin. It follows that a person with an abundance of opsonin in his blood will have good immunity, for his leucocytes will have relish for and devour any invading microörganisms.

An *agglutinin* is a substance which causes bacteria to gather together into clumps, *i.e.,* to agglutinate. It does so by imparting a stickiness to the surface of the bacteria. The presence of agglutinins in the blood is of great advantage in defense against bacteria, because it causes them to stick together and to the surrounding tissues, so that they are unable to spread to a distance before the leucocytes arrive on the scene and devour them with the assistance of the opsonins. Agglutinins are greatly increased in amount as the result of infection. This is well seen in typhoid fever, where the Widal test for that disease is in essence a test for the presence of agglutinins.

ALLERGY

A few unfortunate individuals suffer from a peculiar hypersensitiveness to proteins of various kinds, a condition which is the reverse of immunity and which is known as allergy. Frequently the allergic disposition or constitution has a strong hereditary basis. The offending proteins may be those of bacteria, of foods, of animal emanations, or of plant pollens. In such persons even the most minute quantities of the particular protein may produce a violent reaction. The manifestations vary in different people, depending on which particular tissue happens to be hypersensitive. If that tissue is the lining of the nose and eyelids the result is hay fever, if it is the musculature of the bronchi the result is asthma, if it is the wall of the bowel the result is abdominal cramps and diarrhea, if it is the skin the result is urticaria or nettle rash. The same protein may produce effects on different tissues. Thus plant pollen may cause both hay fever and asthma in the same individual, whilst certain foods such as shellfish (shrimps, oysters) and strawberries may cause eczema and urticaria as well as gastrointestinal disturbance.

Hay Fever.—Hay fever is one of the most clear-cut of the allergic diseases. The attacks are strictly seasonal, occurring in spring, summer, or autumn, depending on whether the patient is hypersensitive to the pollens of trees,

grasses, or such a fall plant as ragweed. The symptoms are itching and congestion of the eyes, violent paroxysms of sneezing, and a profuse watery discharge from the nose. The particular protein responsible can usually be determined by means of skin tests, *i.e.*, scratching the arm and rubbing in the suspected protein; if an inflamed area or wheal is produced, the patient is hypersensitive to that protein. When the protein is known the patient may be desensitized against it by means of repeated small injections of the protein before the onset of the hay fever period. In about two-thirds of the cases this is followed by marked improvement.

Many sufferers from hay fever obtain marked benefit from the use of antihistamine drugs. There are many of these materials now available. They counteract the effect of histamine which is liberated in the tissues following exposure to the offending protein material. In some people, these drugs have a marked sedative action producing drowsiness which must be watched for if these drugs are taken while the patient is carrying on his usual activities.

Asthma.—Asthma is an allergic condition in which there is hypersensitiveness of the walls of the bronchi either to foreign proteins of external origin or to bacteria which have their habitat in the respiratory passages. The foreign proteins (*i.e.*, foreign to the body) may be the pollens of plants, the dander and emanations of animals (especially horses), vegetable dusts such as face powders containing orris root, and certain foods such as eggwhite, especially in children. The walls of the bronchi consist mainly of a lining of mucous membrane and layers of plain muscle. In an allergic attack the muscle contracts and the mucous membrane becomes swollen. The patient therefore suffers great difficulty in breathing, even more in expiration than inspiration, and wheezing is a marked feature of the respiratory distress. The treatment of an acute attack of asthma is best carried out by the use of epinephrine by hypodermic injection, or by inhalation of epinephrine spray. Aminophylline and ephedrine are also valuable drugs in the alleviation of an attack of asthma. In severe attacks ACTH has been of value in many instances. The general principles of treatment of asthma from the standpoint of prevention of attacks should be concerned with the removal of any materials to which the patient may be sensitive, but only too often all attempts in this direction end in failure. In addition, many attacks of asthma are precipitated by emotional disturbances, and assistance to prevent this factor may be of great help in this disease. The continued use of drugs such as aminophylline and ephedrine are frequently of value in preventing attacks. The use of the antihistamine drugs in the treatment of asthma is generally disappointing.

Food Allergy.—Many persons are hypersensitive to such articles of diet as oysters, fish, strawberries, pork, cereals, eggs, and milk. In these persons a very small amount of the food in question may produce an immediate attack of vomiting and diarrhea accompanied by collapse, of urticaria and other skin eruptions, or of asthma. The fault lies in the person, not in the food, clearly illustrating the old adage that "what is one man's meat is another man's poison." The search for the article at fault may tax the the detective powers of the physician to the utmost. It may be accomplished by means of skin tests, or even more reliably by eliminating one article after another from the diet.

Chapter

6

SOME BACTERIAL INFECTIONS

THE subject of bacteriology is a vast subject in itself, and for detailed information textbooks on bacteriology must be consulted. In an Introduction to Medical Science reference can only be made to some of the more common bacterial infections. Bacteria may take the form of bacilli (rod-shaped), cocci (spherical), or spirilla (spirals). Some bacilli contain spores, round bodies which make them highly resistant. The various forms are shown in Figure 19. Only a few bacteria are disease-producing or pathogenic (*pathos*, disease). The vast majority are non-pathogenic. Most of these are able to live only on dead matter and are therefore called saprophytes (*sapros*, decayed), in contradistinction to parasites which exist on living matter. Saprophytes are not only harmless, but are essential to

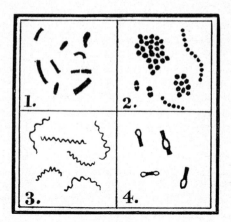

FIG. 19.—Various bacteria. 1, Bacilli; 2, staphylococci and streptococci; 3, spirilla, small spirals—spirillum of syphilis; 4, spore-forming bacilli.

life on this planet, for they keep the supply of food in constant motion. They prepare food materials for plants, which are eaten by animals, which are eaten by man, and finally the dead bodies of animals and men are broken down by bacteria into their original elements, which are returned to the soil. The new antibiotics such as penicillin and streptomycin, which are prepared from microörganisms (fungi) in the soil can kill bacteria with startling rapidity, but if they kill off the useful bacteria they may leave a vacuum which is soon occupied by pathogenic organisms. What is potent for good may be powerful for evil.

In the following pages a brief outline is given of some bacterial infections which are not described in connection with individual organs.

STAPHYLOCOCCAL INFECTIONS

The staphylococcus is a Gram-positive round organism which grows in small clusters like a bunch of grapes. There are two principal forms, Staphylococcus aureus (golden) and Staphylococcus albus (white), depending on the color of the colonies on solid media. The white form is always present on the skin, and is usually, though by no means always, harmless. It is the cause of the stitch abscesses of the skin which sometimes follow a surgical operation.

The staphylococcus is a pyogenic organism, a pus-producer, and is a common cause of acute inflammation. It enters the body through cracks in the skin often as the result of local irritation, such as the rubbing of a hard collar-stud on the neck. The mere pricking of a pimple may start the infection. In contrast to streptococci, the staphylococcus usually produces inflammation which remains localized.

The chief lesions may be external or internal. External lesions occur in the following places: (1) *Skin; pimples* are staphylococcal infections in the surface layer of the skin, *boils* are in the deeper layer, whilst a *carbuncle* is a large collection of pus in the subcutaneous tissue which communicates with the surface by several openings. *Infected wounds and stitch abscesses* are caused by staphylococci. (2) Boils on the *upper lip and nose* are of especial importance, as the infection is apt to pass back along the facial vein (which has no valves) into the cavernous venous sinus in the base of the skull, with a resulting *thrombophlebitis*, a condition of grave danger. (3) On the *eyelid* staphylococci may cause a *stye*. Internal lesions take the form of abscesses principally in the bones (osteomyelitis) and kidneys.

Some persons, especially when young, are subject to repeated staphylococcal infections, especially boils. In these cases injections of a vaccine may gradually make the patient resistant to infection.

STREPTOCOCCAL INFECTIONS

The streptococcus is a Gram-positive spherical organism identical in appearance with the staphylococcus except that it grows in chains of varying length instead of in clusters. It is more difficult to grow than the Staphylococcus, and flourishes best on media enriched with blood (blood agar). Streptococci can be divided into two groups, depending on the reaction on blood agar. In the first group, *hemolytic streptococci*, the bacteria cause hemolysis or breaking down of blood in the medium, so that the colonies are surrounded by a pale colorless halo. In the second group the bacteria produce a green color on the blood agar, so that the group is called *Streptococcus viridans*. The hemolytic group causes much more acute and virulent infections than the viridans group. Streptococcus viridans is of low virulence and does not cause a sharp, acute reaction. Nevertheless it is an important cause of disease. It gives rise to focal or

limited infection in the tonsils, at the roots of teeth, and in the sinuses of the nose and face.

The habitat or natural home of the streptococcus is the mucous membrane of the respiratory and intestinal tracts. It is found less often on the skin. It tends to produce spreading inflammation which extends widely throughout the tissues in comparison with the circumscribed lesions caused by the staphylococcus. Some of the most widespread infections, such as septicemia and peritonitis, are caused by streptococci. It is the commonest cause of puerperal sepsis, the frequently fatal infection which used to follow childbirth. Most cases of septic throat, tonsillitis, and ear infections are due to streptococci.

Streptococcal infections may start in two different ways: (1) Cocci already present on the mucous membrane may invade the underlying tissue owing to some lowering of resistance. It is in this way that tonsillitis, streptococcal pneumonia, and appendicitis may be produced. (2) Virulent streptococci may be introduced from outside the body through the skin or mucous membrane. It is in this way that a surgeon's hand may be infected whilst operating on a septic case, or that the uterus may be infected owing to lack of care during or after labor.

Erysipelas is an acute spreading inflammation of the skin caused by streptococci. The usual site is the face or scalp, the bacteria probably entering from the nose. The inflamed skin is of a bright red color and curiously firm. Like other streptococcal and staphylococcal infections it is accompanied by fever and an increase in the leucocytes of the blood (leucocytosis).

Scarlet fever is caused by a special variety of streptococcus, and is characterized by a high temperature, sore throat, and a widespread rash, often followed by complications in the ear, kidneys, and lymph glands of the neck. The throat is always actively inflamed, and this is probably the starting point of the infection which may spread along the Eustachian tube (the communication between the throat and ear) and cause acute inflammation of the ear. The lymph glands of the neck are swollen, and sometimes abscesses are formed in them. The tongue shows a rash like that of the skin, so that is has a strawberry appearance (strawberry tongue).

The symptoms are caused by the toxin of the scarlet fever streptococcus. This toxin is used in the *Dick test* for susceptibility to scarlet fever. The diluted toxin is injected into the skin, and the appearance of a red area in the course of a few hours shows that the patient has no natural antitoxin in his blood, *i.e.*, he is susceptible to scarlet fever. In early childhood nearly everyone shows a positive reaction, but with increasing years the number of susceptible individuals steadily decreases, due to the fact that most persons are exposed to infection too slight in degree to cause the disease but sufficient to stimulate the formation of antitoxin.

RHEUMATIC FEVER

Rheumatic fever is an acute infection affecting principally the joints and the heart, and accompanied by sore throat. It is difficult to speak with certainty as to its cause, but it may be regarded as a manifestation of in-

fection with hemolytic streptococci which are located in the throat or tonsils. These bacteria are not found, at least in any numbers, in the organs attacked by rheumatic fever, such as the joints and the heart. It is assumed, therefore, that these organs have become hypersensitive or allergic to the streptococci, so that minute quantities of these organisms or their toxic products may produce acute inflammation when they are carried by the blood to the hypersensitive tissues.

The most striking and obvious clinical feature is acute inflammation of the joints, which become so excessively tender that the slightest movement of the joint produces excruciating pain. Nevertheless the inflammation is not a suppurative one, there is little destruction of tissue, and when the infection subsides the joints return to their normal condition. The acute joint symptoms such as swelling and pain are greatly relieved by the use of sodium salicylate, which is practically a specific remedy for this infection.

The same is not true, however, of the heart. During the acute illness there may be no evidence of any cardiac lesion, but months or years later symptoms of these lesions may make their appearance. Rheumatic fever is the commonest cause of heart disease. Both the heart valves and the heart muscle are attacked, but the lesions need not be described here, as they will be considered in connection with diseases of the heart. It is evident that the heart lesions of rheumatic fever are much more serious than the joint lesions, although it is the latter which first claim the attention of the patient and the doctor. For this reason one of the important elements in the treatment of rheumatic fever is prolonged rest in bed, so that the affected heart may have every chance of recovering to the greatest extent possible. Moreover in some persons, particularly in children, the inflammation in the joints may be so slight that the disease is not diagnosed as rheumatic fever, yet the heart may be seriously affected. Patients with rheumatic heart disease may therefore give a history of repeated sore throats, but not of acute joint pains. From all this the truth of the saying becomes apparent that "rheumatic fever licks the joints, but bites the heart."

Rheumatic fever belongs to the group known as the *collagen diseases.* Collagen is another name for the connective tissue of the body, and the chief characteristic of the collagen diseases is degeneration and necrosis of connective tissue fibers and of the ground substance or cement which binds them together. The lesions are found chiefly in the vascular system (heart and arteries), the joints, the serous membranes and the skin. The lesions are controlled to a remarkable degree by cortisone, one of the hormones of the adrenal cortex, or by ACTH, the pituitary hormone which stimulates the production of cortisone.

Treatment.—During an attack of acute rheumatic fever damage may occur to the heart valves and to the heart muscle, which may progress unrecognized at first. During the period in which any activity of the rheumatic process is suspected the patient should be kept at rest in bed until the signs of the acute stage are past. This may require many weeks or months. The use of salicylates, and more recently of cortisone, during this acute phase relieves the symptoms and may prevent some of the progress of the disease, although the use of cortisone has not been over a suffi-

ciently long period, as yet, to enable an adequate assessment to be made. The great value of rest lies in the fact that the greater the strain on the heart the longer will the inflammation take to subside and the greater will be the subsequent damage to the valves and heart muscle. But this does not mean that rest must be prolonged indefinitely; as the heart muscle recovers from exhaustion and resumes its tone, graduated exercise can be resumed and soon the patient may be able to live a normal life again. Something may be done in the way of prevention of further attacks of endocarditis by removal of foci of infection, such as infected tonsils and abscessed teeth, although opinion is divided as to the value of these procedures. It is now believed, also, that recurrent attacks of rheumatic fever can be prevented by the prophylactic use of small doses of sulfonamide, particularly during the winter months when respiratory infections are more likely to occur.

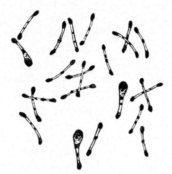

FIG. 20.—Diphtheria bacilli showing granules and Indian clubs.

DIPHTHERIA

The diphtheria or Klebs-Loeffler bacillus (Corynebacterium diphtheriæ) is a thin Gram-positive bacillus, often slightly curved. It stains irregularly with methylene blue, some parts appearing dark, whilst others remain light; for this reason the bacilli may have a granular appearance. There is apt to be pleomorphism, *i.e.*, variation in structure, and some of the bacilli may have an expanded end, giving an Indian-club appearance (Fig. 20). The bacilli are easily stained and easily grown in culture within twenty-four hours. Loeffler's blood serum (solid) is the standard medium for this purpose. Under the microscope the bacilli present an arrangement which suggests a box of split matches.

Unlike many of the other pathogenic bacteria the diphtheria bacillus does not invade the tissues of the patient. It remains on the surface of the mucous membrane of the throat and produces a powerful toxin which kills the cells with which it comes in contact. It also excites a plentiful production of fibrin. The dead or necrosed cells are not shed off, but are bound together by the threads of fibrin to form a tough leathery layer known as the *false membrane*, so-called because it is not one of the natural or true membranes of the body. The name diphtheria is from the Greek meaning leather. Sometimes the nose and rarely the ear, conjunctiva of the eye and

even wounds may be affected. In each of these instances a diphtheritic (false) membrane is formed, which is swarming with bacilli. The incubation period is from two to seven days.

The danger to the patient is twofold: (1) he may die of suffocation owing to the false membrane obstructing the air-passages, especially the glottis; (2) the toxin may be absorbed into the blood and cause paralysis either of the heart or of the peripheral nerves.

Infection may be *spread* directly, *i.e.*, from person to person, or indirectly by infected articles such as cups, handkerchiefs, and even books. Direct infection may be from a patient, but often it is from a healthy carrier, *i.e.*, a person carrying diphtheria bacilli in his throat but not suffering from the disease; often, indeed, he has never had a previous attack.

Immunity against diphtheria may be natural or artificial. About 85 per cent of nursing babies have natural immunity which comes from the mother. This disappears after eight months. Most children are therefore susceptible, and 80 per cent of the deaths occur under five years of age. Susceptibility can be shown by means of the *Schick test*. A minute quantity of diphtheria toxin is injected into the skin. If a red area develops, the person is susceptible to diphtheria. If it does not, he is immune, because his blood contains antitoxin which neutralizes toxins. Susceptible children can be immunized by means of diphtheria *toxoid*. This is diphtheria toxin which has been rendered harmless by the addition of formalin. The immunity is of variable duration, but usually lasts for several years. These procedures are of value both for persons who have been exposed to infection and for children during an outbreak of diphtheria. It can be stated with confidence that the use of toxoid in conjunction with the Schick test has placed in the hands of the physician a weapon with which diphtheria can be finally eradicated. During the year 1940 there was not a single case of diphtheria in Toronto, a city with a population of 800,000. This remarkable result was obtained by wide-spread immunization of young children.

WHOOPING COUGH

Whooping cough or *pertussis* is believed to be due to a minute Gram-negative bacillus known as Bacillus pertussis (Hemophilus pertussis). Although this is found in enormous numbers in the bronchial secretion, it is not certain that this is the causal agent, and some people believe that the disease is due to a virus. The laboratory diagnosis is made by means of a "cough plate"; the patient coughs on to a plate of blood agar, and this is examined next day for colonies of the bacilli.

Whooping cough is a far more dangerous and widespread disease than is generally recognized. The mortality rate for whooping cough is higher than for measles, scarlet fever, and even typhoid fever. It is the pulmonary complications that follow on the initial infection which are responsible for the deaths, and it is the subacute and chronic inflammations of the lung which lead to prolonged illness and pave the way for tuberculosis.

As with diphtheria, it is children who are in danger. About 33 per cent of the cases and 90 per cent of the deaths occur in children under three years of age.

The disease tends to come in periodic epidemics, especially in early spring and late summer. Susceptibility seems to be almost universal. Transmission is either direct from a sick person to a healthy one, or by the common use of freshly contaminated utensils.

Prophylactic inoculation with a vaccine has been tried extensively, but it cannot be said that there is unanimity as to its merits. It seems to be of marked value in one epidemic and of almost no use in another.

TUBERCULOSIS

Tuberculosis is a chronic inflammation caused by Bacillus tuberculosis (Mycobacterium tuberculosis), and is one of the most widespread of all diseases. Amongst the poorer classes of the large cities it is hardly too much to say that after middle life nearly everyone shows evidence of having had tuberculous infection. This is not the same as saying that they are suffering from the disease. The lesions may be extremely small and quiescent, and the presence of the infection may only be demonstrable by means of laboratory tests, but it is there none the less, and the sword of Damocles hangs over the unsuspecting victim's head, occasionally falling where living conditions are unfavorable. It is evident that the natural defensive power of the body against tuberculous infection is sufficiently great to hold it in check in the majority of cases. This defense may be broken down on the one hand by an infection such as influenza which undermines the health,

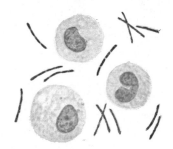

FIG. 21.—Tubercle bacilli in sputum, showing acid-fast character.

by overwork, poor hygienic conditions, insufficient food, etc., and on the other hand by a fresh overwhelming dose of tubercle bacilli.

The *tubercle bacillus* is a thin curved rod which does not grow on the ordinary culture media. It can be stained in a specific way, being colored red by carbol fuchsin and retaining the color after treatment by acid which removes the color from other bacteria (Fig. 21). Bacteria with this property are called acid-fast, a rather misleading term which really means acid-resisting. They are coated with a sheath of waxy material, and it is this sheath which prevents the acid removing the red fuchsin, whereas other bacteria not so protected lose their color. Another example of an acid-fast organism is the bacillus of leprosy. On account of its waxy sheath the tubercle bacillus is an exceptionally hardy germ. It may live for six months if not exposed to sunlight. Direct sunlight, however, will kill it in a few hours, a fact of obvious importance in the prevention of spread of the disease.

The laboratory diagnosis is made by direct microscopic examination of the infected material (sputum, urine, etc.) rather than by culture as is done with most bacteria, because the bacilli do not grow readily on culture media and several weeks may need to elapse before the colonies can be seen.

Inoculation of a susceptible animal such as a guinea-pig is also of great value, but again several weeks must pass before the animal develops evidence of the disease. There are two forms of tubercle bacilli, the human and bovine, the latter causing disease in cows as well as in man. They are identical under the microscope, but can be differentiated by special culture methods and by the inoculation of animals.

Tuberculosis used to head the list of the killing diseases, so that Osler called it the "Captain of the Men of Death." During the nineteenth century, man slew on the battlefield 19 million persons, but during the same period the tubercle bacillus slew 34 millions. The disease is steadily becoming less common as well as less dangerous, even though no specific weapon has yet been discovered with which to fight it. The reduction in the tuberculosis rate is due to the following factors: (1) improved social living conditions with better nutrition, fresh air and sunlight; (2) education in hygiene, so that people lead more healthful lives as regards exercise and fresh air; (3) segregation of the sick in sanatoria and destruction of tuberculous sputum; (4) people seek medical advice earlier; and (5) improved methods of treatment.

Methods of Infection.—In trying to prevent a disease it is essential to know the method of infection. In the case of tuberculosis infection may occur in a number of ways: 1. *By Inhalation.*—The only likely source of infection from man is the sputum of a patient with tuberculosis of the lungs. There is practically no danger of infection from tuberculosis of any other organ. The bacilli may be inhaled from sputum which has dried and been changed into dust. They are soon killed by sunlight, but may survive a long time in the dark. When a patient with pulmonary tuberculosis coughs he infects the air in the immediate neighborhood with millions of tubercle bacilli contained in tiny drops of moisture. It has been estimated that a moderately advanced case may expel from 2 to 4 billion bacilli in twenty-four hours. This gives some idea of the infectivity of such a patient. This is probably the most important method of infection in the adult, for the "dose" of bacilli will be much larger than in the case of inhaled dust, and a large dose has much to do with breaking down the resistance of the exposed person. It is evident how vitally important it is to instruct the patient with pulmonary tuberculosis how to conduct himself so that he will not be a source of danger to those with whom he comes in contact. Attention to certain rules of hygiene, which are also rules of polite behavior, such as coughing into a handkerchief, never expectorating on the floor, etc., remove practically all the danger from living in close contact with a patient suffering from active tuberculosis. The technique of prevention, however, must be as unremitting and relentless as the similar technique in an operating room. Bacilli may also be inhaled from the mouth into the lungs in minute droplets of fluid. It is probable that many children become infected through the introduction of bacilli into the mouth by contaminated hands followed by inhalation into the lungs. The danger to a child crawling about the floor on which tuberculous sputum has been expectorated is self-evident. There are thus three principal methods of infection by inhalation, *e.g.*, dust infection, droplet infection, and mouth infection.

2. *By Swallowing.*—Children frequently acquire tuberculosis by drinking infected cow's milk. Here, of course, the bacillus is of the bovine type, and the lesions are naturally abdominal, either in the bowel or in the abdominal lymph glands. But the glands in the neck may also be infected by bacilli passing through the tonsils. The amount of infection with the bovine tubercle bacillus in a community depends on the strictness of the milk inspection. The danger of milk infection is greatest in the first five years of life, and remains marked to the age of sixteen. It is comparatively slight in adults, who are relatively insusceptible to bovine infection. The importance of the rigid sanitary control of milk supplies to children is self-evident.

3. *Through the Skin.*—Although this method is rare it is of importance to the nurse and the laboratory technician because the disease may be acquired by handling infected material, and is therefore liable to develop on the hands of nurses, orderlies and pathologists, the latter being infected in the post-mortem room. A warty lesion develops on the hand, and the infection may spread up the arm to the lymph glands in the axilla, but there is little danger of general infection or infection of the lungs.

Methods of Spread.—The tubercle bacillus is like the streptococcus, as it causes a spreading infection and may invade the blood stream. The infection may spread in three ways: (1) *Through the tissues.* In the organ infected, unless the defense forces gain the mastery, the disease will gradually spread until the greater part of that organ is destroyed. (2) *By the lymphatics.* The bacilli tend to spread from the site of infection along the lymphatic vessels to the lymph glands which drain the part, where they set up tuberculous disease. Thus the glands in the neck are infected from the tonsil, the glands in the chest from the lung, the abdominal glands from the bowel. (3) *By the blood stream.* A breaking-down tuberculous lesion may perforate the wall of a vessel and discharge millions of bacilli into the blood stream. These are arrested in every organ in the body, where they cause the formation of numberless minute lesions the size of a pin's head; these are called miliary tubercles and the condition is known as *general miliary tuberculosis.* In addition to this massive infection, occasional bacilli may enter the blood stream and set up a single tuberculous focus in one organ such as kidney or bone.

The Lesions.—Tuberculosis is a chronic inflammation. The characteristic cell of the inflammatory exudate is the macrophage, which becomes changed in character so that it has a swollen pale body and indefinite outlines. These characteristics are due to the fact that the fatty envelope of the bacilli is dissolved and taken up by the cells, which in their new form are called *epithelioid cells* (epithelial-like) and are the most characteristic single feature of the tuberculous reaction. The bacilli are surrounded by a mass of these cells which are actively phagocytic. Sometimes a number of epithelioid cells will fuse together to form a large *giant cell,* with as many nuclei as there are cells concerned with its formation. Further out there is a zone of lymphocytes, also called small round cells. There is none of the dilatation of bloodvessels nor exudation of serum which is so characteristic of acute inflammation, and for this reason the heat and redness of acute inflammation are also absent.

The collection of inflammatory cells around the clump of tubercle bacilli forms a little mass which becomes visible to the naked eye and is called a *tubercle* or *miliary tubercle* (*milium,* a millet seed) (Fig. 22). This is the standard lesion of tuberculosis, and is found in whichever organ the disease occurs, be it lung, kidney, or brain. Indeed, it is the tubercle which originally gave the disease its name. As the bacilli spread throughout the organ large numbers of tubercles are formed, and these grow ever larger, fuse together, and thus come to form extensive tuberculous areas.

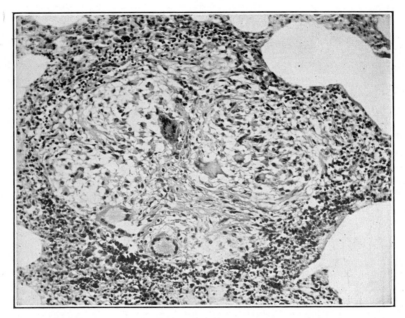

FIG. 22.—A miliary tubercle in the lung, showing epithelioid cells, giant cells, and peripheral lymphocytes. × 150. (Boyd, Textbook of Pathology.)

Meanwhile a further change takes place in the center of the tubercle. The cells are killed by the bacilli, undergo necrosis, and finally lose all vestige of structure and fuse together to form a cheesy mass which is called caseous (cheesy) material, the process being known as *caseation.* In the course of time the caseous material may become liquefied, so that a cavity or cavities are formed in the organ.

Organs Involved.—Practically every organ of the body may be involved by tuberculosis. It is exceptional, however, for more than one or two organs to be attacked at the same time, except in general miliary tuberculosis. Although such a bone as the femur must necessarily be infected from the blood stream, it is nevertheless unusual for other bones to be involved in the same case. It is difficult to give a satisfactory explanation for this behavior.

The *lungs* and *pleura* are most frequently attacked, and pulmonary disease accounts for 85 to 90 per cent of all deaths from tuberculosis.

Lymph glands come next, most often those in the neck, less frequently the abdominal glands. Tuberculosis of the *larynx* is a serious form, secondary to pulmonary tuberculosis. The *intestine* may be the seat of tuberculous ulcers, due in children to drinking infected milk, in adults to swallowing tuberculous sputum. The bacilli may spread from these ulcers to the *peritoneum* and cause tuberculous peritonitis. Tuberculosis of the *kidney* is not uncommon, and it tends to spread down to the *bladder*, and in the male may infect the *prostate* and *testes*. In the female the *Fallopian tubes* are often infected, a condition known as tuberculous salpingitis. The *bones* and *joints* are often involved, especially in children; in the *spine* the condition is called Pott's disease. Tuberculous *meningitis* is the most fatal form. Other organs may also be attacked, but the above-named are the commonest.

Possible Outcome.—Tuberculosis is a fight in which the forces of attack and defense, of destruction and conservation, are usually fairly evenly balanced. The outcome depends on two main factors, the resistance of the tissues and the size of dose of the bacilli. If the resistance is good and the dose small there is a proliferation of fibrous tissue around the tubercle which limits the spread of the infection and eventually invades the tubercle and converts it into a mass of scar tissue known as a *healed tubercle*. This process of encapsulation and scarring is seen particularly well in the lung, and may occur even when the tuberculous area is of considerable size. Tuberculous scars are commonly found at the apex of the lung, and these scars often contain calcium which is deposited in the caseous material as healing occurs, and which can be detected in roentgen-ray pictures. Healing of the tuberculous lesion is by far the most common outcome.

When the dose of bacilli is larger or the resistance of the patient is lowered by overwork, etc., the disease tends to progress slowly, but fibrous tissue formation is continually going on, so that the destruction of tissue is gradual, and the process may be halted after it has lasted for a long time. Halting, however, is not synonymous with recovery, and unless the patient pays strict attention to the rules of hygiene the process may light up again, with recurrence of the severe symptoms. He is metaphorically sitting on a barrel of gunpowder and he must not forget that fact.

Finally, the infection may be overwhelming and resistance at a minimum. In these cases there is almost pure destruction with practically no attempt at limitation; the disease rages like a fire throughout the lung, huge cavities are formed, and the patient dies in the course of a few weeks or months. These are the cases which are popularly and justifiably known as galloping consumption.

Though particular mention has been made of the lung, because it is the organ most commonly attacked by tuberculosis, it will be understood that the same variations of the disease may occur in any organ with the same caseation, cavity formation, fibrosis, calcification, etc.

Many years ago Osler illustrated the possible outcome in tuberculosis by reference to the parable of the sower. "Some seeds fell by the wayside, and the fowls of the air came and destroyed them"; these are the bacilli which are scattered broadcast from an infectious case, but few are inhaled by

other persons, and the majority of these bacilli die. "Some fell on stony places"; these bacilli fail to grow in immune persons, or form only small lesions which wither away "because they have no root." "Some fell among thorns"; these seeds grow, but the protecting forces serve to choke them. "But others fell on good ground and sprang up and bore fruit a hundred-fold"; these are the cases where the dose is overwhelming and resistance at a minimum.

In the *prevention* of tuberculosis two factors must be considered: the infection and the resistance of those exposed to the infection. There are two sources of infection: the human patient with pulmonary tuberculosis and infected cows' milk (bovine infection). The latter, which is of special importance in children, can be combated by testing dairy cows with tuberculin, pasteurization of milk, and other public health measures. Spread of infection from the patient can be prevented by careful disposal of the sputum, and education in the dangers of unguarded coughing and spitting. Tubercle bacilli can live outside the body as long as they have food and moisture and are protected from direct sunlight. Under these conditions they may survive for months. Sputum cups which can be burned are preferable. If these are not available, the regular cups and their contents should be boiled for ten minutes. Gauze used for the collection of sputum can be burned. If the patient does not go to a sanatorium, the other members of the household should undergo a periodic check-up by the tuberculin test and roentgen-ray examination for the development of infection.

Principles of Treatment.—We have seen that tuberculosis is a struggle in which the defense forces have an excellent chance of victory. Treatment is directed not towards a frontal attack on the tubercle bacillus but to assisting the forces of conservation. In this task the master word is Rest. The rest must be both local and general. Some organs or parts can be rested, whilst others, of course, cannot. A tuberculous joint can be put completely at rest, and in the earlier stages of the disease the power of recovery is remarkable. The seemingly impossible feat of resting the lung has been made possible by means of artificial pneumothorax, which consists in the introduction of air into the pleural cavity between the lung and the chest wall; the pressure of the air causes the lung to collapse so that it can no longer move when the patient takes a breath. Breathing is done with the other lung. On the other hand nothing can be done to rest such an organ as the kidney, and in this case the only satisfactory treatment is removal of the diseased organ. General rest including mental rest is just as important as local rest; that is why sanatorium treatment is so valuable. Rest is, of course, only one factor in the regimen, which includes good food, fresh air, absence of worry, and sleep.

In the past the direct attack against the tubercle bacillus by means of antibacterial drugs has been completely unsuccessful, largely on account of the sheath of waxy material which surrounds the bacillus like an armored plate. Experimental work on tuberculous infections in animals with new chemotherapeutic agents holds out hope that this defense may be broken down in the not too distant future. If such proves to be the case, the result will be one of the most notable triumphs in the history of medical science.

SYPHILIS

Syphilis, like tuberculosis, is a chronic inflammatory disease of long duration, but differs in being one of the venereal diseases. It is acquired by contact with a syphilitic lesion in a patient suffering from the disease, usually but by no means invariably during sexual intercourse, so that the first lesions to appear are on the genital organs. Sometimes, however, the primary lesion may appear on the finger, as in the case of a doctor examining a syphilitic patient, or on the lip from kissing an infected mouth.

Although syphilis has been the subject of study for hundreds of years, our modern knowledge of the disease is based on three great discoveries which were made in the course of five years at the beginning of the twentieth century, for its cause was discovered in 1905 by Schaudinn, an invaluable test for its presence was introduced by Wassermann in 1906, and a specific

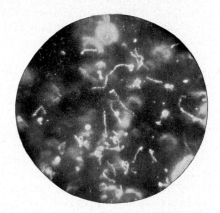

FIG. 23.—Treponema pallidum as they appear under the dark-field microscope. Magnification × 600. (Park and Williams.)

cure in the form of arsenic ("606") was given to the world by Ehrlich in 1910. By means of the *Wassermann test* on the blood we have learned that many manifestations of disease which previously were mysterious and baffling are in reality due to syphilis.

Cause.—The cause of syphilis is a delicate spiral-shaped organism, the Spirochæta pallida (Treponema pallidum). It cannot be grown on any of the ordinary culture media nor stained by ordinary staining methods. It is best demonstrated by the dark-field method, in which a special attachment to the microscope enables the organisms to be seen as bright white threads against a dark background (Fig. 23). The early lesions, both on the genital organs and in the mouth, contain enormous numbers of spirochetes, so that these lesions are highly infectious.

Wassermann Reaction.—The Wassermann reaction is a test for the presence of syphilitic infection. Its special value lies in the fact that it is positive even in the absence of any clinical evidence of syphilis, so that with its assistance latent cases of the disease can be detected. This is of the

greatest importance in any campaign designed to stamp out this cursed disease.

The reaction is based on the principle of *complement fixation*. It has been pointed out in the section on Immunity that antibodies or immune bodies are produced by the tissues in response to infection by bacteria. Any substance which calls forth the production of an antibody is known as an antigen. The antibody cannot unite with and neutralize the antigen unless the two are linked together by a third substance known as complement. When the three are linked together the complement is said to be *fixed*, for it is unable to enter into combination with another antigen-antibody pair. Complement can therefore be used as an indicator of the presence of an antigen and its corresponding antibody. If antigen and complement are placed in a test-tube and the blood serum of a patient is added, the complement will be fixed if the serum contains the corresponding antibody, but it will remain free if the antibody is absent. If the antigen added to the test-tube is syphilitic antigen, it is evident that the reaction can be used to detect the presence or absence of syphilitic antibody in the patient's blood, to show, in other words if the patient does or does not suffer from syphilitic infection.

The test consists of two steps. The first has just been indicated. The second step consists in showing whether the complement has been fixed or if it is still free. This is done by adding another antigen-antibody mixture of such a character that a color change occurs if union takes place owing to the presence of complement. This mixture consists of the red blood cells of a sheep (antigen) and the serum of a rabbit into which sheep's red cells have been injected so that an antibody to the sheep's cells is produced by the rabbit. If the sheep's red cells and the rabbit's serum are placed in a test-tube they do not unite because there is no complement present to link them together. The sheep's cells are unaffected and fall to the bottom of the tube leaving a colorless fluid above. If complement is added the antigen and antibody unite, and the red cells are dissolved or hemolyzed, so that they disappear but color the contents of the tube red. It is evident that if the colorless contents of the first tube (syphilitic antigen, antibody and complement) are added to the second tube, the presence or absence of hemolysis will indicate whether or not complement has been fixed in the first tube. This in turn will show whether or not the patient's blood contained the syphilitic antibody. A positive and a negative reaction are illustrated diagrammatically in Plate I.

Other tests are used either as a check for the Wassermann reaction or in place of it. Most of these, as for example the well-known *Kahn test*, depend on precipitation rather than on complement fixation. The antigen is added to the patient's blood serum, and the occurrence of a precipitate indicates the presence of syphilitic infection. It is evident that the technique of this type of test is much simpler than a test based on complement fixation, but this does not mean that it requires any less skill or accuracy than the Wassermann reaction. In all laboratory tests for syphilis the results of a wrong report are so far-reaching and disastrous that the most meticulous care is needed not only in the performance of the test but also in the collection and labelling of the sample of blood.

PLATE I.—WASSERMANN REACTION

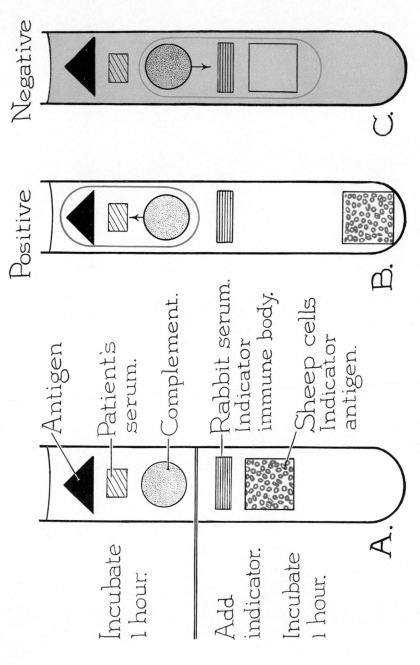

Antigen

Patient's serum.

Complement.

Rabbit serum. Indicator immune body.

Sheep cells Indicator antigen.

Incubate 1 hour.

Add indicator.

Incubate 1 hour.

A.

Positive

B.

Negative

C.

In the positive tube the sheep's cells have fallen to the bottom; in the negative tube they have been hemolyzed.

Course of the Disease.—What may be called the natural history of the disease is peculiar and highly interesting, and can be divided into three stages known as primary, secondary, and tertiary. For three or four weeks after infection the person feels perfectly well and shows no evidence of the disease. Then a lesion known as the *primary sore* or *chancre* appears at the site of infection. It takes the form of a curiously hard nodule, quite painless, which may become ulcerated, enormous numbers of spirochetes being discharged from the raw surface. The lesion consists of masses of chronic inflammatory cells, with no sign of acute inflammation. In the course of a few weeks it heals and may or may not leave a tell-tale scar. The regional lymph glands, *i.e.*, those which drain the part, are enlarged and hard in the primary stage. Usually these are the glands in the groin, but if the primary lesion is on the lip the glands below the jaw will be involved. At the end of the primary stage the patient appears to have recovered, but the Wassermann test in the blood has now become positive, and shows that although he seems to be so well he is really suffering from active syphilis.

The *secondary lesions* appear after two or three months, and are due to the spirochetes having been carried far and wide by the blood stream from the primary lesion throughout the body. The skin, mucous membranes, and lymph glands are principally affected. A great variety of *skin rashes* may appear, which may easily be mistaken for some other skin disease. White patches appear on the mucous membrane lining the mouth, tongue, and tonsils; they are called *mucous patches*, and as they discharge countless spirochetes they are highly infective. The *lymph glands* all over the body become slightly enlarged. All of these secondary lesions finally disappear without leaving any trace, and the patient again appears to be well, although the Wassermann test in the blood is still positive.

The *tertiary lesions* appear after an interval of one or many years. They are essentially destructive, and even if they do heal they leave the organ damaged and badly scarred. Tertiary lesions are so widespread that to enumerate them would be like giving the list of the ships in *The Iliad* or the names of the kings of Judah, but one or two may be mentioned. Ulcers followed by *scarring in the upper third of the leg* below the knee are often syphilitic. Syphilis frequently attacks the arteries; in the brain the small arteries become thickened and narrowed so that thrombosis is apt to develop; in the main arteries such as the aorta the wall becomes so weakened that the diseased part of the vessel dilates and forms a bulging known as an *aneurysm*. The most serious of all the tertiary lesions are those in the nervous system, which may develop many years after the original infection. The spinal cord may be involved with the production of *locomotor ataxia*, also known as *tabes dorsalis*, or the chief lesions may be in the brain causing *general paralysis of the insane*.

The *laboratory diagnosis* in the primary stage is made by dark-field examination for the spirochetes in the discharge from the primary sore, and in the secondary and tertiary stages by the Wassermann test on the blood.

Prevention.—The prevention of venereal diseases is a matter of special difficulty, because they possess social and moral features which are peculiar to them alone. The very names of syphilis and gonorrhea have been banned

in the past. Their economic importance is enormous. Our mental hospitals are filled with the victims of syphilis. But the most grievous burden falls on the innocent, particularly on women and children. Fortunately there are signs that governments are awakening to the menace of these most prevalent of diseases; they cripple the manpower of a nation in war time, and nothing is better calculated to stir a modern government to activity than the discovery of that fact.

Of the two diseases, syphilis is much the more far-reaching in its effects because it attacks such vital organs as the heart, the arteries, and the brain. It is also much more readily preventable. One of the most urgent public health problems at the present day is the prevention of this disease. Speaking of the United States, Dr. Thomas Parran, head of the United States Public Health Service declares that syphilis attacked and disabled more than half a million persons in 1935, that it is more common than measles, twice as common as tuberculosis, and a hundred times as common as infantile paralysis. It disables five times as many persons as are permanently disabled by automobile accidents. It is responsible for 10 per cent of all cases of insanity, 18 per cent of all diseases of the heart and arteries, and for many stillbirths and deaths of babies in the first few weeks of life. It ranks with cancer, tuberculosis, and pneumonia as one of the four great killing diseases.

In the past the public and governing bodies have not only imitated the ostrich by burying their heads in the sand, but have insisted on washing their hands while in that comforting position. "The wages of sin is death; let the sinner die." Funds are donated by governments and philanthropists for fighting every disease from yellow fever to the common cold, but no one hears of money being given for waging war against syphilis. The problem of syphilis, however, must not be confused with the problem of prostitution. From the statistics of large clinics it appears that only about 25 per cent of cases can be traced to the commercial prostitute, a large number are due to clandestine love affairs, and in the remainder the infection is conveyed from husband to wife, or is due to a kiss, a soiled drinking cup, or other methods of transmission. If we wish to do so, we can stamp out syphilis quite as effectively as typhoid fever has been stamped out; indeed from the purely scientific point of view the task is much simpler, for the spirochete of syphilis is a delicate organism which cannot live outside the body like the typhoid bacillus for any period of time. But if the task is to be accomplished, the same means must be employed which have been found effectual in controlling the other great killing infections. In Scandinavian countries, where compulsory measures have been adopted, syphilis has been controlled to a remarkable degree. Thus, in Sweden there were only 431 new cases in one year, whilst in the state of New York (excluding New York City), with the same population, there were 1836 new cases in one month. In Great Britain the syphilis rate has been cut in half since 1920.

The main lines of attack on this great plague are: (1) Prompt treatment, (2) examination of the family of the patient by means of the Wassermann test, (3) the detection of syphilis in the numberless cases where the infection may mimic other diseases, and (4), most important of all, educa-

tion of the public and a consideration of the advisability of teaching social hygiene in schools. If treatment is delayed for a few weeks until the Wassermann reaction in the blood becomes positive, the chances of permanent cure are greatly lessened. In an obstetrical clinic a Wassermann test should be done on every patient, for if the pregnant woman is treated before the fifth month there is an excellent chance that the baby will be born free from disease. It is true that these are therapeutic measures, and that prevention is better than cure, but in the war against syphilis the most powerful weapon for prevention is adequate and universal treatment of the infection. In conclusion we may again quote Dr. Parran: "Syphilis must be the next great plague to go."

Treatment.—The treatment of syphilis has been revolutionized in recent years. With modern methods the disease can be cured in the majority of cases, provided that an early diagnosis is made and vigorous treatment is started at once. For centuries mercury was the sheet anchor, but this merely stimulated the natural defense forces of the body which are never sufficient in themselves. In 1910, Ehrlich showed that certain preparations of arsenic attacked spirochetes directly and he named his preparation salvarsan or "606" because he had previously tried 605 other preparations which proved unsatisfactory. Preparations of bismuth were also used in combination with arsenical compounds. However, with the advent of penicillin, treatment of syphilis has been further changed so that now penicillin is used almost entirely in the treatment of all forms of syphilis with more satisfactory results than have been obtained with any previous method of treatment. It would appear from recent observations throughout the country that syphilis may become a disappearing disease because of the effective control of it with penicillin. Occasionally in some forms of nervous system involvement the addition of artificial fever treatment is of help.

Congenital Syphilis

Syphilis may be either acquired or congenital. In congenital syphilis the child is infected with the disease from the mother before birth, although it does not necessarily show signs of the disease at birth. Indeed there are three possibilities: (1) The child may be born dead, usually showing well-marked evidence of syphilis. Syphilis is an important cause of stillbirth. (2) The child may be born alive with external evidence of syphilis. The skin shows inflammatory patches on the buttocks, the spleen is enlarged, and the mucous membrane of the nose is ulcerated with subsequent destruction of the bridge of the nose (saddle-nose of congenital syphilis). (3) The child may appear healthy at birth, but lesions appear later. These lesions are on the whole similar to those of acquired syphilis, but in addition the teeth may be small and peg-shaped, and the cornea of the eye may become hazy and opaque.

ANTHRAX

The anthrax bacillus is a large square-ended, Gram-positive bacillus, which outside the body forms spores (Fig. 24). The spores are extremely

resistant to chemical disinfectants and also to heat. They may remain alive in the soil for many years, and when they finally get a chance to enter the body again develop into bacilli. The organisms grow readily in culture.

Anthrax is a disease of animals, principally cattle and sheep. It is very prevalent in European animals, but is much less common in North America, so that in this country the human disease is correspondingly uncommon.

Man is infected from animal material, not from other persons; usually from the hides of cattle or the wool of sheep. The skin is the common site of infection, and the disease may be acquired by using infected shaving brushes, working with the hides of diseased cattle, etc. The spores may be inhaled into the lungs, usually in the process of the "carding" of wool; the pulmonary form is known as "woolsorters' disease."

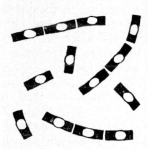

FIG. 24.—Anthrax bacilli showing spores.

The skin lesion is called a *malignant pustule* and is easily recognized. A pimple appears on the surface of the hand, forearm, or face, which develops into a boil and then a pustule containing blood-stained fluid swarming with anthrax bacilli. The surface turns black, and then presents a highly characteristic appearance. If it is recognized and promptly excised, recovery follows. If not, the blood stream is invaded, the bacilli multiply with frightful rapidity, filling the capillaries of all the organs, and death soon results. A specific antiserum gives good results when used in conjunction with early excision of the lesion. The pulmonary form is always fatal. Penicillin and aureomycin have been used with beneficial results in anthrax infections in recent years.

PLAGUE

The disease is caused by Bacillus pestis (Pasteurella pestis), a small Gram-negative extremely virulent organism. There is no more terrifying chapter in the story of disease than that of plague. The great plagues of the Middle Ages were worse than any wars. The Black Death came the nearest to exterminating the human race, for it killed 25 million people in Europe at a time when the population of that continent was very small. Zinsser, in his delightfully written *Rats, Lice and History*, refers to plague and typhus as "those two calamities sharing with human ferocity the greatest responsibility of wholesale sorrow, suffering and death throughout the ages."

The bacillus usually enters the body through the skin by means of the bite of a flea which carries the infection from the rat to man. Indeed plague is primarily a disease of rats. A human epidemic is accompanied or preceded by a rat epidemic. When a rat dies the infected fleas leave it and go in search of a new and preferably a human victim. A patient with plague is not infective unless fleas carry the infection from him to others.

There is no inflammation at the site of the flea bite, but the nearest lymph glands become swollen and acutely inflamed, forming masses called

buboes. It is these which give the disease its name of bubonic plague. The bacilli then invade the blood stream and are found in enormous numbers in the internal organs. The patient dies of an overwhelming septicemia before their is time for marked lesions to develop. The mortality is extremely high, and the patient may be dead in less than twenty-four hours.

Sometimes an epidemic takes a pneumonic form, in which the infection is spread by droplets of sputum. Pneumonic plague is one of the most deadly and rapidly fatal of all infections.

The control of plague consists in the extermination of rats, and in preventing them from leaving a ship coming from a country where plague is prevalent. This is done by placing large discs on the ship's cables, which prevent the rats running down the ropes. The problem of the flea has also to be kept in mind. The deadly triangle of the rat, the flea and man must be broken.

Treatment with sulphadiazine and streptomycin has resulted in some improvement in the outlook in cases of plague. Measures to control the flea have been increasingly effective since the introduction of D.D.T. during World War II. The use of D.D.T. in areas infested with rats and also the dusting of persons exposed to fleas are important in the control of this menace.

TULAREMIA

Tularemia is a plague-like disease which affects animals principally, but which may be spread from them to man. Ground squirrels and jackrabbits are the animals most often affected. The name comes from Tulare County in California, where an epidemic disease killed large numbers of ground squirrels, the causal organism being named Bacterium tularense. Infection is carried from animals to man (1) by biting flies, (2) by ticks, and (3) most often by contact with skins of infected rabbits. It is seen, therefore, in farmers, hunters, butchers, housewives, and others who are likely to skin rabbits. In man the disease is fortunately not nearly so fatal as in animals.

The bacteria enter through cuts and cracks in the skin, and an ulcer develops at the site of infection. In this respect the disease differs from plague. The regional lymph glands are swollen and tender, as in plague. There is prolonged fever and prostration. Recovery is the rule, but convalescence may take some months. In fatal cases areas of necrosis are found in the internal organs.

UNDULANT FEVER

This disease is caused by a very small organism midway in form between a coccus and bacillus. For this reason it is called neither, but is given the name of its discoverer, Sir David Bruce, and is known as Brucella. Infection with Brucella (brucellosis) is essentially an animal disease, attacking particularly cattle and goats. The germs infecting these two kinds of animals are of slightly different strains, although indistinguishable under the microscope. That infecting goats is known as Brucella melitensis,

6

because it was first discovered by Bruce in the goats on the island of Malta. The strain infecting cattle is called Brucella abortus, because it produces contagious abortion in these animals; it also infects swine. Man acquires the infection by drinking cows' milk or goats' milk. In North America the only infecting agent which need be considered is Brucella abortus.

The disease is extraordinarily prevalent in cattle. In some parts of the Eastern States 90 per cent of the herds are infected. Fortunately the abortus infection is not so pathogenic for man as the melitensis form. Most of the persons who drink infected cows' milk show no sign of the disease, though they may have agglutinins in the blood, indicating that they have been infected. But the disease is undoubtedly very much commoner than is usually thought. Its great importance lies in the fact that it is apt to be confused with such long-continued fevers as typhoid, miliary tuberculosis, and subacute bacterial endocarditis. These are all apt to be fatal diseases, whereas in undulant fever the mortality is less than 2 per cent.

The disease begins insidiously with an evening rise of temperature, and the patient may be ill for some time without knowing that he has any fever. The fever may come in waves, hence the name undulant fever, although this feature is often absent. Its most striking characteristic is its remarkable persistence; three months is an average duration, but it may last for years. Persistent weakness, muscle pains, joint pains, and marked perspiration with a peculiar sweet sickly odor to the sweat are some of the common features of a disease which may easily pass unrecognized. The patient may feel extraordinarily miserable, and one doctor remarked on recovering from the disease: "If the cows felt as miserable as I did, I do not blame them for aborting." Strange to say, there are no characteristic lesions, merely those of any septicemia.

The most reliable means of diagnosis is the test for agglutinins in the blood against Brucella abortus, a test identical with the Widal test for typhoid. Agglutination in a dilution of over 1 in 100 indicates active disease; agglutination in a dilution of 1 in 80 in the absence of clinical symptoms indicates a past infection.

Recently, the use of aureomycin and a combination of streptomycin and sulfadiazine have resulted in improvement and often cure of this infection.

ANAEROBIC BACTERIA

All the bacteria which have been considered so far are able to live and multiply in air, or rather in oxygen. There is a group, however, which cannot do so, and these are called the anaerobes. They are all Gram-positive bacilli, and are of large size. Three of this group demand special consideration; two are important in wound infection and the third in food poisoning.

Bacillus Welchii (Clostridium Perfringens).—This anaerobic bacillus was discovered by the great American pathologist William Welch in 1891. It occurs in the intestinal tract of men and animals where it does no harm, but wounds may become infected either by soil containing animal manure or from contaminated clothing. It is in war wounds that Bacillus welchii infection is of the greatest importance. The bacillus is short, plump, Gram-

positive, produces spores, and is surrounded by a capsule which gives it a characteristic appearance (Fig. 25).

Unlike ordinary disease-producing bacteria it does not invade living tissue, growing only in dead or injured tissue where there is a sufficiently low supply of oxygen to meet its requirements. It is therefore a saprophyte. It flourishes in muscles which have been torn up by bullets or fragments of shrapnel, have been deprived of their blood supply, and are thus anaerobic.

The chief characteristic of Bacillus welchii is that it produces gas from the muscle sugars, so that it is commonly called the "gas" bacillus, and the disease itself is known as *gas gangrene*. The gas is the result of fermentation, which may be defined as the splitting of a complex organic compound (in this case muscle sugar) into simpler elements. The gas spreads along the muscle sheaths, separating these from the muscles, and bubbles of foul-smelling gas and blood-stained fluid can be pressed up and down the length of the muscle. This fluid is highly toxic, so that it kills the muscle fibers which are then invaded by the bacteria. The process is one of putrefaction or breaking down of muscle, and is marked by a terrible odor. A toxin is also produced, which poisons the patient. Against this toxin an antitoxin has been prepared.

The most important part of the *treatment* of gas gangrene is to reduce the likelihood of anaerobic environment for the organisms by adequate surgical treatment to remove dead tissue and blood clots. The use of antiserums and large doses of penicillin have also been effective in controlling this type of infection in wounds.

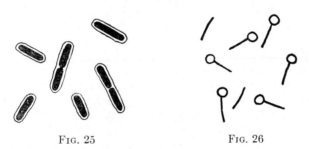

Fig. 25   Fig. 26

Fig. 25.—Bacillus welchii showing capsules.

Fig. 26.—Bacillus tetani showing terminal spores.

Bacillus Tetani (Clostridium Tetani).—The tetanus bacillus is a slender anaerobic organism with a spore at one end, giving it an appearance like a drum-stick which is highly characteristic (Fig. 26). It lives in the intestine of horses, and occurs in about 15 per cent of horses' feces.

It is the cause of a highly dangerous wound infection, which results when infected soil, the dirt of streets, etc., gains entrance to a wound. The spores can live in dust for long periods. Another source of infection in surgical wounds is catgut, which is prepared from the intestine of the horse, not the cat. If this is imperfectly sterilized, the spores may persist, and later cause infection in the operation wound.

The organism remains localized in the wound and does not invade the tissues. As it is anaerobic, it grows best when other bacteria are present which kill the tissue so that the supply of oxygen diminishes.

The tetanus bacillus is dangerous because it produces one of the most powerful toxins known, far more virulent than the most deadly snake venom. The toxin gradually passes along the nerves from the wound to the spinal cord. There it becomes anchored to the motor nerve cells, which it stimulates so that the muscles become rigid and the patient is thrown into terrible convulsions. The jaw muscles are early involved by stiffness and the mouth cannot be opened, so that the common name of the disease is *lockjaw*.

The incubation period, *i.e.*, the time between infection and the first appearance of symptoms, is considerable, for the toxin travels along the nerves only slowly. The average time is seven to ten days. In wounds of the face it is shorter, as there is less distance for the toxin to travel. In other cases it may be several weeks. This long incubation period is fortunate, because it makes preventive inoculation possible. When the possibility of tetanus is suspected, and this should be the case in all street accidents or contaminated wounds, a prophylactic injection of tetanus antitoxin is given. This neutralizes the toxin before it has time to reach the nerve cells in the spinal cord. After that it is usually too late to do much good, as the toxin is firmly anchored to the nerve cells. In war time every wounded man received a dose of antitetanic serum on the chance that the wound might have become infected with tetanus.

Bacillus Botulinus (Clostridium Botulinum).—This anaerobic bacillus is entirely different in its action to anything so far considered. We are really not concerned with the organism itself, for it does not grow in the human body. But it does grow in spoiled sausage (*botulus*, a sausage), preserved meat, canned vegetables, ripe olives, etc. Its spores are very resistant, and if the temperature employed in home canning is insufficient, the bacilli will produce a very potent toxin, which if taken in even very small amounts, may cause death. The condition is called *botulism*. The toxin does not produce any inflammation in the stomach or intestine, but is absorbed and acts on the brain, producing eye disturbances such as double vision and squint, and finally coma and death. The symptoms are apt to be mistaken for those of encephalitis, so that the correct diagnosis of food poisoning may be missed. Prevention is the best treatment, and this means proper attention to detail in the matter of home canning.

FUNGUS DISEASES: THE MYCOSES

Fungi constitute a group, including molds and yeasts, of what are called the higher bacteria. These are more highly developed than the simple cocci and bacilli which have so far been considered. Most of the fungi consist of branched filaments known as *mycelia* which form *spores*. The vast majority are non-pathogenic, but as they are omnipresent in the air they are apt to contaminate culture media, to grow as molds on food, and to be generally troublesome. A few are disease-producing.

Most pathogenic fungi have very slight invasive power, so that they are confined to the skin; at least one attacks the mucous membrane of the mouth, and two or three may invade the internal organs with disastrous results. The diseases produced by fungi are known as the *mycoses* or mycotic diseases.

Dermatomycoses.—As the name implies, this is the group of fungus diseases of the skin. They are also known as *ringworm*, a name which suggests a single disease marked by the formation of rings due to widening of the area of infection; in reality it is a group of diseases, in many of which there is no ring formation. These infections are all markedly contagious, and are communicated by means of contaminated clothing and structures such as the floors of rooms. Although not dangerous, they are notoriously difficult to treat. The following are some of the more common forms.

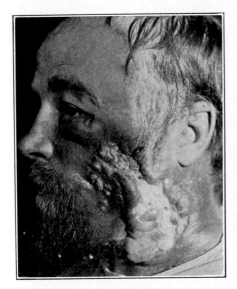
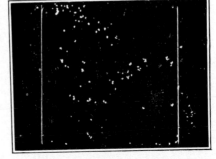

Fig. 27   Fig. 28

Fig. 27.—Actinomycosis of the neck.   (Bell, Textbook of Pathology.)

Fig. 28.—Sulphur granules, photographed on slide with black background.   (Boyd, Textbook of Pathology.)

Ringworm of the Scalp.—Also known as *tinea* (not to be confused with tænia or tapeworm).   For some reason it affects only children.   It is highly contagious, and in schools and institutions it may assume epidemic proportions.   The fungus, known as *trichophyton* (Greek *thrix*, hair; *phyton*, plant) invades and lives in the hair and the roots of the hair; this explains why it attacks the scalp, why it produces bald patches, and why it is so difficult to eradicate.

Ringworm of the Groin.—Not nearly so common.   The fungus invades the epidermis, and is therefore known as an *epidermophyton*.

Interdigital Ringworm.—This form occurs between the fingers and toes. and has recently become very common indeed, because of the increased use of gymnasiums, locker rooms, showers, swimming pools, etc. The frequency of the disease has in places assumed epidemic proportions. The association of the disease with various sports is the reason for its common name, "athlete's foot." The fungus usually responsible is *epidermophyton*.

Mucous Membrane Mycoses.—The only fungus infection of mucous membrane which need be considered is known as *thrush*. This is a localized disease of the mouth which occurs most frequently in children suffering from malnutrition, and is characterized by white patches on the mucous membrane, especially that of the tongue. The fungus is known as *Oidium albicans*.

Mycoses of Internal Organs.—In this group there is one not uncommon disease, actinomycosis; another a good deal rarer, blastomycosis; and some so rare that they will not be mentioned.

Actinomycosis.—The disease is a chronic inflammation, not unlike tuberculosis, but differing from that disease in that there is pus production. The infection, which is much commoner in domestic animals (cattle, horses, pigs) than in man, is caused by the *actinomyces* or *ray fungus*. The common site is the head and neck. A firm mass develops, usually under the lower jaw; this breaks down to form abscesses, which discharge on the skin (Fig. 27). The pus contains tiny yellow bodies known as *sulphur granules;* under the microscope these are seen to consist of a mass of ray fungus, and therefore form an important means of diagnosis. There is a rarer *abdominal form* of the disease which starts in the bowel in the region of the appendix.

Penicillin and the sulphonamides, together with surgical treatment, where necessary, have effected improvement and cures in many cases, particularly the more localized infections.

Blastomycosis.—A rare fungus infection of the skin and underlying tissues caused by *blastomyces*. There is marked destruction of tissues and a tendency to invade the blood stream and internal organs with fatal results.

VIRUS DISEASES

There is a large group of diseases affecting not only man but also animals, insects and plants, which have all the characteristics of infectious diseases, yet in which no microörganisms have been discovered either with the microscope or by means of culture. We know that these diseases are infectious. because they can be transmitted from one animal to another by inoculating diseased tissue. If an extract of this tissue be made and passed through the finest filter known, the pores of which are small enough to hold back all bacteria, the filtrate which comes through the filter is still as infective as ever when injected into a living animal. To this infective material the name of virus has been given; it is called ultramicroscopic because it is beyond the range of the most powerful microscope, and filterable or filter-passing because no filter can hold it back. By means of the electron microscope, which gives very much higher magnifications than the ordinary microscope, it is now possible to obtain photographs of many of the viruses.

One of the most important points of difference between viruses and ordi-

nary bacteria is that the bacteria grow readily on culture media which are composed of dead material, whereas a virus will only grow on living cells. It penetrates the cell and establishes a parasitic existence in its interior. The most convenient living medium for the culture of viruses is the yolk sac of a hen's egg.

It must be obvious that the study of viruses is very much more difficult than ordinary bacteriological studies; neither the ordinary microscope nor the culture tube can be used. A virus can only be recognized by the effect which it produces in the living body; just as the presence of electricity can only be recognized by the effect it produces. Thus the virus of poliomyelitis (infantile paralysis) can be recognized by the fact that when human material containing the virus is injected into a monkey, the animal becomes paralyzed.

Some of the commonest and most widespread diseases are now known to be due to ultramicroscopic or filterable viruses, as well as others which are no longer common because they have been brought under control in various ways. The following list of virus diseases illustrates this truth: the common cold, influenza, measles, mumps, poliomyelitis, encephalitis, rabies (hydrophobia), herpes zoster (shingles), smallpox and yellow fever. This list of human virus diseases could be greatly enlarged, and it must be remembered that viruses cause many important diseases of animals, such as dog distemper, and even attack plants (tobacco, potato, etc.).

There is much uncertainty as to the true nature of viruses. From the fact that they can multiply indefinitely (although only within living cells) it has been thought that they are living particles, very much smaller than bacteria. This may be true for some viruses, but not for others, which appear to be rather of a chemical nature. Suffice it to say that viruses are the most mysterious of all disease agents, and appear to have a place in the dim borderland between the living and non-living.

Smallpox.—This disease, also called *variola*, is one of the most virulent of infectious diseases. All races of men are susceptible, and no one from childhood to old age is exempt. Actual contact, direct or indirect, with a patient is not necessary for transmission. It will sweep through a country with the speed of a prairie fire. (Other virus diseases, such as influenza, may travel with the same terrifying speed). Small wonder, then, that in bygone years nearly everyone, high or low, rich or poor, bore the marks of "the pox" on his or her face. The picture in seventeenth century England is drawn thus by the vivid pen of Macaulay: "The smallpox was always present, filling the churchyards with corpses, tormenting with constant fears all whom it had not stricken, leaving on those whose lives it spared the hideous traces of its power, turning the babe into a changeling at which the mother shuddered, and making the eyes and cheeks of a betrothed maiden objects of horror to the lover." Now almost no doctor living in countries where this book is likely to be read has ever seen a case of smallpox. Surely this is the greatest triumph in the whole of preventive medicine.

The portal of entry of the infection is not known for certain, but it is believed to be the respiratory tract. Headache and persistent pain in the back are characteristic symptoms. After an incubation period of about

twelve days the skin lesions appear. At first these are solid papules, but in a few days they become converted into pustules which may cover the face and the entire body. Scabs are formed over the pustules, and as the scabs dry they are cast off and changed into dust, each particle of the dust being covered with the virus. From this it will be seen how important the problem of nursing is, especially in a community which has not been adequately vaccinated. As the pustules heal, scars of varying depth are left in the skin. Thus the dangers of smallpox are twofold: (1) death, (2) disfigurement.

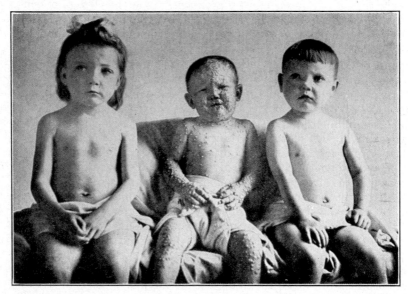

Fig. 29.—The value of vaccination. Three of a family exposed to smallpox; the middle one unvaccinated, the other two vaccinated one year before. (Schamberg and Kolmer.)

The patient must be isolated, and contacts are quarantined for fourteen days and vaccinated. Discharges from the nose, mouth, and mucous membranes are disinfected or burned. The skin is covered with petroleum jelly to prevent scaling and dissemination of the infection. The usual general precautions are taken, such as the use of a mask and gown, washing the hands, separate dishes for the patient, the disinfection of the bed and body linen.

Vaccination, however, is the chief means of prevention (Fig. 29). The vaccine employed is the virus of cowpox, the corresponding disease in the cow but much milder. We owe the method to the English physician, Jenner, at that time a country practitioner, who observed that milkmaids who had had cowpox were immune from smallpox. The virus is inoculated into the skin, and this is followed by the development of a papule, then a watery vesicle, and finally a pustule, looking to the eyes of Jenner like "a pearl upon the rose leaf." Immunity following vaccination lasts a number of years, but it is not lifelong. To insure complete immunity

the child should be vaccinated before the age of seven, again at the age of fifteen, and once during adult life. When there is no smallpox in the country these extreme measures are hardly necessary. If the nurse has to attend cases of the disease it is safer to be re-vaccinated every few years.

Measles.—Also known as *morbilli.* This is another example of a highly infectious virus disease. All races and all ages are susceptible. Practically all city dwellers acquire the disease during childhood, and are subsequently immune. In rural districts it is not so common, but when young adults from such districts are brought together in military or other camps they are very apt to develop the disease. In aboriginal communities where the disease has been unknown it behaves with the fury of smallpox, and the mortality is high.

The virus is contained in the nasal secretions, and it is probably acquired through the respiratory tract. The average incubation period is from ten to fourteen days. Unfortunately the patient is infective for five days before as well as for five days after the appearance of the rash. It is this which makes the disease so difficult to control. The chief symptoms are fever, the characteristic rash, and signs of an acute catarrhal inflammation of the upper respiratory tract and eyes. The rash covers the face and the whole body, but as there is no tissue destruction, it leaves no scars when it clears up. The mouth shows lesions which are of value in diagnosis in difficult cases; these are known as *Koplik spots,* and are small white areas on the mucous membrane due to thickening of the epithelium. The great danger the patient must be guarded against is bronchopneumonia, which is often fatal. Even if he recovers from the bronchopneumonia, he is in danger of developing an acute form of pulmonary tuberculosis owing to lowered resistance.

Poliomyelitis.—The disease infantile paralysis is more readily understood when considered in connection with diseases of the nervous system (page 265).

Yellow Fever.—Our last example of a virus disease is a tropical infection, but very widespread and of great importance to trade and commerce. The chief symptoms are fever, vomiting, diarrhea, and intense jaundice, so that the skin turns yellow. In epidemics there is a mortality of 80 per cent, so it is little wonder that it was dreaded by Europeans. A vivid but accurate account of the disease with be found in *Anthony Adverse.* As with other virus diseases, if the patient recovers he has a lifelong immunity. Natives living in the tropics develop an acquired immunity.

The real interest, indeed romance, of yellow fever is not so much the virus which causes it, as the means by which the virus is transmitted. Until 1900 it was believed that the disease was due to unsanitary conditions, the infection being probably conveyed from the sick to the healthy by intestinal discharges. In that year the American Yellow Fever Commission under Walter Reed determined to put to the test the theory that a mosquito might carry the infection, as had already been shown to be the case in malaria. At that time no animal was known which was susceptible to the disease, so human volunteers had to be used. These allowed themselves to be bitten by mosquitoes which had already fed on yellow fever patients. One member of the Commission, Dr. Carroll, developed yellow

fever and nearly died; a second, Dr. Lazear, became even more desperately ill and finally died.

The centuries-old problem of yellow fever had at last been solved. The disease was transmitted by a mosquito, the female stegomyia, (a different variety from the anopheles which carries malaria.) If the stegomyia could be destroyed, the scourge of the tropics could be eradicated. How this was done by General Gorgas cannot be related here, but success was complete. The control of yellow fever has opened up South and Central America, has made Rio de Janeiro habitable, and the Panama Canal possible.

Chapter
7
SOME ANIMAL PARASITES

An animal parasite is a member of the animal kingdom (the bacteria being vegetable) which has acquired the power of living in the body of another animal known as the host. The parasite may or may not produce disease in the host. Here we are only concerned with the human host and with pathogenic (disease-producing) parasites. Most parasites have developed one very remarkable habit: they spend one part of their life cycle in one host (man) and another part of the cycle in another host (an animal). The second host may be of any size, from a cow to a mosquito, but each parasite has its own particular animal host; the cow and the mosquito are not interchangeable. Moreover, the second host is a necessity, not a luxury; unless it can be found the race of that particular parasite will die out. It is evident that this invaluable knowledge places a very powerful weapon in the hands of those engaged in the prevention of parasitic diseases. Finally, the second host may be responsible for conveying the disease to man, as in the case of the mosquito and malaria.

THE MALARIAL PARASITE

Malaria is caused by a minute unicellular parasite, *i.e.*, one consisting of a single cell. Part of the life cycle is spent in man and part in the anopheles mosquito. Destruction of this type of mosquito will therefore be followed by the disappearance of malaria. The disease is the most widespread serious malady affecting the human race, although necessarily confined to those parts of the world infested by the anopheles. Greece, a land of heroes, fell in a few centuries to be a land of slaves, largely because the shaking finger of malaria had touched the people. The disease still constitutes the greatest public health problem in the world. In certain tropical regions everyone is infected with malaria from the time he is a few days old until he dies. Such persons never know for a single day the feeling of perfect health. Malaria is responsible, either directly or indirectly by weakening resistance, for about 2 million deaths every year in India alone, and it is estimated that about 100 million suffer annually from the disease in that country.

When an infected mosquito bites man it injects the parasites into the blood stream. Each parasite enters one red blood corpuscle and multiplies inside it until it destroys the corpuscle, which then bursts and liberates the new parasites into the blood. These attack new red corpuscles, multiply inside them and destroy them. It is obvious that in this way

billions of parasites may be produced, and billions of red blood corpuscles may be destroyed, so that the patient will develop a profound anemia. The time taken by the parasite to multiply in the blood cells is always the same, so that the billions of blood cells all burst at the same time and liberate the new parasites into the blood stream at the same time. This massive discharge of parasites into the blood produces sudden high fever and an attack of shivering known as a *rigor*. The temperature rapidly falls, and may remain normal until the next batch of parasites are liberated. One form of parasite completes this part of its life cycle every forty-eight hours, and so the fever and chill occur every other day; as this is every third day (counting the day of the attack), this form is known as *tertian* malaria. In another form the life cycle occupies seventy-two hours, the attack of fever occurs on the fourth day (counting the day of the attack), so that the disease is known as *quartan* malaria.

The human part of the life cycle is asexual, *i.e.*, two sexes are not necessary for reproduction. But this can only go on for a certain time. Unless rejuvenation of the parasite occurs by sexual reproduction, for which the mosquito is necessary, the parasite will die out. Sexual forms, male and female, are present in human blood, but they are unable to unite. Their chance comes when the mosquito bites a malarial patient and sucks his blood into her stomach (it is only the female of the species that does the biting). The male and female forms now unite and the fruit of the union is a fresh brood of rejuvenated parasites, which make their way to the mosquito's proboscis and await their chance to enter the blood of the next man the insect happens to bite. Thus the mosquito not only carries on the life cycle of a parasite but conveys it from person to person.

Diagnosis.—The diagnosis of malaria is suggested by the chills and regular repeated attacks of fever, but it can only be made with certainty by finding the parasites in a smear of the patient's blood. The best time to make the blood examination is just before the onset of a chill.

Treatment.—The control of malaria in the districts of the world in which it is common has been aided by intensive campaigns against the mosquito by measures such as drainage of marshes, the treatment of stagnant water with oil or D.D.T. to kill the larva of the mosquito, etc.

There are many drugs which are used in the treatment of a patient with malaria, and these have been improved greatly during the past few years. The common drugs in use are quinine, chloroquine, pentaquine, mepacrine, and pamaquine. An important advance has been the introduction of mepacrine and chloroquine as means of suppression of the disease during times of exposure in malarial countries.

TAPEWORMS

We now pass to a very different type of animal parasite. The parasites of malaria and dysentery are minute microscopic forms of life. Tapeworms, on the other hand, are many yards in length. Yet they are infinitely less dangerous to health than the minute parasites. Tapeworms are of various kinds, but they also pass part of their life cycle in man and part in another animal. A tapeworm gets its name from its shape, for it is

long and narrow like a piece of tape (Fig. 30). The head is very small and the body very long. There are four tapeworms of importance in human pathology. Three of these pass the sexual or adult stage in man and the asexual or cystic stage in an animal. The fourth passes the adult stage in an animal (dog) and the cystic stage in man. The fourth alone is capable of producing serious disease in man. The easiest way to remember the somewhat difficult names of tapeworms is by the name of the animal which acts as the second host. All of these worms are known by the generic term, tænia.

The *beef tapeworm* (Tænia saginata, Tænia mediocanellata) is the common tapeworm of the United States and Canada. It may be 30 feet long, but its head is only 2 mm. in diameter. It lives in the intestine, and the body of the female is crowded with eggs which are discharged in the stools. If these are swallowed by cattle they are carried to the muscles, where they pass through a second phase of the life cycle and develop into cysts. If the beef from an infected cow is eaten imperfectly cooked, human infection will result, and the cystic parasite will grow into the full-length adult in the intestine. The diagnosis is made by examining the stools for fragments of the worm (segments) which become broken off and discharged.

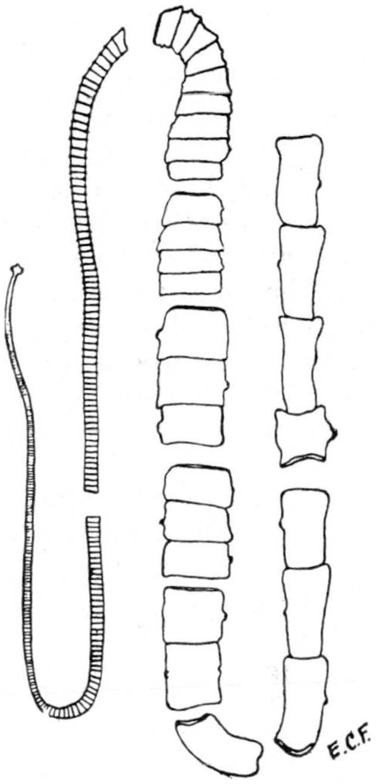

The *pork tapeworm* (Tænia solium) is a similar but smaller worm only 10 feet long. The second host is the pig, and human infection results from eating infected pork which contains the tiny cysts.

The *fish tapeworm* (Diphyllobothrium latum) is very long, and passes the cystic stage in some of the larger fresh-water fish, such as pike and perch. There is no

FIG. 30.—Tapeworm showing the small head and some of the segments. (Faust's Human Helminthology.)

danger in eating these fish provided they have been properly cooked, and the same is true of the beef and pork.

The *dog tapeworm* (Tænia echinococcus) is entirely different from the other three in the following respects: (1) It is extremely small, only $\frac{1}{4}$ inch long. (2) It is the cystic stage which is passed in man; the adult stage occurs in the dog. (3) The cysts often cause serious symptoms in man and may prove fatal. Human infection is usually due to eating unboiled vegetables soiled by the excreta of dogs. The disease in man, which is most prevalent in Australia, the Argentine, and Iceland where infected dogs and men come into close contact, is called hydatid disease, and the cysts are known as *hydatid cysts*. These cysts are formed principally in the liver, but may oc-

cur in any of the organs. They may attain a large size, and sometimes cause the death of the patient.

HOOKWORM (ANKYLOSTOMA DUODENALE)

Hookworm disease or ankylostomiasis is one of the most prevalent diseases in the world. It has been estimated that there are some 100,000,000 cases. It is a disease of warm and tropical climates and is very prevalent in the southern part of the United States. The worm, which is less than 1 inch in length, occurs in large numbers in the duodenum, the first part of the intestine. The mouth is armed with four teeth or hooklets which serve to attach it to the wall of the duodenum and which give it its name (*ankylos*, hooked, *stoma*, mouth). The method by which it reaches the duodenum is one of the romances of medicine. The young embryo worm lives in warm moist ground, bores through the skin of the bare feet of natives, enters a vein, and is carried by the blood to the lung where it is arrested. Here it escapes into the bronchi and starts to climb up the trachea. When it reaches the upper end it descends the esophagus, passes through the stomach and reaches the end of its long journey in the duodenum. Large numbers of hookworms arrive here, and fasten themselves to the wall of the bowel. In time they produce a marked anemia with profound lassitude and weakness. No animal host is required for the development of the hookworm.

ROUNDWORM (ASCARIS LUMBRICOIDES)

The roundworm resembles the earthworm in size and shape, and is a common inhabitant of the intestine, especially in children. It usually produces no symptoms in the adult, but in children it may cause nervous disturbances. Infection is due to swallowing the eggs of the worm on uncooked vegetables.

THREADWORM (OXYURIS VERMICULARIS)

Threadworms, also known as pinworms, are very common parasites in the intestine of children. The worm is only $\frac{1}{4}$ inch long, and when passed in the stools it resembles a moving piece of white thread. They cause marked irritation and itching of the skin around the anus, and in weakly children they may excite nervous disturbances and convulsions. Infection is due to swallowing contaminated vegetables, fruit, etc.

Treatment of Intestinal Worms.—In the treatment of intestinal worms the general principle is to stun or paralyze the worm by means of a drug and then use a cathartic to sweep it out. The drug is known as a vermifuge, and its action is assisted by a preliminary cleansing of the bowel by means of a twenty-four-hour fast and a mild purge.

In the case of *tapeworm* the vermifuge is extract of male fern, a potent drug which may sometimes produce collapse in the patient, a danger to be guarded against by keeping the patient in bed while the treatment is in progress. The best cathartic is magnesium sulphate. Castor oil must not

be used, as the vermifuge is soluble in it and would be absorbed with the production of toxic symptoms. After the cathartic careful search must be made in the stool for the head of the worm. For *round worms* the vermifuge used is santonin combined with calomel. This is given for three days in succession, and repeated in ten days if the stools still show eggs. For *thread-worms* the use of gentian violet in capsules by mouth is usually an effective treatment. Careful cleansing of the anal region followed by application of ammoniated mercury ointment is important. The main purpose of this treatment is to try to prevent reinfestation by the patient himself.

For *hookworm* the best vermifuge is tetrachloroethylene.

Chapter

8

TUMORS

THE normal organs and tissues of the body are composed of cells which are strictly under the control of the laws of growth. An organ like the liver or a bone increases in size not by the individual cells of which it is composed becoming larger, but by continual division and multiplication of these cells. In youth this multiplication is rapid, but in adult life it is only sufficient to make good the slow wastage which is continually occurring. Hypertrophy of an organ may occur in response to a demand for more work. Thus if one kidney is removed the other kidney doubles in size in order to do double the amount of work; if one-half the thyroid gland is excised the remaining half replaces that which has been removed. This growth of new cells performs a necessary function and is governed by the laws of growth.

A tumor or *neoplasm* is a mass of new cells which proliferate without control and which serve no useful function. This lack of control is particularly marked in malignant tumors (cancer). Cancer cells are the gangsters of the body, for they know no law, pay no regard for the commonweal, serve no useful function, and cause disharmony and death in their surroundings. It used to be thought that cancer was a peculiarly human disease, but we now know that it occurs throughout the entire vertebrate animal kingdom. Nor is the popular idea that cancer is rapidly increasing founded on fact. Much of this increase is due to improved methods of diagnosis, and also to the fact that more people now live to the age at which cancer is likely to develop.

INNOCENT AND MALIGNANT TUMORS

Tumors can be divided into two great classes: the one *innocent*, simple or benign, the other *malignant*. Malignant tumors form the group known as *cancer*. Sometimes an innocent tumor may develop into a malignant one. A malignant tumor differs from an innocent one in the following particulars.

1. A malignant tumor if untreated will kill the patient wherever it occurs, even in the hand or foot. An innocent tumor will only cause death if it happens to grow in a vital organ such as the brain.

2. A malignant tumor infiltrates the surrounding tissue. It sends claws into it like a crab (Fig. 31). The word cancer means a crab. An innocent tumor grows by expansion, as a toy balloon does when blown up, and is usually separated from the surrounding tissue by a capsule so that it can be shelled out, or at least readily removed.

(100)

3. When a malignant tumor is removed it may recur. This is because some of the outlying parts have not been completely removed; they are so minute that they cannot be seen by the surgeon, but they may soon grow to the size of the original tumor.

4. Speaking generally a malignant tumor grows much more rapidly than an innocent one, although some cancers are remarkably slow in growth, especially in old people. The rapid growth is due to the fact that the tumor cells are dividing rapidly. This cell division is called *mitosis*, and it can be recognized under the microscope by the fact that the nucleus of the cell becomes divided into small particles which are grouped together to form *mitotic figures*. Thus the presence of numerous mitotic figures indicates to the pathologist that the tumor is almost certainly a malignant one.

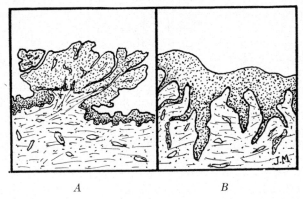

A   *B*

Fig. 31.—*A*, Innocent tumor (papilloma); *B*, malignant tumor, (epidermoid carcinoma.)

5. A malignant tumor sets up secondary growths or *metastases* in lymph nodes and in distant organs. This is because the cancer has invaded the lymph vessels or the bloodvessels and the tumor cells are carried by the lymph or blood stream to other parts of the body, where they settle down and form new tumors. When this happens no operation can hope to save the patient.

There are microscopic differences which are of great importance to the pathologist in the task of determining whether the tumor removed by the surgeon is or is not cancer, but they need not be detailed here. Suffice it to say that an innocent tumor tends to reproduce the structure of the organ from which it grows, whereas a malignant tumor, being beyond the pale of the law, fails to do so.

THE CAUSES OF TUMORS

In this discussion only malignant tumors will be considered. Cancer consists in the abnormal multiplication of the cells of an organ. Its cause must therefore be either something which stimulates cells to abnormal growth or something which breaks down normal growth restraint. The

7

exact cause of cancer is not known. It is doubtful indeed if there is any
one universal cause of all cancers, any more than we would expect to find
any one universal cause of all infectious diseases. Again, just as it would
be absurd to expect to discover one method of treatment which would cure all
infections, so it is probably useless to hope for a single cure of all cancers. The
alliteration of "the cause of cancer" and "the cure of cancer" is unfortunate,
because it has implanted deep in the mind of the public the fixed idea that
there must be *one* cause and *one* cure, so that they tend to reject the information that great advances have been made both in our knowledge of the
causation and the treatment of malignant disease. As a matter of fact
there are many chronic pathological conditions such as arteriosclerosis,
heart disease and Bright's disease which are far more incurable than cancer.
Tumors form a group, just as do the infectious diseases, and each one has
to be considered by itself. We do know a good deal about certain factors
which play a part in the production of cancer, just as we do know a good
deal about treatment of the disease. These factors may be divided into
two groups, the internal and the external.

Internal Factor.—The internal factor is the constitution of the patient,
which in turn is determined by heredity. Most of our knowledge of this
subject has been gained from breeding experiments on animals, particularly
mice, for cancer is not confined to man but occurs throughout the animal
kingdom. It is possible to breed a race of mice by careful selection of the
parents in which 100 per cent of the offspring will develop and die of cancer.
It is also possible to breed another race of mice which are entirely immune
from cancer. Still more remarkable is the fact that a race of mice can be
bred in which all the members will die of cancer of one particular organ,
such as the stomach or the breast. It is not possible to say with certainty
what part heredity plays in the production of human cancer, because human
beings cannot be bred in pure strains like animals, but it is probable that it
is a predisposing factor of importance. If both parents have died of cancer
of the same organ there is a greater chance of one of the children developing
cancer of that organ than in the case of a child of healthy parents. Further
than this it would not be wise to go.

External Factor.—The external factor is chronic irritation. This is most
conclusively shown by experimental work on animals. If the skin of a
mouse is repeatedly painted with tar for several months, cancer may develop at the site of tarring. If the mouse belongs to a cancerous strain this
is much more likely to occur. Men employed in tar works and paraffin
works are liable to develop cancer of the hand. The same used to be true
of roentgen-ray workers before the danger was recognized and proper
precautions taken. Chronic irritation of many different kinds may start
the cancerous process, and recognition of this fact is of great value in the
all-important matter of the prevention of cancer. It is hardly too much to
say that in parts of the body which are under observation, such as the skin
and the mouth, cancer does not start in perfectly normal tissue. In the
skin cancer may start in the scars of old burns, in chronic ulcers and in
areas exposed to the irritation of intense sunlight (hands and face). In
the mouth the irritation of excessive smoking may start cancer of the lip,

the irritation of a jagged tooth or an ill-fitting plate may start cancer of the tongue or the gums.

The irritation has usually to be long continued. This is particularly well seen in experimentally produced cancer, where tar may have to be applied to the skin of a mouse for six months, about one-sixth the entire life of the animal, before cancer is produced. This may have some bearing on the fact that the cancer age is middle age and onwards, although the disease may occur in young people, and some forms develop in early childhood.

It is not possible to apply the theory of mechanical irritation to internal organs such as the brain. This illustrates the fact that there is probably no one universal cause of cancer. It seems likely that abnormal stimuli from the ductless glands may in some cases break down the growth restraint and give rise to cancer. Thus it is possible to produce cancer of the breast in male mice by repeated injections of extract of the ovary (ovarian hormone). We know that the normal development of the female breast at puberty is due to ovarian stimuli, and it is quite possible that the abnormal cell growth which constitutes cancer is caused by abnormal or perverted stimuli.

The germ theory of cancer has always held an attraction, especially for the public. Cancer does not resemble ordinary bacterial disease in any particular, and no bacteria are constantly associated with cancer. The case for viruses is much stronger. It is known definitely that certain animal tumors contain viruses which, when injected into other animals of the same species, are able to reproduce the tumors in the new animals. It is not possible to demonstrate a virus in human cancer, because the only way to demonstrate it would be to inoculate the material into another human being. When we remember that viruses live inside cells, and that some virus diseases of the skin (the poxes) are marked by great multiplication of the epithelial cells, it is more than possible that viruses may play a part in the production of some human cancers.

Viruses may even be responsible for some forms of apparently hereditary cancer. Bittner found that when newborn mice of a high breast cancer strain were fostered with mothers of a low cancer strain the tumor incidence was greatly reduced. Conversely newborn mice of a low cancer strain when fostered by mothers of a high strain showed an increased incidence of cancer. Apparently something is transmitted through the mother's milk which determines the incidence of breast cancer. This was at first called the Bittner milk factor, but it has now been shown to be a virus. This virus enters the animal's body with the mother's milk during the earliest days of life, and when the mouse reaches maturity cancer of the breast develops.

One last point in this discussion of the etiology of cancer: The influence which starts a tumor to grow is not necessarily the same as that which keeps it growing. The former may well be external, the latter internal. The application of tar to a normal cell may change it into a cancer cell, but the cancer continues to grow after the tar is removed, so that some factor other than tar is now at work. It is the same with a fire. This may be started in many ways, *i.e.*, by many factors, mechanical, electrical, chemical, etc., but once the spark is kindled the conflagration continues by virtue of an internal factor, the constitution of the material involved. If the spark is

lacking, if the material is non-inflammable, there will be no fire. Both factors must be present. So it is with cancer.

THE SPREAD OF TUMORS

This subject has already been referred to. An innocent tumor increases in size but can hardly be said to spread. A malignant tumor, on the other hand, spreads locally and to distant parts. The local spread is due to the invasive character of the growth, the cancer cells worming their way into

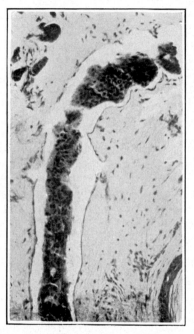

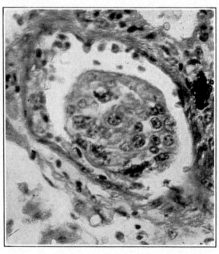

Fig. 32   Fig. 33

Fig. 32.—Lymphatic permeation by carcinoma. × 125. (Boyd, Textbook of Pathology.)

Fig. 33.—Tumor embolus in bloodvessel.

the surrounding tissues, and growing along the lymphatics. This *permeation* of the lymphatics is particularly well seen in cancer of the breast (Fig. 32). This presents a serious problem for the operating surgeon, for if he takes out merely what he can see of the tumor he is certain to leave behind many tumor cells, and soon the patient will return with a *recurrence*.

The other method of spread is by *tumor embolism*, the cancer cells forming emboli and being carried by the blood stream to distant parts in the same way as thrombi may become detached and converted into emboli (Fig. 33). If the *lymphatic vessels* are invaded the tumor cells are carried to the nearest (regional) lymph glands, where they are arrested and form new tumors similar to the primary one. In the surgical treatment of cancer of the

breast the lymph glands in the axilla, which receive the lymph from the breast, are removed together with the breast. This is done even though they are not enlarged, for they may contain cancer cells which have not yet had time to form a visible tumor.

In embolism by the *blood stream* the tumor cells are carried to some other organ where they are arrested in the capillaries and start secondary growths or *metastases*. In abdominal organs such as the stomach the secondary growths are usually in the liver, because the blood from the digestive tract is carried first to the liver. In the case of other organs the metastases commonly occur in the lungs.

TREATMENT OF TUMORS

Innocent tumors are treated with complete success by local removal; that is to say, only the tumor itself needs to be removed and none of the surrounding tissue. With malignant tumors the reverse is the case. Not only the tumor but as much of the surrounding tissue as is feasible must be excised, for it may harbor cancer cells which cannot be detected by the eye or hand but only by the microscope. A cancer of the breast may be no larger than a pea in size, yet the whole breast has to be removed. The regional lymph nodes may also have to be removed, but cancer of each organ must be considered as a separate entity, and what is true of one is not necessarily true of another. Thus the regional lymph nodes, although apparently normal, are always removed in cancer of the breast, but not necessarily in cancer of the lip. The presence of distant metastases (blood spread) is an indication that surgical treatment can offer no hope of cure.

It should be emphasized that every cancer is curable in the early stage before it has begun to spread. This is particularly true of cancer of the skin, lip, and other places where it can be readily seen. Other tumors may eventually recur after, say, five years, but to give a man or woman of sixty years another five years of life is surely something worth while. The great difficulty at present is to diagnose cancer of the internal organs before they have extended too far to be operable.

Radiation.—Radiation is a comparatively new and very valuable method of treating certain forms of cancer. It may be used either in the form of roentgen rays or radium. This treatment is made possible by the fact that radiations have a greater destructive action on rapidly growing cells than on normal cells. They therefore have a *selective action* on cancer cells compared with that on the surrounding tissue. It is possible, however, to kill *all* the tissue by radiation and this danger has constantly to be borne in mind by the doctor. His aim is to use the maximum amount of radiation on the cancer, but to stop just short of damaging the normal tissue. This requires quite as much skill and special training as it does to cut the tumor out with a knife.

Radium gives off radiations (gamma rays) which are similar in nature to *x*-rays and have a similar action on tumor tissue. Both may be used for attacking some tumors, but in most cases one or the other is preferable. *X*-rays may be of low voltage (50,000 to 100,000 volts) or high voltage (usually around 220,000 volts, though in some machines very much higher).

PART II.

THE ORGANS AND THEIR DISEASES

Chapter

9

DISEASES OF THE HEART AND ARTERIES

Structure and Function.—The heart is a hollow muscular pump whose function it is to cause the blood to circulate throughout the body. It sends impure venous blood to the lungs, where fresh oxygen is taken up and carbon dioxide given off, and then pumps the oxygenated blood to the tissues where the oxygen is used. The essential meaning of respiration is this delivery of life-giving oxygen to the tissues. It is evident, therefore, that the heart is concerned with respiration just as much as are the lungs, so that the principal symptom of heart disease is shortness of breath or *dyspnea*.

The general structure of the heart has already been considered in Chapter 1. It is composed of muscle and valves (Fig. 37). The valves consist of an extraordinarily thin and delicate membrane, the *endocardium*, which also lines the cavity. Although so thin, they prevent a single drop of blood leaking through when closed. On the right side of the heart the *tricuspid valve* divides the

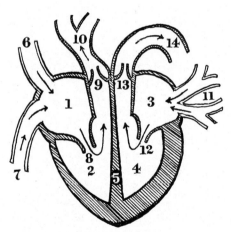

FIG. 37.—Interior of heart. 1, Right auricle; 2, right ventricle; 3, left auricle; 4, left ventricle; 5, septum; 6, superior vena cava; 7, inferior vena cava; 8, tricuspid valve; 9, pulmonary valve; 10, pulmonary artery; 11, pulmonary veins; 12, mitral valve; 13, aortic valve; 14, aorta. (After Rabin, Pathology for Nurses; courtesy of W. B. Saunders Company.)

chamber into an auricle, which receives the venous blood from the body, and a ventricle, which sends the impure blood to the lungs by the pulmonary artery, whose mouth is guarded by the *pulmonary valve*. The left side is divided by the *mitral valve* into an auricle, which receives the purified blood from the lungs, and a ventricle, which sends this blood out into the great

(113)

artery, the aorta, whose mouth is guarded by the *aortic valve*. Valvular disease of the heart nearly always affects the mitral and aortic valves. The function of the valves is to prevent backflow of blood between the beats. These functions are gravely interfered with in valvular disease.

Just as the interior of the heart is lined by the endocardium, so its outer surface is covered by a similar delicate membrane, the *pericardium*. The part of the chest in which the heart is situated is lined by a second layer of pericardium, so that between the two layers there exists a space, the *pericardial cavity*, in which the heart can contract and expand.

The heart muscle or *myocardium* must have an abundant blood supply. This is much more important than in the case of other muscles, because unlike them, it can never for a moment rest. This blood supply is provided by two arteries, the right and left *coronary arteries*, which arise from the aorta immediately above the aortic valve, and which carry blood to every part of the heart muscle. Contrary to what might be expected, very little of the blood which is continually flowing through the chambers of the heart takes any part in supplying the muscle with blood.

The *rate* of the heart beat, *i.e.*; the *pulse*, varies. The normal rhythm of the heart is dependent on the balance of two sets of nervous impulses, one tending to slow, the other to accelerate the heart's action. Both nerves belong to the involuntary or autonomic nervous system. The vagus nerve is responsible for the *retarding impulses*, and we now know that a chemical substance, acetylcholine, is liberated at the nerve endings of the vagus and that this acts on the heart muscle. The *accelerating impulses* pass along the sympathetic nerve fibers, and another chemical substance is probably liberated at their nerve endings. The quickening of the heart beat which results from emotion, the feeling that your heart is in your mouth or in your boots, is due to an upset of the exquisite balance which normally exists between these two sets of influences.

The rate of the heart also depends on the demand of the tissues for oxygen. The runner's heart beats faster and he breathes more quickly in response to an increase in this demand. Muscular work is an expenditure of energy, and energy is obtained from the burning of food. As food cannot be burnt without oxygen, the heart beat is quickened and breathing becomes deeper and faster to supply this need.

The condition of the bloodvessels must also be taken into account in any consideration of the heart's action. When the heart pumps blood into the arteries it does so against a certain amount of resistance. This is called the *peripheral resistance*. As the result of disease this resistance may become too high or too low. Both have an injurious effect on the heart's action. The resistance is increased by prolonged contraction of the muscular walls of the small arteries, the arterioles, resulting in the condition known as *high blood pressure* or *arterial hypertension*. No organ works at its maximum capacity; it has a large amount of *reserve force* in order to cope with emergencies. When hypertension develops the heart becomes larger and more powerful so that it can cope with the increased amount of work, a process known as *compensation*. In the course of time or because of disease of the heart muscle this power may fail, and *decompensation* sets in.

There are three main ways in which the action of the heart may be interfered with, three ways in which heart disease may be produced: (1) The valves of the pump may be damaged by inflammation, a condition known as endocarditis. (2) The muscle of the pump may not receive sufficient nourishment owing to narrowing of the coronary arteries, sometimes associated with thrombosis. (3) The pump may have too much work to do and finally give way through exhaustion. This is apt to occur in long-continued arterial hypertension.

Heart disease heads the causes of death. Its mortality is twice that of cancer, its nearest rival. There are four common types of heart disease: (1) Rheumatic; (2) syphilitic; (3) arteriosclerotic; and (4) hypertensive. *Rheumatic fever* attacks principally the heart valves, although the heart muscle may also suffer. *Syphilis* involves the aorta primarily rather than the heart, but infection spreads from the root of the aorta to the aortic valve, and the efficiency of that valve is seriously damaged. *Arteriosclerotic* heart disease is primarily disease of the coronary arteries, the heart muscle being damaged as the result of the arterial lesions. *Hypertensive* heart disease implies damage to the muscle on account of having to work against the high blood pressure. The four common forms may be divided into three age groups: (1) Below forty years of age the cases are mostly rheumatic; (2) between forty and fifty come most of the syphilitic cases; (3) over fifty there is an increasing incidence of arteriosclerotic and hypertensive cases.

ENDOCARDITIS

We have already seen that the heart valves are formed of a thin membrane, the endocardium, which also lines the chambers of the heart. Each valve is composed of flaps or *cusps* which open when the blood flows through them, but close tightly when the blood is not being forced onward. Bacteria in the blood may settle on the cusps and set up inflammation, a condition naturally called endocarditis. This usually happens on the valves on the left side of the heart (mitral and aortic). Those on the right side (tricuspid and pulmonary) are seldom involved. There are two chief kinds of endocarditis, rheumatic and subacute bacterial.

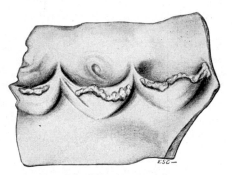

Fig. 38.—Small firm vegetations in rheumatic endocarditis.

Rheumatic Endocarditis.—In our discussion of rheumatic fever we have seen that the great danger to the patient lies not in the joints but in the heart. The products of hemolytic streptococci attack all parts of the heart, endocardium, myocardium (muscle), and pericardium. As a result of the infection the valves (commonly the mitral) become inflamed, and

from the blood flowing over it blood platelets and fibrin are deposited on the inflamed valve. These form little nodules called *vegetations*, each about the size of a pin's head, which form a row along the margin of the cusps (Fig. 38). The inflamed cusps, normally almost as thin as gossamer, become markedly thickened, and tend to adhere to one another, just as do inflamed loops of bowel when brought in contact. As the inflammation subsides, fibrous tissue takes the place of the inflammatory exudate, and this slowly contracts, causing retraction of the cusps.

The result of all this on the function and use of the valve may be of two kinds, although often both are combined. Owing to the adhesions between the thickened cusps they are unable to open properly when the blood flows through the valvular opening, so that this opening becomes permanently narrowed, a condition known as *stenosis* (Fig. 39 *C*). This narrowing may become so extreme that finally the opening is no larger than a button-hole,

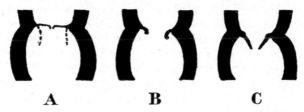

A   **B**   **C**

Fig. 39.—Heart valve lesions. *A*, Normal valve in closed and open (dotted lines) position; *B*, incompetence; *C*, stenosis.

whereas normally it should admit two fingers. The mitral valve is the common site of rheumatic endocarditis, and *mitral stenosis* is one of the most serious forms of heart disease, for not enough blood can flow from the left auricle into the left ventricle, and so is dammed back first in the lungs, then in the right side of the heart, and finally in the veins of the body. It is three times commoner than all other rheumatic heart lesions. The second possibility is *incompetence* of the valve (Fig. 39 *B*). Here the retraction of the cusps is much more marked than their sticking together. The result is that the cusps are unable to meet when the valve tries to close, and the blood escapes back from the ventricle into the auricle in the case of the mitral valve, from the aorta into the ventricle in the case of the aortic. From the point of view of the patient incompetence of the aortic valve is more important than incompetence of the mitral. A commoner and even more serious form of *aortic incompetence* is that produced by syphilis. In this condition syphilitic inflammation followed by scarring not only causes retraction of the cusps but also injures the wall of the aorta to which the cusps are attached, so that it gradually dilates to such a degree that the cusps are unable to come together and close the opening.

It is important to realize that a person with chronic valvular disease of the heart is not necessarily an invalid, nor should he be encouraged to consider himself as such. The evidence of a valvular lesion is a murmur heard by the stethoscope over the heart, but a person with a cardiac murmur may lead a full and vigorous life. If the heart muscle is healthy it is able

to compensate for the valvular lesion, unless the latter is marked and progressive.

In addition to causing inflammation of the valves, rheumatic fever also damages the heart muscle and pericardium. Small areas of inflammation and destruction are scattered through the muscle, and later these become converted into scar tissue. Such a scarred myocardium cannot fail to be weakened. On account of the damage to the wall of the auricle the peculiar condition known as *auricular fibrillation* is apt to develop, especially in mitral stenosis. Normally the auricles beat at the same rate as the ventricles; this is natural, because normally the wave of muscular contraction starts in the auricles and passes on to the ventricles; it is the beat of the ventricles which produces the pulse. In auricular fibrillation the auricles no longer contract in a regular manner; they seem to be trembling instead of contracting. The result is that the ventricles contract in a rapid and irregular manner, this irregularity being reflected in marked irregularity of the pulse. The ventricles tend to become exhausted, with resulting heart failure, the symptoms of which are palpation and dyspnea. The administration of digitalis prevents the irregular impulses from the auricles reaching the ventricles, which then commence to beat in a much slower and more regular manner, with immediate relief to the patient.

The pericardium also becomes inflamed, a condition of *pericarditis*, and the two inflamed layers of pericardium may stick together and form adhesions which may seriously cripple the heart's action. The truth of the remark made in the general discussion of rheumatic fever will now be evident, that it is a disease which licks the joints but bites the heart, for the patient is left with permanent lesions which may cripple his heart to the day of his death, although that day may be far removed. "The moving finger writes, and having writ moves on."

Subacute Bacterial Endocarditis.—This form of endocarditis is much less common that the rheumatic form but very much more fatal. Until the introduction of antibiotic therapy the mortality was practically 100 per cent.

The disease runs its course in a number of months, sometimes a year. It is caused by a variety of streptococcus (Streptococcus viridans) which reaches the heart from the throat. One peculiarity is that the disease is usually superimposed on an old rheumatic endocarditis, previously healthy valves being seldom affected. The inflammation is very much more severe than in the rheumatic form, the *vegetations* are large and extremely friable (Fig. 40), and the cusps of the valve are sometimes destroyed. The vegetations are teeming with streptococci, and these are discharged into the blood stream where they can be detected by blood culture, so that this procedure is of great value in the diagnosis of difficult cases.

The most striking feature of the disease is the formation of large numbers of *emboli* due to the breaking off of fragments of the friable vegetations. These sail off in the blood stream and stick in various organs where they give rise to some of the characteristic symptoms of the disease. Some of the emboli are large, and if these lodge in the brain they may cause paralysis, etc., whilst in the kidney they may cause blood to appear in the urine. Sometimes they are minute, but if these tiny emboli should lodge in the smallest vessels of the skin they will cause these vessels to rupture, with

8

the formation of multiple pin-point hemorrhages known as *petechiæ*. The petechiæ in the skin, the blood in the urine, and the streptococci in the blood culture, together with enlargement of the spleen and long-continued fever are some of the principal clinical features. Signs of heart failure will develop sooner or later.

Treatment.—Until the advent of penicillin the outlook in this disease was uniformly fatal. However, early recognition of the condition and prompt institution of penicillin treatment has resulted in arrest of the process and at least temporary disappearance of the signs of infection in about 50 to 60 per cent of cases. Other antibiotics may be necessary, depending upon the type of organism involved. It must be remembered, however, that there is still present the underlying heart disease upon which the bacterial

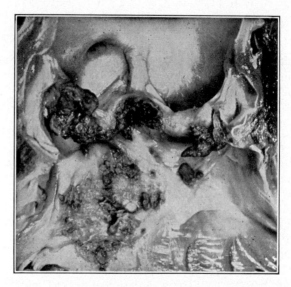

Fig. 40.—Subacute bacterial endocarditis. The friable vegetations, the mural spread, and the old thickening of the aortic cusps are all very characteristic. (Boyd, Textbook of Pathology.)

endocarditis developed, and recurrence of the endocarditis may take place. Treatment with penicillin must be in large doses and administered for a period of from four to six weeks.

In cases of rheumatic heart disease with valvular involvement and in cases of congenital heart disease it is advisable to use antibiotics for a short time before and after any tooth extraction or operation on the nose and throat. This is believed to prevent the occurrence of subacute bacterial endocarditis in many instances by adequate treatment of the transient bacteremia which is known to occur under these circumstances.

Acute Ulcerative Endocarditis.—This is a much rarer form of endocarditis caused by enormous numbers of pyogenic bacteria such as Staphylococcus aureus and Streptococcus hæmolyticus. The cusps of the valves

are rapidly destroyed (hence the terms acute and ulcerative), and the patient usually dies in less than six weeks.

CORONARY ARTERY OCCLUSION

In a previous chapter we studied the effect of cutting off the arterial blood supply to an organ not provided with a good collateral circulation, and we found that the effect depended on whether the closure of the artery was slow or sudden. Gradual closure due to narrowing of the lumen of the artery by atheroma led to slow atrophy and death of the specialized cells of the part (*e.g.*, heart muscle) and their replacement by scar tissue. Sudden closure by embolism or thrombosis caused the formation of an infarct, an area in which all the tissue was killed by the sudden ischemia.

The coronary arteries supplying the heart muscle with blood are unfortunately amongst the vessels most subject to *atheroma* with consequent narrowing of the lumen. This is very common after middle age, but may occasionally occur before the age of thirty. The scarring of the heart muscle caused by the cutting off of the blood supply leads to great weakening of the heart's action.

Frequently *thrombosis* is added to the atheroma, the thrombosis suddenly closing the already narrowed vessel. Two things may happen: (1) The patient may die suddenly, sometimes in his bed; this is likely to happen if the main branch of the left coronary is occluded. (2) If a smaller branch is blocked the patient may survive, but an infarct of the heart is produced which severely cripples the organ. The infarct, consisting of dead tissue, is a weak spot in the heart wall which may in time bulge outward and finally rupture, causing sudden death. Or the patient may have several attacks of thrombosis in different branches of the coronary arteries, any of which may prove fatal.

Although the public speaks of a " coronary attack," from the standpoint of the patient the essential feature is the presence or absence of an infarct. An infarct may occur without thrombosis, the lumen of the coronary artery being greatly narrowed by atheromatous thickening of the inner coat (intima), and the final obstruction produced by rupture of the soft atheromatous material into the lumen. Or thrombosis may occur without the production of an infarct, because the area of cardiac muscle is supplied with blood from one of the other coronary arteries, such a supply being designated as a collateral circulation. It is the infarct of the heart muscle, not the thrombosis of the coronary artery, that produces the symptoms and distress from which the patient suffers. The infarct is a soft, yellow area of dead muscle in the wall of the left ventricle, varying greatly in size (Plate II). The softness of the dead tissue makes it a weak spot in the wall of the ventricle which may rupture during the first week of the attack, or at a later date may bulge outward and rupture, in both instances resulting in sudden death.

When the blood supply to a muscle is suddenly cut off, very *severe pain* will be experienced if the muscle continues to be used. In the case of the heart complete rest is impossible, and the result is the agonizing pain known as *angina pectoris*, and a sense of suffocation as if the chest was held in a

vise.   The sudden pain is felt in the region of the heart and frequently passes down the left arm.   It may, however, be felt in the epigastrium, the upper part of the abdomen, and when not too severe is often mistaken for acute indigestion.   When a person suffers a supposed attack of acute indigestion and dies shortly afterwards, he is almost certain to have had coronary occlusion.   The victim of an anginal attack experiences a feeling of impending dissolution, one of the most terrible accompaniments of the disease.   His face is an ashy gray, and is bathed in a cold sweat.   Occasionally pain is absent, but the patient still has a sense of suffocation and marked *dyspnea* or shortness of breath, which, indeed, is the most constant of all the symptoms.   Sometimes the attack of pain is sudden and short; in other cases it may last for many hours.   The explanation of these differences is difficult, and cannot be entered into here.

The outlook in coronary artery occlusion varies greatly, depending on the size of the artery that is blocked, the extent of the damage to the heart muscle, and the question of collateral circulation.   The patient may die instantaneously; this, indeed, is the commonest cause of sudden death. But if the heart survives the shock, as is frequently the case, the neighboring arteries pour blood into the ischemic area and a collateral circulation is in time established.   When this occurs the patient may make a reasonably satisfactory recovery, but the heart will be permanently crippled, and his future life must be adjusted with this fundamental fact in mind.   The immediate mortality of coronary thrombosis varies from 15 to 25 per cent. If the patient survives the attack the infarcted area needs at least six weeks to become strengthened by scar tissue.   The patient must therefore be kept at complete rest in bed for this period and in some cases for a good deal longer.   Once the infarct has healed the patient may live for fifteen or twenty years in good health provided he observes the rules of the game.

Treatment.—The patient who has suffered an acute occlusion of the coronary artery requires complete rest for four to six weeks.   During the early part of this time, depending upon the severity of the attack, he should do as little as possible in the way of physical exertion.   This may require that he be fed, and nursing care should be such that he will be required to do the least possible with respect to physical exertion.   The use of anticoagulants, heparin and Dicumarol, have recently been introduced into the treatment of this condition in an attempt to decrease the tendency to the formation of blood clots within the heart and veins during the period of treatment.

In *angina pectoris* the patient should be advised to live within his exercise tolerance, *i.e.*, he should do no more activity than he can perform without production of anginal pain.   The use of nitroglycerin may give relief to the anginal pain at the time of its occurrence, but does nothing toward relieving the underlying cause.

HYPERTENSIVE HEART DISEASE.   ARTERIAL HYPERTENSION

If the heart pump has to work for years against a greatly increased resistance in the shape of high blood pressure it will gradually become exhausted and fail.   The strain naturally falls principally on the left ventricle, and

PLATE II

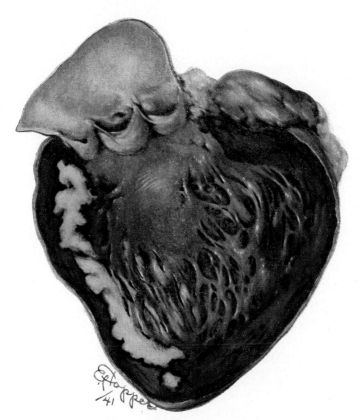

Recent Infarct of Heart

The yellow necrotic tissue in wall of left ventricle is edged by a narrow dark red border

for a time the wall becomes thicker (hypertrophied) so as to be able to overcome the increased resistance. Finally, however, this power is lost, the heart fails, the ventricle becomes dilated, and the end picture is very much like that of other forms of heart failure. The condition is known as hypertensive heart disease. The symptoms are similar to those of heart failure from other causes such as valvular disease and coronary artery disease. It must be pointed out, however, that very many persons with hypertension live vigorous lives for many years without developing signs of heart failure. Such people would be happier if they were ignorant of the fact that they had high blood pressure.

The cause of hypertension is a mystery. Certain forms complicate other diseases such as goiter and Bright's disease, but the common form of high blood pressure is called *essential hypertension* because no obvious cause for it can be demonstrated. Recent work suggests that an imbalance between hormones of the adrenal cortex and the kidney may be connected with the production of this mysterious condition. The small arteries throughout the body are contracted with narrowing of their lumen, and this leads to increase of the peripheral resistance to the blood flow so that the pressure of the blood in the large arteries rises. The patient with hypertension may not die of heart failure, but as the result of the bursting of a bloodvessel in the brain (cerebral hemorrhage, apoplexy). The narrowing of the small arteries to the kidneys may lead to atrophy of those organs, and the patient may die of renal failure. Death in hypertension may thus be due to disease of the heart, the brain, or the kidneys.

SYPHILITIC HEART DISEASE. AORTIC ANEURISM

Syphilis attacks the aorta rather than the heart, but aortic disease is apt to involve the heart secondarily. The origin of the aorta from the heart and the ascending aorta are the principal sufferers from the attack of the Spirochæta pallida. A destructive inflammation is produced, and this inflammation may extend to the aortic valve, the cusps of which become scarred and contracted so that they are no longer able to close, with incompetence as the result. But aortic incompetence may be produced without involvement of the cusps. These cusps are attached to the root or origin of the aorta, which contains much elastic tissue. Syphilis destroys the elastic tissue, and this leads to dilatation of the aortic wall. The result of this dilatation is that the cusps of the valve, even though healthy, are unable to meet and close the opening, so that blood escapes from the aorta back into the left ventricle, a condition of aortic incompetence. The escaping blood produces a loud murmur heard over the aortic valve.

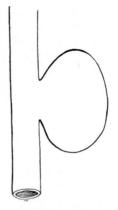

Fig. 41.—Aneurism of the aorta.

Aortic Aneurism.—An aneurism is a localized dilatation or bulging of an artery due to weakening of the wall of the vessel (Fig. 41). In the

thoracic aorta the common cause of aneurism is syphilis; in the abdominal aorta it is atheroma. The spirochetes of syphilis may damage the wall of the aorta to such an extent that it develops a localized bulging, such as may be seen in a bicycle tire or a toy balloon when it is inflated. As the bulging increases the wall becomes weaker and weaker until finally the aneurism bursts, causing sudden death of the patient. Before it bursts it causes pressure on the surrounding structures, giving rise to symptoms from which a correct diagnosis can be made. The aneurism can readily be seen in a roentgen-ray picture. If the reader is interested in the state of mind of a person who knows that he carries an aortic aneurism within his chest ready to burst at any moment, he will find it in Joseph Conrad's "The Shadow Line."

THE BASIS OF SYMPTOMS OF HEART DISEASE

Of all the ailments which may blow out life's little candle heart disease is the chief. But it will be realized from the foregoing discussion that the symptoms may be very varied. These symptoms may be those which point to the heart itself, or they may be the result of failure of the circulation, which again may be chiefly arterial or chiefly venous. In valvular disease such as mitral stenosis or aortic incompetence the heart becomes enlarged both from dilatation and hypertrophy. The *dilatation* of the chambers is to accommodate the increased volume of blood which is either dammed back into the left auricle in mitral stenosis or escapes back into the left ventricle through an incompetent aortic valve. The *hypertrophy* of the heart muscle is a *compensatory* mechanism by virtue of which more work is done in order to overcome the valvular defect. For a while this compensation is successful and no symptoms of heart disease develop, although physical examination of the heart may reveal to the physician the true state of affairs. The compensation may be wonderfully successful and the patient may enjoy good health for many years, especially if he regulates his life with discretion. Sooner or later, however, especially with the approach of age, compensation is likely to fail and a stage of *decompensation* is entered upon, with the development of the symptoms known as congestive heart failure.

Of the *cardiac symptoms* of heart disease the chief are pain, palpitation, and disorders of rhythm. *Pain* has already been discussed in connection with coronary thrombosis. *Palpitation*, a condition in which the patient becomes aware of the forcible beating of his heart, may be a symptom either of valvular or myocardial disease. Frequently, however, it does not indicate any organic heart disease, being caused by purely nervous disorders. *Disorders of rhythm* may take the form of increased rate (tachycardia) or irregularity of rhythm, occasional beats being missed. *Murmurs* may be heart with the stethoscope, caused by the blood leaking back through an incompetent valve or forcing its way through a stenosed one. *Heart block* is a condition in which the pulse rate drops to about one-half the normal, and is caused by scars due to coronary artery disease interfering with the "conduction bundle" which carries the nervous impulse necessary for muscular contraction from one part of the heart to the other.

Of the *symptoms due to interference with the circulation,* the commonest is *dyspnea.* The shortness of breath is due to the fact that the failing heart is unable to purify the blood properly by sending it through the lungs; when the impure blood reaches the brain it stimulates the respiratory center, causing the patient to breathe rapidly and feel short of breath. *Fainting attacks* may occur in aortic incompetence because part of the blood, instead of going to the brain, escapes back into the left ventricle. This causes cerebral anemia (ischemia) which is the essential cause of all fainting attacks. *Congestive heart failure* is a picture presented by patients the right side of whose heart is becoming exhausted, and is particularly well seen in mitral stenosis. There is damming back of the blood in the veins which empty into the right auricle, so that the veins in the neck stand out prominently; the liver is enlarged and tender because the blood accumulates in its substance. The lips, ears and fingers are *cyanosed* or blue because of insufficient oxygenation of the blood flowing through them, for it is the presence of oxygen which imparts to the blood in the arteries its bright red color.

Edema or dropsy is evidence of congestive heart failure, although it may also be caused by other conditions such as Bright's disease. In heart disease it is due to the blood serum which accumulates in the congested veins gradually passing out and collecting in the tissues; it is most marked in the feet and legs where it causes a swelling in which a hole can be made by steady pressure of the finger (pitting on pressure). The reason for this transudation of fluid from the bloodvessels is partly the increased pressure in the capillaries and small veins caused by the back pressure from the heart, and partly damage to the vessel walls with an increase of their permeability owing to an insufficient supply of the oxygen which is necessary for their health.

Finally it must be remembered that no organ is influenced to so marked a degree by nervous stimuli and what are commonly referred to as the emotions. The simple everyday words of our language testify to the truth of this statement. We say that the person is heavy-hearted, hard-hearted, heartless, good-hearted, that his heart aches with loneliness, flutters with alarm or stops with fear. It is evident that cardiac symptoms may have an emotional rather than an organic basis, and to confuse one with the other is a serious matter both for the physician and the patient.

CONGENITAL HEART DISEASE

Heart disease may be congenital rather than acquired. The child is born with cardiac defects due to failure in the process of development. An important predisposing cause is German measles in the mother during the first three months of pregnancy. The condition has assumed practical importance, because surgical operations have been developed for the treatment of three of these defects. A great number of different defects have been reported, but only the three amenable to surgical treatment will be described.

Tetralogy of Fallot.—The essence of this condition is pulmonary stenosis. The pulmonary valve is markedly narrowed, so that the blood is unable to

pass in sufficient quantity from the right ventricle to the lungs.   Fallot described three other changes in addition to the pulmonary stenosis.   (1) The septum which separates the left side of the heart from the right is shifted to the right, thus farther narrowing the pulmonary opening; (2) a gap is present in the septum (patent interventricular septum) through which the blood can pass; (3) the wall of the right ventricle is hypertrophied by reason of the increased work it has to do in forcing the blood through the narrow pulmonary opening.   The combination of these four is the reason for the rather pedantic word tetralogy (*tetra*, four).   The tetralogy of Fallot is the most common cause of the condition known as the "blue baby," a name given because of the extreme degree of cyanosis, the blue color being most marked on the lips, ears, cheeks and hands.   The principle of the operation is to bypass the obstruction at the opening of the pulmonary artery. This is done by anastomosing the left subclavian artery, a branch of the aorta, to the pulmonary artery beyond the obstruction, so that the blood now reaches the lungs, although from the left instead of the right ventricle. Reference to Figure 37, page 113, may make the matter more clear, although the branches of the aorta are not shown in the diagram.   The improvement in the child's condition is immediate and dramatic, the cyanosis and shortness of breath being often improved by the time the patient is returned to bed from the operating room.

Patent Ductus Arteriosus.—The ductus arteriosus is a short vessel which passes from the bifurcation of the main pulmonary artery into its two main branches to the arch of the aorta.   During intra-uterine life the blood from the right side of the heart passes along this channel into the aorta without passing through the lungs, as these organs are not used for respiration while the child is still within the womb.   The ductus should become closed a few weeks after birth.   It may, however, remain open or patent.   In this condition the blood flows from the aorta into the pulmonary artery owing to the pressure being higher in the former than the latter.   The blood therefore receives sufficient oxygen from the lungs, and there is no cyanosis except in cases complicated by other congenital defects.   Although the condition is compatible with a long and active life, in the great majority of cases life expectancy is considerably shortened.   The great danger is the development of streptococcal endarteritis at either end of the ductus.   The treatment is surgical division of the ductus, a relatively simple operation.

Coarctation of the Aorta.—This is a narrowing of the aorta (*coarctare*, to press tog ther) in the region where it is joined by the ductus.   This is beyond the origin of the large arteries to the head and arms, so that there is an abundant flow of blood to these parts and the blood pressure in the arm is high.   Very little blood passes through the narrowed aorta to the abdomen and legs, where the blood pressure is low and the pulse can hardly be felt, although some blood manages to bypass the obstruction through abundant collateral vessels which open up.   Recognition of this collateral circulation greatly assists the doctor in making a correct diagnosis.   The surgical treatment consists in clamping the aorta above and below the obstruction, excising the narrowed segment, and sewing the divided ends of the aorta together.   This dramatic operation is usually attended with complete success.

PRINCIPLES OF TREATMENT OF CARDIAC FAILURE

Perhaps the most important fact to remember is that the majority of people with structural heart disease are able to lead useful lives. Many cases of heart disease are kept in bed quite unnecessarily. The discovery that a cardiac murmur is present does not mean that the patient's whole mode of life has to be changed. A man with valvular disease of the heart may live comfortably for many years on account of the compensating power of the heart muscle. It must be remembered that the essential part of the heart is the muscle, not the valves.

One can do little about the underlying heart disease, but the occurrence of the edema can be prevented in many cases by adequate treatment. The most important part of the treatment is the use of a diet which is low in salt. In heart failure salt tends to accumulate in the body fluids. This results in the retention of water and production of swelling in various regions. The restriction of salt intake to very low levels tends to prevent the accumulation of this swelling. Digitalis is an important drug in the treatment of heart failure, particularly in cases where auricular fibrillation has occurred. Salt and water can be eliminated from the body by the use of diuretics, the most important of which are the mercurial diuretics, which are given by injection. After an attack of heart failure the patient may be again able to resume activity, but he must be instructed to limit his exertion to reasonable limits within his exercise tolerance. Education of the patient with heart disease as to the mode of life best suited to him is a most important item in the treatment. Too great solicitude on the part of the patient can be almost as unfortunate as too great recklessness.

DISEASES OF THE ARTERIES

Diseases of the arteries are among the most common causes of invalidism and death in those of middle age and later life. These diseases belong to two great groups: (1) degenerative (arteriosclerosis) and (2) inflammatory (arteritis).

Arteriosclerosis.—Sclerosis or hardening of the arteries may take either of two common forms: atheroma or atherosclerosis and arteriolosclerosis. *Atheroma* has already been described on page 47. It is in essence a patchy or nodular thickening of the intima of the artery with a great accumulation of cholesterol crystals and resulting narrowing of the lumen at one or more spots (Fig. 42). The blood supply may be cut down to the danger point, and a thrombus is apt to form on the diseased wall and obstruct the narrowed lumen. This is the mechanism of production of coronary thrombosis, cerebral thrombosis, and thrombosis in the arteries of the leg. Atheroma is an extremely common condition and is the chief cause of ischemia of the heart muscle, the brain and the leg. We are completely ignorant as to the cause or causes of atheroma. This is very unfortunate, because this lack of knowledge has proved an insurmountable obstacle to devising some method of preventing this crippling and often fatal condition which is the curse of the declining years of life.

Arteriolosclerosis affects the arterioles, the smallest arteries, particularly those of the kidney. There is a diffuse thickening of the wall of the arterioles (in contrast to the nodular thickening of atheroma) with accompanying narrowing of the lumen. There is none of the cholesterol accumulation which is so characteristic a feature of atheroma. Arteriolosclerosis is a common accompaniment of hypertension, but it may also occur in old age even though the blood pressure remains normal. In younger persons hypertension and arteriolosclerosis often go hand in hand.

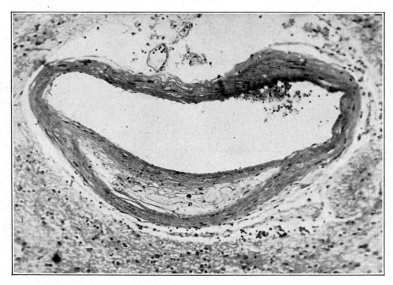

Fig. 42.—Atheroma of a cerebral vessel. The thickened intima shows degeneration in its deeper layers, and there is some atrophy of the media underlying the thickened plaque. × 125. (Boyd, Textbook of Pathology.)

Arteritis.—Inflammation of the arterial wall may occur for a variety of reasons. It used to be due to bacterial infection, particularly after surgical operation, but asepsis and antibiotics have made this a thing of the past. A number of forms of acute arteritis appear to be manifestations of allergy or hypersensitivity, although little or nothing is known about the substances to which the person is allergic. Three of these will be described, namely Buerger's disease, periarteritis nodosa, and its first cousin disseminated lupus erythematosus. All of these diseases are uncommon.

Buerger's disease is also called *thromboangiitis obliterans*, because it affects both arteries and veins and is associated with thrombosis which leads to obliteration of the lumen. The sex incidence is striking, for the disease is practically confined to men. It is a disease of young adult life, is particularly common in Jews, and usually affects the arteries of the legs, although those of the arms may also be involved. The cause is unknown, but it is believed that there is a condition of allergic hypersensitivity in the arterial wall. as a result of which an acute inflammatory reaction develops.

Patients seem to be specially hypersensitive to tobacco, and the sufferer is often found to be a very heavy cigarette smoker. In the treatment of the disease one of the most important points is to give up tobacco. The disease has an acute and a chronic stage. It is the chronic form which is more likely to give rise to serious symptoms, because the vessels are more widely and seriously involved by that time. The walls both of the arteries and the veins are inflamed, and the lumen of both these vessels is blocked by thrombi. The result is ischemia of the more distant parts of the leg and foot.

The first symptoms are usually indefinite pains in one foot or cramp-like pains in the calf after walking a short distance, a condition known as intermittent claudication (*claudicare*, to limp). No pulse can be felt at the ankle. When the foot hangs down it becomes bright red and throbs painfully. When the foot is raised it becomes more blanched than normal. Later in the disease ulcers and gangrene of the feet may develop, so that amputation may have to be performed. The tragedy of the condition is that the process tends to extend upwards along the leg so that amputation may have to be done at an ever higher level.

Periarteritis nodosa is a much more acute inflammatory condition than is Buerger's disease, and it affects the small arteries to the viscera rather than those to the limbs. The cause is unknown, but it is not unlikely that this disease also represents a type of hypersensitivity. The disease often runs an acute course with fever and prostration ending fatally in the course of a few weeks or months. The symptoms are extremely varied, depending on which arteries are involved. The principal vessels affected are those of the gastrointestinal tract, the kidney, and the heart. There may be acute abdominal symptoms due to involvement of the mesenteric arteries, acute cardiac symptoms from coronary artery involvement, or neuritic pains due to lesions of the arteries supplying the peripheral nerves.

Disseminated lupus erythematosus is a rare condition similar in many ways to periarteritis nodosa, for it involves the small vessels to the viscera. The heart, kidneys, skin and serous membranes are also involved. A butterfly-like red rash over the bridge of the nose and both cheeks is a common and striking feature. A peculiar occurrence is the finding of what are known as LE (lupus erythematosus) cells. These are polymorphonuclear leucocytes containing a large homogeneous inclusion mass. The LE cells were first found in the bone marrow of patients suffering from the disease, but it is now known that the phenomenon depends on the presence of some factor in the patient's blood serum which acts upon the cells. When a test is made for the LE phenomenon, the patient's blood serum is mixed with the bone marrow cells of an animal such as a rabbit, and a smear is made and searched for the development of LE cells.

Both periarteritis nodosa and disseminated lupus belong to the group of conditions known as the *collagen diseases*. These are closely related to rheumatic fever and rheumatoid arthritis, and are therefore benefitted at least temporarily by the administration of cortisone.

Chapter

10

DISEASES OF THE LUNGS

Structure and Function.—The essential business of the lungs is purification of the blood, a business in which the heart and lungs are partners. The impure blood laden with the waste products of the body in the form of carbon dioxide is brought to the lungs where the carbon dioxide gas is given off into the air and fresh oxygen is taken up into the blood. The purified blood returns directly to the heart, and is then sent through the arteries to supply the needs of the body. The lungs constitute the great mixing place of air and blood, and they have a corresponding structure.

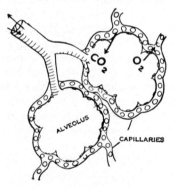

FIG. 43.—Bronchiole going to two alveoli. The small circles in the capillaries are red blood cells. (Best and Taylor, The Human Body; courtesy of Henry Holt & Co.)

Each lung is a honeycomb, with air in place of honey in the cells of the comb, and an infinite number of blood capillaries in their walls. These walls are so thin that gases (carbon dioxide and oxygen) can readily pass through in either direction (Fig. 43). The air is carried to the air spaces or *alveoli* by the bronchi and their terminations, the bronchioles, which subdivide and ramify throughout the entire lung.

Owing to the rhythmic movements of the chest during respiration air is being continually sucked into and expelled from the lungs. One great disadvantage of this arrangement is that the interior of the lungs is in communication with the outside air, so that infecting germs are liable to enter and cause inflammation, although most of them are held back in the nose and throat. This is not the case with any of the other organs of the body, and for this reason inflammation and tuberculosis are far commoner in the lungs than in organs like the heart and kidney.

The lung, like the heart, is covered by a thin membrane, the *pleura*, and a similar membrane lines the chest wall. Although a potential space, the *pleural cavity*, exists between the layers, in health these layers are in contact with one another. It is evident that inflammation of the lung may easily extend to the pleura and set up inflammation in that membrane, a condition known as pleurisy.

The limits of this book make it impossible to consider diseases of the nose, throat, larynx, and trachea, which form the upper part of the respiratory

apex downwards, so that the oldest and most advanced lesions are at the top. In a case with extensive lesions there may be cavities in the upper part of the lung, consolidation in the middle, and separate tubercles at the base. Pleurisy is always present, and adhesions are formed between the two layers of the pleura.

3. **Acute Tuberculous Pneumonia.**—Here the infection overwhelms the resistance, and runs through the lung like a forest fire, giving rise to the clinical picture of galloping consumption or acute phthisis (wasting). There are no discrete tubercles, but in their place a diffuse pneumonic process. There is no fibrosis, no attempt at limitation of the infection. Acute cavities are formed. The disease may prove fatal in a few months or even weeks.

Acute miliary tuberculosis is a fourth possibility, but this may be regarded as a complication of any of the previous three. The tuberculous process may penetrate the wall of a bloodvessel and discharge large numbers of bacilli into the blood stream. These are carried throughout the body, where they cause the formation of an infinite number of miliary tubercles in all the organs. The lungs are no exception, so that in addition to a small lesion at the apex of one lung, both lungs may be peppered with fine miliary tubercles.

The Basis of Symptoms.—The *general symptoms*, such as fever, loss of weight, weakness, etc., are due to the absorption of toxins. They become more marked when secondary infection with pyogenic bacteria is added to the pure tuberculous infection (again an example of the seven devils). *Cough* is a bronchial symptom due to irritation of the larger bronchi. *Pain* in the side is due to tuberculous pleurisy. The character of the *sputum* depends on the nature of the lesions. In acute miliary tuberculosis there may be no sputum. Until cavities have formed it is scanty and may contain no bacilli. After cavity formation it is copious, purulent owing to secondary infection, and contains large numbers of bacilli. The more rapid the disease the more bacilli will there be, the more stationary the disease the fewer are their numbers.

Hemoptysis, the coughing up of blood, is due to erosion of a bloodvessel. It has been said that hemoptysis marks the end of the beginning or the beginning of the end of the disease. At the beginning there may be erosion of a small vessel in the early process of softening, and the sputum becomes blood-streaked. In the advanced stage a large artery crossing a chronic cavity may give way causing a severe and possibly fatal hemorrhage.

Principles of Treatment.—It has already been pointed out in the general discussion on tuberculosis that good hygiene and rest, physical and mental, are the most important factors in the treatment of the disease. In the case of pulmonary tuberculosis one lung can be put at least partially at rest in a number of ways, and if the disease is confined to one lung the benefit of this treatment may be very marked. The simplest method is by means of *artificial pneumothorax*, a procedure in which air is introduced into the pleural cavity between the lung and the chest wall. The pressure of the air causes the lung to collapse like a sponge that has been squeezed and prevents it from moving with respiration. In time the air is absorbed, but the procedure can be repeated. This method is not feasible when the pleural

cavity is obliterated by adhesions which bind the lung to the chest wall·

The lung can also be rested by *dividing the phrenic nerve* in the neck. The phrenic nerve supplies the diaphragm, the muscular partition between the thorax and abdomen which rises and falls with every breath a person takes. When the nerve is cut the diaphragm is paralyzed on that side and the lung is given at least partial rest.

The third and most drastic method of putting the lung at rest is by the operation of *thoracoplasty*. The lung does not expand and contract during respiration by virtue of its own motive power, but because the muscles of the thorax cause the chest to expand and contract, and the lung follows these movements passively. Thoracoplasty consists of a plastic or moulding operation on the thorax in which a number of ribs are removed, so that the side of the chest falls in and is unable to move. The lung also becomes immobile, and the tuberculous lesions at last have an opportunity to heal.

Streptomycin, alone or in combination with para-aminosalicylic acid, has been of value in arresting some types of pulmonary tuberculosis. It is particularly valuable in cases where there is an acute spread of the disease; also in cases of tuberculous bronchitis and it has been of value in arresting cases of miliary tuberculosis. This method of treatment should be used along with the other principles of treatment outlined above. The duration of streptomycin treatment is usually for a period of about three months. The use of para-aminosalicylic acid tends to lessen the development of insensitivity to streptomycin on the part of the tubercle bacillus.

It must not be forgotten that the patient with pulmonary tuberculosis is a potential source of danger to those with whom he comes in contact. This danger may remain potential and not become actual if he is educated in the principles of hygiene. The two sources of danger are sputum and coughing at close quarters. If sputum is safely disposed of and the danger of coughing infected droplets in the direction of another person recognized, the tuberculous patient need not be a source of infection to those with whom he lives. But the danger is always present, and precautions must not for a moment be relaxed. The price of safety is eternal vigilance.

THE DUST DISEASES

The long-continued irritation of certain dusts may cause a chronic interstitial pneumonia known as pneumoconiosis (*konis*, dust). These dusts are encountered as the result of certain industrial processes. The dangerous element in the dust is silica.

Silicosis.—Silicosis is the most widespread, the most serious and the oldest of all occupational diseases. It provides a serious hazard in the gold-mining industry in certain districts such as the South African Rand and northern Ontario. If, in coal mining, hard rock has to be drilled through, coal miners may also suffer. Other occupations in which there is danger are tin mining, stone working, metal grinding, and sand blasting. In all of these cases, dust containing fine particles of silica may be inhaled over long periods of time.

The silica dust is carried by phagocytes from the bronchioles into the septa of the alveoli. There the dust acts as an irritant which stimulates

the formation of large amounts of connective tissue. This fibrosis goes hand in hand with destruction of the lung structure. At first there are discrete nodules of fibrous tissue, but in the course of time these coalesce to form large fibrous areas, which are completely useless from the point of view of respiratory function. These fibrous areas give a characteristic *x*-ray picture, by means of which an accurate diagnosis can be made.

The condition is a progressive one and the patient continues to get worse even after he has been removed from the source of dust for a number of years. There is gradually increasing shortness of breath, with developing heart failure owing to the difficulty which the right ventricle has in pumping blood to the densely fibrosed lungs. This is one of the few conditions for which there is absolutely no treatment, and it is evident that in this case prevention is all-important. This can be done by paying attention to adequate ventilation of factories, etc., and providing miners with masks which will filter out the dust. Silicosis, however, remains one of the great industrial hazards.

Other Dust Pneumonias.—*Anthracosis* is a condition in which the lung becomes filled with coal dust. If the coal is hard coal damage will result, because the rock from which the coal was mined contains a certain amount of silica. *Asbestosis* is an important disease due to the inhalation of asbestos dust. The disease may be acquired either during the crushing of asbestos rock or in the process of the manufacture of asbestos. As the great bulk of asbestos comes from the province of Quebec, it is natural that most of the cases should be found in this locality. The lung shows the same airless and fibrous condition which is so characteristic of silicosis. Both in asbestosis and in silicosis there is a marked tendency to the development of pulmonary tuberculosis.

CANCER OF THE LUNG

Carcinoma of the lung is one of the common forms of cancer, although it is only within recent years that this has come to be recognized. Much of this advance in knowledge is due to roentgen-ray examination. The condition is known as *bronchogenic carcinoma*, because the tumor arises from a bronchus and not from the lung tissue itself. The factors which cause this form of cancer are not known, but it is interesting to note that the disease is exceedingly common amongst workers in certain mines rich in radium and radioactive substances, particularly Schneeberg in Saxony and Joachimsthal in Bohemia. For some reason the disease is very much commoner in men than in women. In some statistics the proportion has been 8 to 1. The excessive use of cigarettes in recent years has been blamed, rightly or wrongly.

The tumor grows into and surrounds one of the main bronchi, gradually narrowing the lumen until it becomes completely blocked (Plate III). Two results follow from this blockage. In the first place the part of the lung supplied by the bronchus is cut off from a fresh supply of air, the air in this part of the lung is gradually absorbed into the blood, and finally the affected area of the lung undergoes *collapse*. This collapse can readily be recognized in the roentgen-ray picture even though the tumor itself may be

invisible, and by this means a correct diagnosis can be made. The second result is *bronchiectasis* and abscess formation. This is due to the fact that the secretions in the blocked part of the bronchus cannot escape and therefore stagnate and undergo putrefaction, so that the wall of the bronchus is weakened and dilates, a condition of bronchiectasis. Cancer cells from the surface of the tumor which projects into the lumen of the bronchus are shed off and coughed up in the sputum. Examination of the sputum for these cells, either by making smears or by coagulating the sputum into a block of tissue and cutting microscopic sections, is a valuable means of making an early diagnosis, especially in cases where the tumor cannot be seen by the bronchoscope.

One of the chief features of the disease is the formation of *metastases*. Even when the tumor in the bronchus is comparatively small, the cancer cells may spread by lymph vessels to the lymph glands in the chest, where they form a large tumor mass, and by the blood stream to distant organs such as the liver, brain, and bones. The first indication that the patient has a cancer of the lung may be swelling of the abdomen due to a large tumor in the liver, severe headache due to a brain tumor, or a fracture caused by weakening of a bone from the presence of a secondary tumor. The adrenal and kidney are often involved. In addition to distant metastases the tumor may spread widely throughout the lung and involve the pleura.

The Basis of Symptoms.—The symptoms are due to pressure and obstruction. The persistent *cough* is due to irritation of the bronchus by a growth. When a patient in the cancer age, particularly a man, has suffered from a cough and expectoration without obvious cause for more than a few weeks, it is always wise to suspect cancer and to examine the sputum for cancer cells or to pass a bronchoscope and inspect the lining of the bronchi. *Bloody sputum* is caused by the tumor in the bronchus opening into a bloodvessel. *Dyspnea*, one of the commonest symptoms, is due to cutting off of the air from the lung, pressure by the enlarged glands, and interference with the heart's action. *Pain* in the chest and back is caused by pressure on the nerves. *Pleural effusion* is common, and is due to irritation of the pleura by spread of the tumor. Other symptoms may be due to metastases in the brain, etc.

Principles of Treatment.—The only method of treatment which gives any hope of cure in this disease is excision of the tumor by removal of the whole lung. The number of complete cures effected by this means of treatment has not been great, but the possibilities of cure can be increased by early diagnosis of the condition. X-ray treatment does not offer very satisfactory results.

PLEURISY AND EMPYEMA

The pleura, that delicate membrane which embraces the lung so intimately, is naturally involved in the infections which attack the lung. Inflammation of the pleura, or pleurisy, is therefore a common accompaniment both of pneumonia and tuberculosis. Inflammation of serous membranes, of which the pleura is an example, is characterized by the formation of a shaggy inflammatory exudate consisting partly of fibrin and partly of polymorphonuclear leucocytes. This exudate forms a rough layer on the smooth

PLATE III

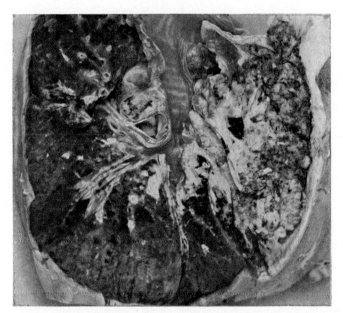

Bronchogenic Carcinoma

The carcinoma is arising from and occluding one of the main bronchi. The corresponding
part of the lung and the pleura are infiltrated with tumor.

surface of the pleura covering the lung and may also involve the pleura lining the chest wall. These two rough surfaces rub together each time the lung moves during respiration, producing sharp stabbing pain in the side. In time the two inflamed surfaces may stick together with the formation of temporary or permanent adhesions. Fluid poured out in the exudate may accumulate in the pleural cavity between the two layers, a condition known as *pleurisy with effusion*. In *dry pleurisy*, a more common condition, there is little or no fluid in the pleural cavity. If the fluid is large in amount it will press the air out of the lung and cause partial or complete *collapse* of that organ (Fig. 47). The fluid exudate of pleurisy with effusion is serous in character, that is to say it consists mostly of blood serum with only a slight admixture of inflammatory cells.

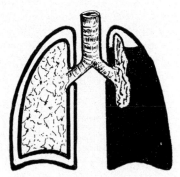

Fig. 47.—Pleural effusion. The left pleural cavity is almost completely filled with fluid causing marked collapse of lung.

Empyema is purulent pleurisy, in which the pleural cavity is filled not with watery serous fluid but with pus. It is therefore synonymous with pus in the pleural cavity. A common cause of empyema is the formation of an abscess of the lung immediately under the pleura; if this abscess should rupture into the pleural cavity with an outpouring not only of pus but of enormous numbers of bacteria, empyema will result. Empyema may complicate lobar pneumonia, especially in children, but is more likely to follow streptococcal bronchopneumonia such as may occur in the course of influenza.

Pleurisy with effusion may clear up by itself, the fluid being gradually absorbed, although when it is large in amount it may have to be drawn off. In empyema, on the other hand, the infection of the pleura is so heavy and so well established that active intervention is necessary. This intervention takes the form of drainage of the pus by various devices which need not be described in detail.

Pleural Fluid.—The pleural cavities are normally empty, but as a result of disease they may contain a large amount of fluid. This fluid may be either an exudate or a transudate. In both cases the fluid comes from the bloodvessels. An *exudate* is formed as the result of inflammation (pleurisy, empyema), which renders the walls of the vessels more permeable so that

an inflammatory exudate pours out. We shall therefore expect an exudate to resemble the blood in containing much albumin and leucocytes (pus cells) and in having a high specific gravity. A *transudate* is formed as the result of back pressure in the veins and capillaries, which causes the watery part of the blood to escape through the vessel walls. This occurs in congestive heart failure. A transudate is more watery than an exudate, contains little albumin and few cells, and has a low specific gravity. In an exudate the albumin is over 3 per cent, the specific gravity is above 1.018, and the fluid may be turbid on account of the presence of large numbers of pus cells. In a transudate the albumin is under 3 per cent, the specific gravity is under 1.015, and the fluid is clear.

Pleural fluid may be a clear transudate, or a fairly clear exudate (pleurisy with effusion), or thick purulent fluid (empyema). Pleurisy with effusion is usually due to pulmonary tuberculosis. As an exudate is caused by bacterial infection, the fluid is cultured in the laboratory, so that it must be collected in a sterile container. It is preferable to add a little sodium citrate to the container to prevent the fluid from clotting.

PNEUMOTHORAX

Reference has already been made to *artificial* pneumothorax, a procedure in which air is intentionally introduced into the pleural cavity in order to put an inflamed lung at rest. Occasionally, however, air may gain access to the pleural cavity as the result of injury or disease. This is known as *spontaneous pneumothorax*. The air may come from the lung, usually as the result of rupture of a tuberculous cavity on the surface. More rarely it may come from the outside, as in a perforating wound of the chest or fracture of a rib. Whatever the cause of the pneumothorax, the air accumulates in the pleural cavity and compresses the lung causing collapse in just the same way as an accumulation of fluid may lead to collapse. The presence of air can easily be detected by the physician by the physical signs which it produces and by the appearance in the roentgen-ray picture.

ATELECTASIS

Atelectasis means collapse of the lung. The lung is a sponge filled with air. When this sponge is compressed it collapses. Before birth there is, of course, no air in the lungs, and they are therefore completely collapsed, a condition of *congenital atelectasis*. As soon as the child breathes after birth the lungs become expanded with air. In medico-legal work the absence of atelectasis is a proof that the child has lived after birth.

Apart from the congenital form, collapse of the lung may be produced in two entirely different ways: by compression of the lung or by obstruction of a bronchus. *Compression of the lung* may be caused by pleural effusion, empyema, or the presence of air under pressure in the pleural cavity (pneumothorax). *Obstruction of a bronchus* may be caused in a variety of ways. A foreign body such as a peanut, coin, or tooth, may pass down the trachea and become lodged in a bronchus. No air can now enter the part of the lung supplied by the blocked bronchus; the air already there is absorbed into

the blood, and the lung collapses. In debilitated children suffering from bronchitis mucus may collect in the bronchi in such large amount that obstruction and atelectasis results; owing to the debility the mucus is not expelled by vigorous coughing. For the same reason areas of collapse may develop after an abdominal operation, because mucus collects in the bronchi owing to the irritation of the anesthetic, and coughing is interfered with by the abdominal wound. In bronchogenic carcinoma the tumor often obstructs a bronchus so that the distal part of the lung undergoes collapse, a condition which can be recognized in the roentgen-ray picture, and which is of great help in making a diagnosis.

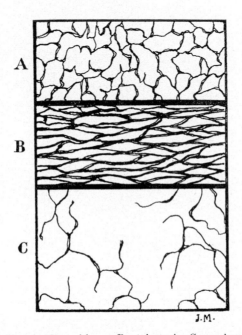

Fig. 48.—*A*, Normal lung; *B*, atelectasis; *C*, emphysema.

In all forms of atelectasis the lung presents the same appearance. A part or the whole of the lung is collapsed like a compressed sponge; it is firm, airless, and dark owing to the air being squeezed out of it. Microscopically the walls of the alveoli are pressed together, so that the lumen is almost obliterated (Fig. 48 *B*).

EMPHYSEMA

Emphysema is the opposite of atelectasis, for the alveoli are distended instead of collapsed. The walls between the air spaces are atrophied and many disappear, so that one large space is formed from many smaller ones (Fig. 48 *C*). The lungs, in contrast to atelectasis, are voluminous and pale, and often present large blebs or bullæ which project on the surface. Em-

physema often complicates chronic bronchitis and asthma, the constant coughing apparently resulting in distention of the air spaces.

The effects of emphysema may be serious and far-reaching. The chest becomes barrel-shaped, respiratory movements are diminished, and expiration is difficult and prolonged. Owing to the widespread atrophy and destruction of the alveolar walls, the small bloodvessels which run in them are obliterated, with resulting obstruction to the flow of blood from the right side of the heart in the pulmonary artery. The back pressure on the heart may become so extreme that great cardiac and respiratory distress develops, with marked cyanosis and finally fatal heart failure.

Chapter

11

DISEASES OF THE UPPER DIGESTIVE TRACT

The digestive or alimentary canal extends from the mouth, through which food enters the body, to the anus through which the residue escapes. Its function is two-fold: (1) To convert the food into a digestible form in which it can be assimilated; (2) to absorb the food thus digested. More briefly, the functions are digestion and absorption. Digestion is commenced in the mouth and continued in the stomach. Absorption is accomplished by the intestine, although digestion also takes place in the upper portion of that tube. We may, therefore, divide the alimentary canal into an upper part, the mouth, esophagus or gullet, and stomach, and a lower part, the small and large intestine. The distinction is convenient on account of the difference in the diseases which affect the two portions. The common diseases of the upper part are inflammation and tumors.

THE MOUTH

The principal structures in the mouth are the lips, tongue, tonsils, and teeth. The teeth will be considered in Chapter 22.

CANCER OF THE LIP

As the lips are covered by skin and gum, both of which are epithelial structures, the common tumor is carcinoma. Cancer of the lip is uncommon in women and extremely rare in the upper lip. It occurs principally in men over middle age, and begins as a thickening at the junction of the skin and mucous membrane (the red part of the lip) which may or may not be raised above the surface (Fig. 49). It is usually preceded by some chronic inflammatory lesion such as an ulcer or crack which may have been present for months or even years. The irritation produced by excessive smoking may be a factor. The most important single fact about cancer of the lip is that it is remarkably amenable to treatment. Surgical removal or treatment by radium usually brings about a complete and lasting cure. The worst thing to do is to apply some form of caustic or irritant with the idea of burning

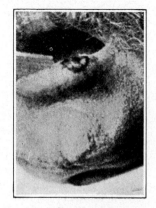

FIG. 49.—Cancer of lower lip.

(145)

off the nodule, for such treatment only serves to stimulate the growth of the tumor. If the condition is untreated it will gradually destroy the lip, and the tumor cells will be carried to the local lymph nodes under the jaw and in the neck, enlargement of which will form a large hard lump. When this occurs the prospects of successful treatment are greatly lessened.

CANCER OF THE TONGUE

As might be expected, the appearance of the lesion and the etiological factors concerned are similar to those of cancer of the lip. Chronic irritation in the form of a jagged tooth or a badly fitting plate is an important factor. The tumor usually begins on the edge of the tongue, and is felt as a lump which finally breaks down to form an ulcer. The tumor spreads much more rapidly than in the case of cancer of the lip, so that the presence of a lump in the tongue, however small, demands immediate attention. The prognosis is much worse than in cancer of the lip, particularly in cancer of the posterior part of the tongue, but radium treatment has served greatly to lighten the gloom of the picture.

CANCER OF THE MOUTH

Carcinoma may arise from the gum of the jaws and cheeks, the palate and the throat. In the front of the mouth the tumor is of the same character as cancer of the lip and tongue, and is again associated with chronic irritation. At the back of the mouth and in the throat the tumor may present two special characteristics: (1) The local lesion may remain small and indeed undiscoverable for a long time, but the lymph nodes in the neck become greatly enlarged; (2) the tumor (mass in neck) is highly radiosensitive, although it is seldom that a cure can be effected by this means.

TONSILLITIS

The tonsils are masses of lymphatic tissue, one on each side of the throat. They are full of little recesses or *crypts*, and as the mouth is teeming with bacteria it is natural that infection should be frequent. The infecting agent is commonly the streptococcus. As a result of the acute inflammation the tonsils become markedly swollen, narrowing the opening of the throat, and causing great pain and difficulty in swallowing. The surface may be covered with pus. *Quinsy* is a very severe suppuration of the entire tonsil, frequently with spread of the infection to the surrounding tissues of the throat and abscess formation. One attack of tonsillitis tends to predispose to another, and a state of chronic infection may be established within the crypts. The danger of such a condition is that the tonsil becomes a constant focus of infection from which streptococci gain access to the blood stream, are carried to distant parts of the body, and there set up chronic inflammatory lesions in the joints and other organs. The infection of chronic arthritis probably originates in the throat and tonsils in the majority of cases. Acute or chronic sore throat, like tonsillitis, is due principally to streptococcal infection.

CANCER OF THE ESOPHAGUS

The only important disease of the esophagus is carcinoma. This usually occurs in men over middle age, although it is also met with in women. The tumor surrounds the muscular tube, producing narrowing of its lumen, so that difficulty in swallowing is the chief symptom. The only treatment is surgical removal of the tumor, and this is possible in very few cases and can only be undertaken by the most skilful of surgeons.

THE STOMACH

Structure and Function.—The stomach is an elongated muscular bag situated in the upper part of the abdomen (epigastrium) under the ribs. Its capacity is about $1\frac{1}{2}$ quarts. The end which opens into the duodenum is called the *pylorus*. At the pylorus there is a circular band of muscle, the *pyloric sphincter*, which is usually contracted, but relaxes to allow food which has been properly liquefied by the gastric juice to pass into the duodenum. If it refuses to relax, the stomach becomes dilated. The most frequent cause of *dilatation of the stomach* is an ulcer or cancer at the pylorus. When an ulcer becomes chronic or heals, much scar tissue is formed, which contracts and narrows the opening (pyloric stenosis). The mere irritation of the ulcer may cause the muscle of the sphincter to go into spasm, thus keeping the opening closed. Sometimes abnormal nervous stimuli will produce the same result even though no lesion can be found in the stomach. This "functional obstruction" is known as *pylorospasm*. The normal stomach should empty itself in from one to seven hours, depending on the nature of the meal. If the stomach is not empty at the end of seven hours as shown by the roentgen-rays, *retention* is said to be present. In marked organic obstruction the stomach may become enormously dilated, and may fill the greater part of the abdomen, causing great distress and continuous vomiting.

The gastric juice contains a digestive ferment, *pepsin*, which acts only on the proteins of the food, and *hydrochloric acid*, which is necessary for the proper functioning of the pepsin. Both are produced by the gastric mucous membrane in response to certain nervous and chemical stimuli. The *nervous stimulus* is brought about by the attractive appearance, taste, and odor of the food. If these are unattractive, or if the eater gives no consideration to the things eaten, this nervous stimulus is lost and digestion suffers. It is not the mouth only which waters at the sight or even the thought of delicious food; the stomach also "waters." Food must be enjoyed to be digested properly, and a good cook is one of the stomach's most valuable assistants. The *chemical stimulus* is a hormone produced at the pyloric end by the action of meat extracts on the mucous membrane. For this reason soups and meat juices form the proper beginning of a dinner. The hydrochloric acid ceases to be produced in cancer of the stomach and in certain grave anemias, particularly pernicious anemia. This absence of hydrochloric acid, as shown by analysis of the stomach contents (gastric analysis), is of great diagnostic value.

Vomiting is the sudden ejection of the gastric contents caused by contraction of the muscular wall of the stomach. This may be brought on by the action of an acute irritant such as concentrated alcohol (cocktails) on an empty stomach. Gastric retention is frequently accompanied by vomiting. Even nervous influences such as a nauseating sight, violent emotion, or the giddiness of seasickness or airsickness may cause the stomach to contract and thus produce vomiting.

Organic disease of the stomach is commonly accompanied by "indigestion" or *dyspepsia*, a feeling of bloating, fulness or actual pain. In many cases, however, these symptoms are caused by lesions in some other organ such as the gall-bladder, duodenum or appendix. These organs are supplied by branches of the same nerves which go to the stomach and the stomach is so sensitive an organ that it may cry aloud in sympathy with its suffering neighbors. Sometimes these cries are so loud that they drown those of the organ really involved, and this sometimes makes the correct diagnosis of abdominal diseases a matter of extreme difficulty. The patient should sympathize with his doctor as well as the doctor with his patient.

The two common organic diseases of the stomach are ulcer and cancer.

GASTRIC ULCER

An ulcer of the stomach is called a *peptic ulcer*, because the peptic or digestive juice plays an all-important part in its production. But a similar ulcer occurs in the part of the duodenum next to the stomach so that *duodenal ulcer* will be considered together with gastric ulcer under the common heading of peptic ulcer.

The *cause* of peptic ulcer can be stated in part, but only in part. When for any reason a small area of gastric or duodenal mucous membrane is injured and becomes necrosed, the acid gastric juice digests the dead tissue just as it would digest any piece of dead meat. In this way a depression or hole is made which extends for a varying depth into the wall of the stomach or duodenum. The chemical conditions are the same in the first part of the duodenum as in the stomach, for the acid gastric juice is poured into that part of the bowel when the pyloric sphincter relaxes. At about 3 inches along the duodenum the pancreatic duct and bile duct open on the mucous membrane, and as the juices from these ducts are strongly alkaline the acidity of the gastric juice is neutralized. For this reason peptic ulcer is confined to the first part of the duodenum. The rôle of the gastric juice in the production of peptic ulcer is easy to understand. But we are still in the dark as to the *cause of the initial necrosis* of the mucous membrane. The two most probable factors are: (1) A focus of bacterial infection in the wall, the bacteria being carried there by the blood; (2) spasm of a small artery in the wall of the stomach caused by nervous stimuli and leading to ischemia and necrosis of the portion of mucous membrane supplied by the vessel. The patient with peptic ulcer is usually nervous and high-strung, restless and irritable, prone to worry and upset by strain. These characteristics are not the result of the ulcer; they are much more probably its cause, and have to be considered by the physician who undertakes the treatment of a case.

The *site* of the ulcer is usually at the pyloric end of the stomach or along the upper border (lesser curvature). In treating an ordinary ulcer of the skin, treatment consists in putting the part at rest and preventing irritation of the ulcer. But in the stomach the organ is made to work every time a meal is taken, and the hydrochloric acid acts as an acute irritant so that the area of necrosis tends to become deeper. This necrotic tissue is in turn digested and in time the hole may penetrate the whole thickness of the wall so that *perforation* into the abdominal cavity occurs (Fig. 50). a condition which will prove fatal if not treated by immediate operation.

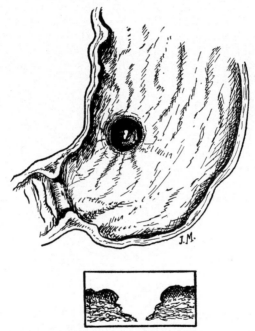

Fig. 50.—Gastric ulcer showing small perforation. Inset shows microscopic appearance and perforation.

Fortunately, however, protective forces are at work which tend to prevent this catastrophe and limit the spread of the ulcer. The continued irritation stimulates the formation of fibrous tissue in the floor of the ulcer and this offers marked resistance to its spread. A chronic peptic ulcer is therefore a circumscribed hole, usually not more than 1 inch in diameter, funnel-shaped, of varying depth, with a hard fibrous base. When the ulcer is still small healing may take place, but when it is deep this is unlikely to occur. The abundant scar tissue at the base of the ulcer may contract to such a degree that obstruction of the pylorus is produced, or if the ulcer is in the middle of the stomach the contraction may divide that organ into two compartments, a condition known as *hour-glass stomach*.

The Basis of Symptoms.—The great symptom of peptic ulcer, whether gastric or duodenal, is *pain*, relieved by the taking of foods and alkalis. The

10

pain may be a mild feeling of discomfort known as *dyspepsia,* or it may be extremely severe. It bears a characteristic relation to food, being relieved by the taking of food for about an hour and then coming on again. The triple rhythm of pain-food-relief shows a remarkable regularity. An alkali such as sodium bicarbonate may relieve the pain to an even greater degree. The usual explanation given for the pain and its relief by food and alkalis is that it is caused by the irritating action of the hydrochloric acid on the raw surface of the ulcer, the acid being neutralized by food and alkali. Muscular contraction of the stomach wall may be even more important in producing pain than the action of the acid. Inflammatory foci in the neighborhood of the ulcer cause contraction of the surrounding muscle and spasm of the pyloric sphincter. This all tends to increase the tension within the stomach and thus excite pain. Food and alkalis cause the stomach to relax for a time and thus relieve the pain. A large gastric ulcer sometimes produces no symptoms until it finally perforates, a state of affairs for which no satisfactory explanation can be offered.

Hemorrhage is a frequent symptom, varying from a slight oozing of blood to a copious flooding which may prove fatal. Severe hemorrhage is due to rupture of a large artery in the base of the ulcer. In gastric ulcer there may be vomiting of blood, the vomitus being not red but "coffee-grounds" in appearance, owing to the action of the gastric juice on the blood. Vomiting of blood is known as *hematemesis.* The patient may not vomit but may pass the blood in the stools, imparting to them a blackish color (tarry stools), a condition known as *melena.*

Perforation is a complication rather than a symptom. A hole is made right through the wall of the stomach or duodenum, through which the gastric contents pour into the abdominal cavity. The patient experiences sudden very severe pain, and soon develops a general peritonitis or inflammation of the lining of the abdominal cavity. The condition will prove fatal unless the opening in the stomach can be closed by immediate operation.

Principles of Treatment.—The majority of cases of *duodenal ulcer* can be well controlled by adequate application of the following principles of treatment. The patient should know as much as possible about the nature of the disease so that he may be able to "live with his ulcer." It should be impressed upon him that the handling of his ulcer is not merely a short-term treatment but rather a lifelong control of the whole situation. Diet always plays a major part in the control of an ulcer; the principles are mainly to use frequent feedings so that the stomach will not remain empty to allow the acid and digestive juice to irritate the ulcer. Certain foodstuffs should be avoided which are known to produce an increase in symptoms. Highly seasoned spiced foods, many raw vegetables and fruits are not to be advised and the patient should not smoke or use alcoholic beverages. The use of antacid preparations are helpful in the alleviation of symptoms but often the patient can be advised to do without these as a routine measure. Mild sedation may be of value at times, if the ulcer symptoms become severe. Antispasmodic drugs, such as atropine and banthine are of value if the simpler forms of treatment are not effective. Surgical treatment of duodenal ulcer by means of partial gastrectomy are required

in a relatively small number of cases. This is indicated if the ulcer produces stenosis and gastric retention. Surgical repair of a perforated ulcer, of course, is required under those circumstances. If an ulcer has produced serious hemorrhage on several occasions surgical treatment is usually required, and if an ulcer fails to respond to an adequate program of medical management surgical treatment should be advised.

In the case of a *gastric ulcer* the same principles of treatment apply. However, the problem of diagnosis of a benign gastric ulcer from malignancy of the stomach is often extremely difficult. It is wise to advise surgical removal of the stomach in case of an ulcer which does not heal, by *x*-ray evidence, following a period of three to six weeks of adequate medical management.

A serious complication of peptic ulcer is hemorrhage. Following any episode of bleeding rest is essential. Sedation may be required and it is most important to replace the blood loss by means of transfusion to prevent the serious consequences of shock from blood loss.

CANCER OF THE STOMACH

Cancer is much commoner in men than in women. Indeed, in men cancer of the stomach is the commonest form of carcinoma. The usual age period is about sixty years, but it may occur much earlier. The tumor is generally situated at the pyloric end of the stomach, but it may occur in any part of the organ. It may form a large mass projecting into the cavity of the stomach (Fig 51) or it may merely constitute a thickening of the wall in the pyloric region (Fig. 52). Gradually, however, this thickening leads to narrowing of the opening until finally complete obstruction may be produced, causing marked dilatation of the rest of the stomach. The tumor in the stomach is best detected by means of the roentgen-rays.

Spread may occur by lymphatics or by the blood stream. Cancer cells are carried to the nearest abdominal lymph nodes by the lymphatics, but sometimes the lymph nodes on the left side of the neck may be enlarged by tumor growth. The cancer cells may be carried by the blood to the liver, brain and other organs. When distant spread has occurred and metastases are formed, no treatment is of any avail.

The Basis of Symptoms.—Unfortunately *pain* is not an early symptom of cancer either in the stomach or in other parts of the body, although it may be marked in the later stages, especially when pyloric obstruction has set in. *Loss of appetite* and a feeling of repletion before the meal is finished is much more characteristic, and should be regarded as a danger signal in a man in the cancer age period who has previously had a healthy appetite, one who frequently states that up to that time he has been able "to digest nails." *Absence of hydrochloric acid* in the gastric contents obtained by the stomach tube is a sign of great importance. So also is the presence of *blood*. This blood is most easily tested for by examination of the stools. It cannot be seen with the naked eye as it is too small in amount, but it is readily detected by a simple chemical test. Blood which can only be detected by such a test is known as *occult blood*, because it is hidden from the eye. *Anemia* or bloodlessness is a common symptom. This is only due in part

to the loss of blood. The ulceration and infection of the tumor which occur in the later stages interfere with blood formation and thus lead to anemia. When pyloric obstruction has developed *vomiting* from the dilated stomach may be a distressing symptom. The vomitus may be of a *coffee-ground* character owing to the presence of altered blood, as in the case of gastric ulcer. It will be noticed that nothing has been said about the presence of a lump or tumor which can be felt by the doctor. Such a lump can only be felt in the later stages when it is too late to hope for cure of the patient.

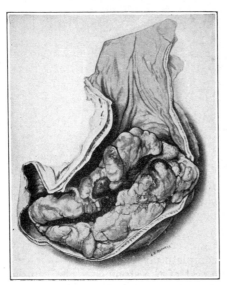
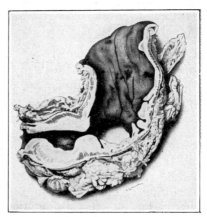

Fig. 51   Fig. 52

Fig. 51.—Cancer of the stomach, papillary form.
Fig. 52.—Cancer of stomach, infiltrating form.

Principles of Treatment.—The only hope of cure is early diagnosis and early operation. The tumor and a large part of the surrounding stomach wall are removed. But even if real cure is impossible, operation may give the patient several years of life and comfort. Even in advanced cancer when it is impossible to remove the tumor much relief may be afforded by the operation of gastro-enterostomy. This enables food to escape from the stomach into the intestine and overcomes the gastric dilatation which is one of the chief causes of distress.

GASTRIC ANALYSIS

The examination of the gastric contents gives three valuable pieces of information: (1) The emptying time of the stomach, *i.e.*, whether or not there is obstruction at the pylorus which prevents the food passing into the duodenum; (2) the presence or absence of hydrochloric acid (HCl), which is secreted by the normal stomach when food is taken; (3) the presence of

blood. Various methods may be employed by the clinician, but the simplest is to give a standard test-meal and remove the stomach contents an hour later by means of the stomach tube. Sometimes a thin tube is left in the stomach for two and a half hours, samples being withdrawn by aspiration every half-hour. If the "fasting contents" are to be examined, the stomach tube is passed first thing in the morning before the patient has taken any food.

Interpretation.—In the normal stomach there should be practically no fasting contents. Any considerable *accumulation of fluid* and food particles indicates pyloric obstruction, which may be caused by cancer at the pylorus or by the fibrotic contraction which accompanies a chronic gastric ulcer. *Blood* may be seen with the naked eye diffused throughout the contents. It may be red or brown in color. The brown color is due to conversion of the hemoglobin to acid hematin by the acid in the stomach and indicates that the blood has been in the stomach for some little time. Blood in the stomach in any considerable amount is due to bleeding from a gastric ulcer or cancer. A few streaks of fresh blood are of no significance, being caused by the passage of the stomach tube. For the same reason delicate chemical tests for blood are of no value, as a trace of blood is very likely to be present.

The *free hydrochloric acid* which should normally be present after a test-meal is absent (achlorhydria) in pernicious anemia, primary hypochromic anemia, and cancer of the stomach. In pernicious anemia the absence is complete, but in cancer of the stomach a small amount may be present. In certain normal persons the nervous excitement of the passage of the stomach tube is sufficient to suppress the secretion of hydrochloric acid. For this reason an addition to the test may be employed, usually the injection of histamine. If after this procedure no free HCl is found, a true achlorhydria is present. In ulcer there is usually an increase in the amount of HCl. This is not due to an increased secretion of acid, but to spasm of the pylorus produced by the irritation of the ulcer, thus preventing the normal regurgitation of alkaline fluid from the duodenum into the stomach which occurs normally and serves to lower the gastric acidity.

Lactic acid may be present in the stomach contents. This indicates that fermentation is going on in the stomach on account of the food being unable to escape into the duodenum. It is usually a sign of cancer obstructing the pyloric end of the stomach.

To Sum Up.—Examination of the gastric contents is of value in three diseases, gastric ulcer, gastric cancer, and severe anemia of both pernicious and primary hypochromic type. In gastric ulcer there may be blood, an excess of hydrochloric acid, and perhaps gastric retention. In cancer there will be little or no hydrochloric acid, blood will probably be present, together with gastric retention and lactic acid if the tumor is near the pylorus. In pernicious and primary hypochromic anemia there will be a complete absence of hydrochloric acid even after the use of histamine, but with no blood, gastric retention, or lactic acid.

(2). The *intestinal symptoms* are abdominal discomfort, constipation or diarrhea. In those cases in which diarrhea occurs the feces may have an appearance described by the rather unpleasantly vivid term "pea-soup stools." *Hemorrhage* from the bowel may take place owing to one of the ulcers having opened into a bloodvessel. The hemorrhage may be very severe and may prove fatal. It usually occurs late in the disease, about the third week, and is accompanied by a sudden drop in the temperature. An even more serious complication is *perforation* of the bowel, owing to an ulcer having penetrated the entire thickness of the intestinal wall. This also usually occurs in the third week. The intestinal contents are poured into the abdominal cavity, and will cause a fatal peritonitis unless an immediate operation is performed. The recognition of the symptoms of perforation is the nurse's duty, and it is no exaggeration to say that the patient's life is literally in her hands. Perforation causes a sudden, sharp,

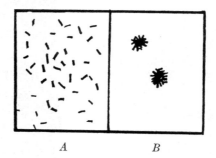

A   B

Fig. 58.—Widal test.   *A*, Negative; *B*, positive.

intense abdominal pain quite different from any he may have experienced hitherto, but it only lasts a few seconds, and is quickly followed by a feeling of complete relief. This remarkable relief will cause the ignorant observer to fall into grave error, but to the instructed mind it is a clear indication of the intense gravity of the situation. The subsequent peritonitis produces very few symptoms, because of the dulled condition of the patient's mind.

(3). The *blood* and blood-forming organs show important changes. There is *enlargement of the spleen*. In most acute infections the number of leucocytes in the blood is markedly increased, a condition of leucocytosis. The opposite is the case in typhoid fever, for not only are the leucocytes not increased in number, they are actually diminished, so that there may be less than 3000 instead of the usual 6000 or more. This condition of *leucopenia* is of great value in making the diagnosis. It is probably due to the fact that the bone-marrow, the factory of the leucocytes, is damaged by the bacilli. The examination of the blood provides two other valuable methods of diagnosis. *Blood culture* shows the presence of bacilli in the blood during the first week of the disease. Blood is taken from a vein in the arm by means of a needle and syringe, placed in a flask of culture medium, and the bacilli allowed to grow there. The *Widal test* is equally useful, but is entirely different in principle. That principle is the deter-

mining whether or not *agglutinins* are present in the blood. Agglutinins are antibodies produced by the patient against the typhoid bacillus; they cause the bacilli to become clumped together or agglutinated. A few drops of blood are taken from the finger or the ear, allowed to clot, and a drop of the serum is then added to a drop of a broth culture of typhoid bacilli and examined under the microscope. If the test is positive the bacilli will be seen to become agglutinated into little clumps; if it is negative they remain separate (Fig. 58). The test usually does not become positive until the second week of the illness. Blood culture shows the presence of the bacilli themselves in the patient (direct evidence); the Widal test shows that they are there by demonstrating a characteristic change which they produce in the blood (indirect evidence).

Principles of Treatment.—The treatment of typhoid fever is largely a matter of nursing, and it is much more important to have a good nurse than a good doctor. The nurse has two main duties: The first is to prevent the spread of the infection to herself and to the rest of the family or to other patients in the hospital; the second is the care of the patient. To prevent the spread of infection demands unceasing and scrupulous attention to detail; a single slip may be disastrous. The stools and urine are the initial source of danger, and have to be disinfected with carbolic acid, lysol, etc., before they are disposed of. But every dish and utensil, bed linen, towels, etc., may be infected by the bacilli, and have to be treated accordingly. The nurse's hands naturally require the greatest attention.

The care of the patient is a heavy task, for owing to his weakness and the clouded state of his mind he can render little assistance. Bed-sores are a constant threat, because he may lie for hours in one position on a bed which may be wet or soiled. The mouth requires constant care. The continued temperature is controlled by various forms of hydrotherapy such as cold sponging, cold packs, and cold baths. The patient is encouraged to drink large amounts of cold water, with the object of eliminating the toxins in the urine. It used to be the custom to starve the typhoid patient, but it is now known that the most important thing to do is to replace the tremendous loss of protein and tissue wastage caused by the long-continued fever. The diet must be of high caloric value and rich in protein, fluid in character, easily digested, and low in residue so as not to irritate the ulcers in the bowel. It therefore consists mainly of milk, cream, and eggs in soft form. When hemorrhage has occurred nothing is given by mouth except small quantities of water. Perforation must be treated by immediate operation with the object of closing the hole in the bowel wall. There has been no method of specific treatment of typhoid fever until the use of chloromycetin was found to be effective in producing marked improvement in many cases. It would appear now that the use of this drug will shorten the duration of the disease.

Prevention.—In the prevention of typhoid fever the patient and the carrier present two separate problems. There are also questions of water purification, sewage disposal, and regulation of milk supply.

The typhoid carrier presents a difficult public health problem. He is naturally unconcious of the fact that he is a carrier and may be unaware that he has had typhoid fever. His discovery results from the fact that

he has been employed in the distribution or preparation of food, *e.g.*, dairymen, cooks, etc. Such occupations are, of course, closed to him. Even when not so employed, he must be educated as to his potential danger to others and the need for careful personal hygiene. Inoculation with typhoid vaccine renders a person immune to typhoid fever for one or two years. It is of great value for those in attendance on cases of the disease, those who may be travelling in countries where typhoid is prevalent, and particularly for military personnel.

DYSENTERY

Dysentery is an acute inflammation of the colon, a colitis, accompanied by very frequent diarrhea and the passage of mucus, pus, and blood in the liquid stools. There are two kinds of dysentery due to entirely different causes, although with rather similar lesions and symptoms. These are amebic dysentery, caused by Amoeba histolytica, and bacillary dysentery, caused by the dysentery bacillus.

Amebic Dysentery.—Amebic dysentery is caused by a unicellular organism, that is to say, a protozoon, called Amoeba histolytica. The parasite is swallowed in infected (uncooked) food or water, and when it reaches the lower part of the intestine (colon) it invades the wall of the bowel, causing the acute inflammation (colitis) known as dysentery. Amebic dysentery is a disease of the tropics but it also occurs in temperate regions.

The chief symptom is profuse and painful diarrhea, the liquid stools containing slimy mucus, pus, and blood. Large numbers of amebæ leave the body in the fecal discharge.

Infection may be the result of fecal contamination of water supply or food. The chief danger is from a carrier rather than from a patient suffering from the active form of the disease. There are two reasons for this. In the first place the danger from the patient is obvious, and precautions can be taken to prevent the spread of the infection, whereas the carrier is unsuspected. The second reason is that the parasites discharged from the carrier are much more resistant to the action of the gastric juice than those from the patient with the active disease. For this reason they are able to pass through the stomach and reach the large bowel, where they are able to set up fresh lesions of the disease.

Another means by which infection may be carried is through the agency of flies. The flies have access to infected discharges from the body, their feet become contaminated, and thus they may transfer the infection to food. It is obvious that this method of spread is of much greater importance in rural districts than in large cities.

The *diagnosis* is made by finding the amebæ in the stools, but in order that they may be recognized they must be living and moving. On being passed from the body they soon lose their power of movement, especially when they are chilled. A specimen of stool (only a very small amount is required) must therefore be placed in a warm receptacle which is then wrapped up so as to prevent chilling and immediately dispatched to the laboratory, where it should be delivered directly to the pathologist, and not merely laid down on a table where it may be overlooked for some

time. Unless these precautions are taken it will be impossible to detect the amebæ.

The *lesions* of both forms of dysentery are very similar. Large and small ulcers are scattered along the length of the colon, and these are responsible for the pain, the diarrhea, and the mucus, pus, and blood in the stools. In the case of amebic dysentery, the amebæ may be found burrowing deeply into the wall of the bowel, and they may invade the branches of the portal vein and be carried to the liver where they set up amebic abscesses of that organ.

The *treatment* of amebic infections depends considerably upon the degree of involvement. If the infection apparently is confined to the intestine, treatment with diodoquin is usually sufficient. If, however, the liver has been invaded the use of emetine by injection is usually required. Recently aureomycin has been found to be very effective in the control of this disease. It may not be possible, however, to eradicate completely the disease in all cases, and some amebæ may remain for a long time, even for years, protected by the bowel wall, and the patient may be subject to repeated attacks of dysentery.

Bacillary Dysentery.—This form of dysentery is caused by a bacillus similar to Bacillus coli and the typhoid bacillus. *Infection* is acquired by eating contaminated food and drinking contaminated water just as in the case of typhoid. The infection may come from a patient suffering from the disease or from a carrier. Like amebic dysentery the disease is very prevalent in the tropics but may also occur in a temperate zone, especially when men are crowded together under poor hygienic conditions. In the past it has been a great destroyer of armies in the field, it is prevalent in large mental hospitals, and it is an important cause of acute diarrhea associated with the passage of pus and blood in children, especially in hot weather.

Treatment.—The sulfonamide drugs have been used against bacillary dysentery, as in the case of so many other bacterial infections. Of these the most successful have been the sulfonamides which are poorly absorbed by the intestine, such as sulfaguanidine, succinylsulfathiazole, and phthalylsulfathiazole.

TUBERCULOSIS OF THE INTESTINES

Tuberculosis of the bowel is usually a complication of tuberculosis of the lungs due to tuberculous sputum being swallowed, but in children it may be due to drinking tuberculous milk.

Lesions.—The lesions, which take the form of ulcers similar to those of typhoid, first appear at the lower end of the small bowel and the beginning of the large bowel, but from there the infection spreads up and down. The affected part tends to become adherent to neighboring loops of bowel, and these adhesions may cause serious intestinal obstruction.

Symptoms.—The symptoms, in addition to those of pulmonary tuberculosis, are abdominal pain, diarrhea, and the presence of pus and blood in the stools. The onset of intestinal tuberculosis adds considerably to the gravity of a case of pulmonary tuberculosis, but if the lung condition can be treated successfully the intestinal lesions tend to clear up.

Treatment.—The general principles of treatment of tuberculosis apply here, that of rest and good sanitorium care. In addition streptomycin may be of help, and if the condition is localized to one part of the bowel surgical removal of that portion may be effective.

CHRONIC ULCERATIVE COLITIS

Bacillary and amebic dysentery are comparative rarities in civilian practice in non-tropical countries. The disease now under consideration is, unfortunately, quite common. It is still very much of a mystery. The lesions, namely, extensive ulceration of the colon and rectum, and the symptoms, namely, diarrhea with mucus, pus, and blood in the stools are those of the other forms of dysentery. But no causative agent has so far been discovered. The patient appears to be hypertensive to certain types of food, and is usually of a high-strung, somewhat neurotic temperament. The disease may last for many years, but is marked by remissions and exacerbations. The latter often occur when the patient is subjected to strain, overwork, worry, et cetera.

APPENDICITIS

The *vermiform appendix* is a small tube about 4 inches long and as thick as the tip of the little finger, which opens out of the cecum close to the spot where the small and large intestine join. If it has a function it does not appear to be of any importance. It is liable to the same diseases as the rest of the bowel, but the one condition that is of supreme importance both from the point of view of frequency and gravity is acute inflammation.

The *cause* of acute appendicitis is bacteria which penetrate the mucous membrane from the lumen, but in some cases they may apparently be carried from the throat or tonsils by the blood stream to the appendix. The principal organisms found are streptococci and Bacillus coli. These are normal inhabitants of the intestine, and the difficulty is to guess at the factors which make them invade the bowel wall. It is undoubtedly a fact that appendicitis is more common than it used to be, and that it is seen more in highly developed countries and cities than in backward countries and rural districts. Natives who live on a diet abundant in cellulose are immune to the disease, but when they adopt the diet of civilization they lose that immunity. These and many other similar facts suggest that habits of life, and in particular modes of diet such as meat-eating, are of importance in predisposing toward appendicitis.

Lesions.—There are all grades of acute appendicitis from the most mild to the most severe, but for purposes of description we shall take the severely inflamed organ which is removed just in time to prevent it from rupturing. Such an appendix is swollen and elongated, sometimes to an extraordinary degree, bright red in color, and covered by an acute inflammatory exudate (peritonitis). The inflammation is usually most marked towards the tip of the appendix. If *gangrene* (death of the tissue) has set in, usually at the tip, the gangrenous part will be green or black. As the process goes on, the wall of the appendix becomes thinned at one or more points and may

rupture (perforation), so that the intestinal contents are poured out into the abdominal cavity causing *general peritonitis* (Fig. 59). A gangrenous appendix is certain to rupture unless it is removed in time.

The picture so far has been painted in the blackest colors—severe inflammation, gangrene, rupture, general peritonitis, death. Fortunately such a sequence is the exception, not the rule. Most attacks of appendicitis are of a mild character and will recover without operation. Unfortunately no one can tell if a given case is going to recover spontaneously or is going to turn into gangrene. Rupture does not necessarily mean a fatal general peritonitis, for adhesions to surrounding structures tend to form before the rupture occurs, and these adhesions limit the inflammatory process so that the peritonitis remains local and an abscess is formed around the appendix. When this abscess is subsequently drained it may be found that the appendix has been completely destroyed. This localization of the inflammation and infection is an excellent example of the beneficent effect of adhesions.

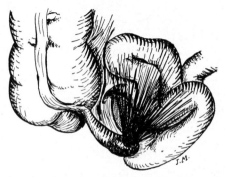

Fig. 59.—Acutely inflamed ruptured appendix. Contents of the appendix are sprayed into the peritoneal cavity.

The Basis of Symptoms.—The principal symptoms of a severe attack of appendicitis are pain and tenderness in the region of the appendix, nausea and vomiting, fever and leucocytosis. The *pain* is at first of a general character, a "stomach-ache," but presently it settles in the right lower segment of the abdomen. *Tenderness on pressure* over the appendix is the most important single symptom. The pain and tenderness are caused by the great inflammatory swelling of the appendix with accompanying tension and pressure on the nerve endings. The pain goes on increasing in intensity until rupture occurs, when it is suddenly, completely, and most unfortunately relieved owing to the tension ceasing suddenly when the pus escapes. The relief is unfortunate because it may persuade the patient, the relatives and even the nurse that all is well, whereas the reverse is the case. The *nausea* and *vomiting* are reflex symptoms due to the fact that the same nerve (vagus nerve) supplies the appendix and the stomach, so that pain stimuli pass from the appendix to the brain and back again to the stomach, where they cause nausea and vomiting. The *fever* and *leucocytosis* are general symptoms due to absorption of bacterial toxins from the inflamed appendix.

The leucocytosis is a very valuable means of distinguishing between true appendicitis and simple colicky pains in that part of the abdomen unaccompanied by inflammation.

Principles of Treatment.—The treatment of acute appendicitis is immediate operation. It is true that a large number of cases would recover spontaneously, but no doctor can tell which case is going to recover and which is going on to rupture and gangrene. Sometimes, although fortunately not commonly, gangrene and rupture may occur within twelve hours of the first attack of pain. The earlier the operation, the safer it is for the patient. Usually when the appendix is removed the abdomen can be closed. If, however, an abscess has formed around the appendix, a drainage tube will be necessary for some time. It often happens that it is not possible for the doctor when he first sees the patient to be certain if the case is one of acute appendicitis. Whilst the patient is being watched he must be kept at rest in bed, and must be given nothing but fluids by mouth (tomato juice, fruit juice, etc.). Morphine and castor oil are banned. The danger of morphine is that it relieves the pain and tenderness to such a degree that the diagnosis may be missed and the patient lose his life. After the diagnosis is made and operation decided on, morphine may, of course, be given to relieve the pain. A purgative such as castor oil is dangerous because the contractions of the bowel which it causes may lead to rupture of the inflamed appendix. This also is the reason for avoiding solid foods. The use of antibiotics has reduced the dangers of peritoneal infection following appendectomy, but the availability of antibiotics should not replace early surgical treatment.

PERITONITIS

The peritoneum is the exquisitely thin layer of serous membrane which lines the abdominal cavity. It consists of two layers, one covering the inner surface of the abdominal wall, the other covering the stomach, intestines, and the other viscera. Between these two layers lies the *peritoneal cavity*. Infection causing inflammation of the peritoneum generally comes from one of the hollow viscera covered by the membrane, but occasionally it is carried by the blood stream. The commonest source of the infection is an acutely inflamed appendix, but rupture of a peptic ulcer in the stomach or duodenum or of a typhoid ulcer will flood the peritoneal cavity with infected material. The common microörganisms are streptococci and Bacillus coli.

Peritonitis may be local or general. *Local peritonitis* is inflammation limited to one region, *e.g.*, the appendix, pelvic organs, etc. The inflamed membrane with its covering of fibrin readily sticks to a neighboring part similarly inflamed. These *adhesions* are at first readily broken down and the parts separated, but they are invaluable in limiting the spread of the infection. This is particularly well seen in the case of the appendix where, if adhesions are formed before rupture occurs, a localized abscess in a walled-off space is the result instead of a spreading fatal peritonitis. *General peritonitis* is the result of an infection which is not limited but spreads throughout the peritoneal cavity. The membrane covering the intestine is red and inflamed, and becomes covered with a sticky inflammatory exu-

date which glues the coils of bowel together. A large amount of fluid may collect in the cavity and between the loops of bowel. This may be thick pus or thin watery fluid, depending on the organisms responsible for the infection.

The great danger of general peritonitis is *acute intestinal obstruction*. When the wall of the bowel (and the peritoneum forms the outer part of this wall) becomes inflamed, muscular movements are no longer able to pass along it, and the extremely serious condition of acute obstruction develops. It is this which will kill the patient rather than the widespread infection, for reasons to be discussed in the next section. The modern treatment of general peritonitis is largely directed towards the acute obstruction which accompanies it.

Tuberculous Peritonitis.—Peritonitis caused by the tubercle bacillus may also be local or general, but it is chronic instead of acute, so that the clinical picture is entirely different from that of acute peritonitis. The infection usually comes from the bowel, but may come from a distant source such as the lungs. The disease is commoner in children and young adults. The peritoneum is covered with tubercles, and in addition there may be a large amount of exudate which glues the coils of bowel together so that a condition of *chronic obstruction* is produced. Sometimes there is a great accumulation of thin watery fluid. This causes a remarkable degree of distention of the abdomen, the tight shiny dome of which overtops the wasted body of the patient. Opening of the abdomen and drainage of the fluid is often followed by remarkable improvement, but the patient is likely to succumb to exhaustion and intestinal obstruction.

INTESTINAL OBSTRUCTION

Intestinal obstruction is a condition in which the contents of the bowel are unable to pass along its length. The obstruction may be organic or paralytic. *Organic obstruction* is due to some material obstacle, such as tumor, twist, or kink, blocking the bowel. The lumen does not need to be blocked for obstruction to be produced. Passage along the bowel is brought about by a series of waves of muscular contraction known as *peristalsis* which, as it were, milk the contents onward. A tumor or other lesion may interrupt the muscle which forms the greater part of the thickness of the bowel wall and thus stop the peristaltic wave and the onward passage of the contents just as effectively as if a plug had been inserted in the lumen. The most important causes of organic obstruction are tumors, adhesions, hernia, intussusception, and volvulus. Each of these will be described in due course.

Paralytic obstruction, usually called *paralytic ileus* because the common site is the ileum or lower part of the small intestine, is due to inflammation of a segment of bowel as a result of which peristaltic movements cannot pass from the segment above to the segment below, the bowels are unable to move, and the practical result is obstruction as complete as if a string had been tied around the bowel. A common cause is the peritonitis which often complicates acute appendicitis with rupture; a loop of ileum hangs down into a pool of pus and becomes completely paralyzed.

11

Intestinal obstruction may be acute or chronic. The difference is fundamental, for in the acute form there is immediate danger to life and urgent need of operation, whereas in chronic obstruction there is no urgency.

Acute Intestinal Obstruction.—This may be organic or paralytic in type. *Organic obstruction* may be caused by a variety of conditions, of which strangulated hernia in the adult and intussusception in the child are the most important; pressure by peritoneal adhesions and volvulus or twisting of the bowel are also important. The common cause of *paralytic obstruction* is general peritonitis, but paralysis of the bowel may result from an abdominal operation. The higher the site of the obstruction, the more dangerous is the condition. Acute obstruction of the large bowel is likely to be due to the chronic obstruction produced by cancer having suddenly become acute owing to an attack of inflammation which by the swelling it produces completely closes the lumen of the bowel that previously was only narrowed; such obstruction is of very different significance to the patient from obstruction of the small intestine.

One of the chief *dangers* in acute organic obstruction of the small bowel is that the blood supply to a segment of bowel is cut off, this segment dies and undergoes *gangrene*, and through the dead wall bacteria pour out causing general peritonitis; or the gangrenous part may rupture, flooding the peritoneum with fecal material. The bowel is attached to the posterior abdominal wall by a long fold of peritoneum known as the mesentery, so that the coils can move about freely in any direction, and it is through the mesentery that the bloodvessels reach the bowel wall and supply it with nourishment. It is evident that if the mesentery becomes nipped as in *strangulated hernia*, or twisted as in the condition called *volvulus*, the blood supply will be cut off and gangrene will develop. In the paralytic form of obstruction there is no direct interference with the blood supply, but the fluid contents of the small bowel stagnate, and the bacteria which they contain proliferate and break down the protein elements of the food with the production of highly poisonous substances. These *intestinal toxins* are absorbed into the blood, and also act on the wall of the bowel, leading finally to gangrene and general peritonitis. From these considerations it is obvious that the patient suffering from acute intestinal obstruction is in a very serious condition and in need of immediate surgical attention. When the abdomen is opened the bowel above the obstruction is seen to be greatly distended with fluid and gas whilst the part below is collapsed. If the blood supply is cut off and the affected part has become gangrenous it will be greenish or black in color.

Symptoms.—The symptoms of acute intestinal obstruction are very important to recognize. There is *complete constipation*. Once the lower part of the bowel has emptied itself no further fecal matter can be brought away even with the assistance of an enema. No gas (flatus) is passed. Peristaltic movements are vigorous in organic obstruction, but as the intestinal contents cannot be forced past the obstruction the peristaltic wave is reversed, moving in the opposite direction, so that *vomiting* takes the place of emptying of the bowel. First the contents of the stomach are vomited, then the bile-stained contents of the upper part of the small intestine, and finally the foul-smelling contents of the lower part of the intestine

(fecal vomiting), depending on the site of the obstruction. The abdomen will become tense and distended on account of the greatly dilated condition of the intestine. *Pain* is at first sharp and spasmodic (colicky); later it becomes continuous. In organic obstruction there are early symptoms of *shock*, as the nerves to the bowel as well as the bloodvessels are pinched. The later symptoms are those of *toxemia and collapse* due to absorption of the poisonous material in the intestine; these symptoms are, of course, present in paralytic as well as in organic obstruction.

Treatment.—Treatment is governed by two principles: to relieve the obstruction and to overcome if possible the damage it has produced. If the obstruction is due to a twist of the mesentery or the strangulation of a hernia, the twist may be undone when the abdomen is opened or the cause of the strangulation removed. Even when this has been done, the surgeon is still confronted with the more difficult task of overcoming the effects of the obstruction. If a loop of bowel has become gangrenous it will have to be excised and the cut ends of the healthy bowel sewn together. If a large part of the small bowel is dilated, partially paralyzed, and filled with intensely poisonous material, an opening will have to be made as low as possible in the ileum (*ileostomy*), and the bowel drained by means of a large rubber tube inserted into the opening. A measure which has proved of great value is drainage of the intestine by the Miller-Abbott tube. This is a thin rubber tube which is introduced into the nose, passed down the esophagus, through the stomach, and finally enters the intestine. By means of suction applied to the upper end of the tube, the toxic fluid which collects in the bowel can be removed at repeated intervals without undue discomfort to the patient, for the tube is allowed to remain in position. One of the most dangerous features of acute obstruction is the great distention of the bowel which it causes. If this can be relieved by "decompression," the life of the patient may be saved in a case which would otherwise prove fatal. It is evident that such decompression can be accomplished both by means of ileostomy and the use of the Miller-Abbott tube.

Chronic Obstruction.—Here the process is slow and there is no interference with the blood supply. The usual causes are cancer of the bowel and pressure by peritoneal adhesions. Although the obstruction is not complete, the bowel above the obstruction is dilated whilst the part below it is collapsed. The obstruction is usually in the large intestine, so that hard masses of feces tend to accumulate above the obstruction. These may irritate the bowel, causing mild attacks of diarrhea. For this reason alternating periods of constipation and diarrhea are very suggestive of chronic intestinal obstruction, and should always arouse a suspicion of cancer of the bowel.

Of particular concern is the question of the restoration of the fluid that the patient has lost by vomiting and by suction. This fluid contains water, protein, hydrochloric acid, sodium chloride, potassium chloride and other substances which are of great value to the body in maintaining a balance between the fluid in cells and the circulating blood in the capillaries.

Because the patient is usually unable to retain oral fluids, his needs are supplied by the intravenous administration of blood, plasma or water solutions containing glucose, for nourishment, sodium chloride and potassium

chloride in carefully calculated amounts designed to replace what he has lost and to allow a little extra for his daily needs, but with due regard for the dangers of overloading his system with fluids.

Two of the causes of acute intestinal obstruction which have already been alluded to will now be considered rather more in detail. These are hernia and intussusception.

Hernia.—A hernia or rupture is a protrusion of a loop of bowel through an opening or weak point in the abdominal wall. The common site for such a protrusion is in the groin (*inguinal* and *femoral hernia*), occasionally at the navel or umbilicus (*umbilical hernia*). Such a protrusion tends to become larger as time goes on. At first the loop can be pushed back or

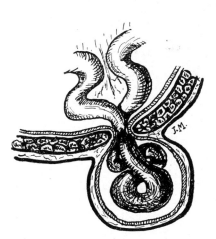
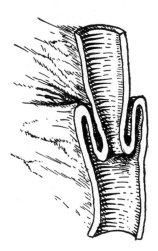

FIG. 60.—Strangulated hernia. The constricted loop is dark and congested.

FIG. 61.—Intussusception.

reduced, although it tends to come down again when the pressure inside the abdomen is increased by coughing, straining, lifting a heavy weight, etc. Eventually adhesions may form and the hernia becomes *irreducible*.

The great danger of every hernia is the possibility of *strangulation* (Fig. 60). The muscular contraction of the bowel may force so much bowel through the narrow opening that acute pressure is exerted by the sharp edges of the opening on the vessels entering the wall of the loop and supplying it with blood. The blood supply is thereby cut off and gangrene will soon develop. At the same time the increasing pressure closes the lumen of the bowel. The patient has therefore developed acute intestinal obstruction, and is in imminent danger of general peritonitis. Strangulated hernia is therefore one of the acute abdominal catastrophes which demand immediate surgical attention.

The sharp edges of the opening have to be divided, the injured loop returned to the abdominal cavity, and the opening closed so that the hernia will not recur. If the loop of bowel is not seriously damaged no more may need to be done. If, however, gangrene has set in the affected part has to

be excised and the cut ends of the bowel sewn together. The success of the operation depends on how early the diagnosis is made and how early the treatment is carried out.

Intussusception.—An important cause of acute intestinal obstruction in children is intussusception. By this we mean that a segment of bowel is pushed into and ensheathed by the succeeding portion, in the same way as the finger of a glove can be pushed down into its hand (Fig. 61). The entering part of bowel is seized by the part it enters and forced along it by peristaltic movements just as a mass of feces might be psuhed along. The usual starting-point is the junction of the small and large intestine at the ileocecal valve. The condition generally occurs in boys under one year of age.

The danger of the condition is *strangulation*. The sheath of bowel grips the entering part so tightly that blood cannot escape by the veins and great swelling of the part occurs. This serves to increase the tension so that the arteries are compressed, the blood supply stops, and *gangrene* sets in. Once more the patient is confronted with the double danger of acute intestinal obstruction and general peritonitis.

Immediate diagnosis and treatment are just as necessary as in the case of strangulated hernia.

Symptoms.—The symptoms are sudden abdominal *pain* in a child and the passage of *blood* and *mucus* in the stools. The reason for the blood is that the greatly dilated veins in the mucous membrane of the bowel give way and hemorrhage occurs into the lumen. Outpouring of mucus is the usual result of any acute irritation of the mucous membrane of the colon. Although blood and mucus appear, no fecal material is passed on account of the intestinal obstruction.

Treatment.—The treatment varies with the stage of the disease. At the beginning it may be possible to undo the intussusception by giving an enema. If this fails, the abdomen must be opened and the entering loop pulled out of its sheath. In the later stages even this may be impossible, and the affected segment of bowel may have to be excised.

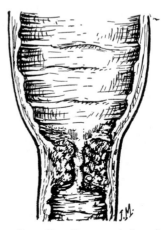

Fig. 62.—Cancer of bowel Bowel above tumor is dilated

CANCER OF THE INTESTINE

The only common tumor of the bowel which gives rise to symptoms is carcinoma, and this is the most important cause of chronic obstruction. It very seldom occurs in the small intestine, the usual sites being the rectum and sigmoid and less commonly the rest of the large intestine, especially at the ileocecal junction. The tumor slowly surrounds the bowel and causes

gradual narrowing of the lumen and *chronic intestinal obstruction* (Fig. 62.) *Cancer of the rectum* remains for a long time confined to the bowel without spreading to neighboring structures or to distant organs, so that if a reasonably early diagnosis can be made the prognosis is quite hopeful.

Symptoms.—The early symptoms are unfortunately vague, *e.g.*, persistent constipation with occasional attacks of colicky pain. Gradually increasing constipation in a man above middle age who previously has been regular in his intestinal habits is a danger signal and suggests a medical examination by which the diagnosis can easily be confirmed or refuted. Blood in the stool is an important sign. Piles may be present owing to pressure on the veins. Alternating attacks of constipation and diarrhea may finally be replaced by complete obstruction. The only *treatment* is surgical removal, which in early cases may give excellent results.

DIARRHEA

In our survey of some of the principal diseases of the intestine diarrhea has been noted as a frequent symptom. It may therefore be worth while briefly to review this important symptom. Diarrhea, the passage of too frequent and too soft stools, is the result of the fluid contents of the small intestine being hurried too rapidly through the large intestine so that there is not sufficient time for the fluid to be absorbed. It is therefore to be expected that diarrhea will be most marked in an inflammatory disease of the large bowel such as *dysentery*. In this condition there is also a copious outpouting of mucus from the glands lining the colon, which makes the stools still more liquid. In *cholera*, an acute inflammatory disease of both small and large intestine which has not been considered on account of its rarity in temperate countries, there is such a copious outpouring of fluid that the stools are known as "rice-water stools." Inflammation of the small intestine, especially when associated with ulcers, may also cause diarrhea. Examples of such diseases are *typhoid fever* and *tuberculosis of the bowel*; it must be noted, however, that constipation is as common as diarrhea in typhoid, and that in tuberculosis there are often lesions in the large intestine.

Irritating foods tend to cause diarrhea. This may be because the food is particularly indigestible and coarse. Or the diarrhea may be caused by *food infections*, bacteria contaminating foods which have been allowed to decompose or "go bad."

Absence of hydrochloric acid in the stomach sometimes causes diarrhea which persists in spite of all treatment until the gastric contents are analyzed. When the deficiency is discovered the diarrhea is soon cleared up by the administration of small amounts of hydrochloric acid at meal time.

Nervous diarrhea is well known, and is due to excessive nervous stimuli causing an undue amount of peristalsis. Some persons always have a looseness of the bowels when going up for examinations and at other similar but equally inopportune moments.

THE FECES

In the course of digestion the food passes from the stomach into the intestines, where it meets in the duodenum two powerful digestive agents, the bile and the pancreatic juice, both of which are necessary for the proper digestion of fat. In the small intestine the food becomes completely fluid, owing to the solid masses of food being dissolved and to the presence of the digestive fluids of the bowel. It now passes slowly along the large intestine, where the greater part of the water is absorbed, so that the stools or feces which leave the body are soft, well-formed, brown, cylindrical masses. If the bowel movements are accelerated to any marked degree, there is insufficient time for the water to be absorbed, so that the stools remain fluid, a condition of diarrhea. It is evident that an examination of the feces will reveal many facts of importance with regard to the gastro-intestinal canal and the process of digestion. To the nurse the gross or naked eye examination of the stool is of particular importance, because she may detect pathological changes (the presence of blood, mucus, parasites, etc.), even though no specimen has been sent to the laboratory.

Color.—The normal color varies from yellow to brown. When the stool is large and pale it contains undigested fat, the commonest cause of which is obstruction to the flow of bile into the duodenum either by a gall stone impacted in the bile duct or by a tumor. A chemical test for bile will give a negative result. In disease of the pancreas the stool tends to be even more voluminous and greasy, due to complete suppression of fat digestion on account of the absence of pancreatic juice.

The stools may be colored by *blood*. This blood may be bright red, dark, or black Red blood comes from the lower part of the intestine. Streaks of bright blood, especially at the end of defecation, are probably due to bleeding piles. Bright blood may come from a carcinoma of the rectum or elsewhere in the large intestine. During the third and fourth weeks of typhoid fever the nurse must watch the stools carefully for bright blood, because a few specks or streaks may be the forerunner of a severe hemorrhage. Acute inflammation of the colon (colitis, dysentery) is often marked by the presence of blood in the fluid stools, associated usually with mucus and pus. Dark or black blood has been altered by digestion so that it comes from high up in the alimentary canal, usually the stomach or duodenum, the lesion being ulcer or cancer. If the bleeding from the ulcer or tumor is only slight, it will not be possible to detect the blood with the naked eye; it is hidden or occult. When these lesions are suspected, a specimen is sent to the laboratory to be tested chemically for *occult blood*. It is important that the patient be properly prepared before this examination by omitting all red meat, meat soups and meat extracts from his diet for at least three days. The inclusion of green vegetables in the diet does not interfere with most of the tests for occult blood. It must be remembered that the stools may be dark and tarry in appearance for other reasons than the presence of blood, especially the medicinal use of iron or bismuth.

Form.—The normal form and consistency of the stools depends upon the extraction of water during their passage through the large intestine. If the time of this passage is shortened owing to the increased irritability

of the bowel which occurs in such a condition as dysentery, water is not absorbed, and the stools are therefore fluid in character. On the other hand, the feces may remain in the large bowel for an undue length of time owing to chronic constipation. In this case the stools take the form of small, hard, round masses known as scybala. When the stools are narrow and ribbon-like it is probable that there is some marked narrowing at the lower end of the large bowel, usually due to cancer of the rectum.

Mucus and pus are found in large amount in acute dysentery and ulcerative colitis, often associated with blood. The mucus is produced by the cells lining the mucous membrane of the inflamed large bowel, just as mucus is discharged from an inflamed nose. The presence of pus is natural in an acute inflammation like dysentery. The mucus can be seen with the naked eye as slimy streaks or shreds. Pus is best detected by means of the microscope.

Parasites.—The common intestinal parasites causing disease may be divided into two groups: (1) The parasitic worms; (2) the amœba histolytica which causes dysentery. The first can be seen with the naked eye, the second requires the aid of the microscope. The worms are of two types, tapeworms and round worms.

A *tapeworm* may be several feet, or even yards, long. It has a minute head about the size of a pin's head by which it attaches itself to the mucous membrane of the bowel, and a long body made up of hundreds or thousands of segments, each of which is filled with enormous numbers of eggs (ova). The segments are detached one by one and passed in the stool, the ova being shed at the same time. The presence of a tapeworm in the bowel can therefore be diagnosed by finding either segments or ova in the feces; the former are seen with the naked eye, the latter with the microscope. Treatment for tapeworm infection consists in giving the patient a drug which will cause the worm to release its hold on the bowel wall, and then expelling it by means of purgatives. The *entire* stool must be sent to the laboratory, in order that a search may be made for the head of the worm, which may be no larger than the head of a pin. Unless the head is removed the entire body with its hundreds of segments can be reformed. Discovery of the head is therefore the only proof that the patient has been cured.

Round worms are not composed of segments. The diagnosis has therefore to be made either by seeing some of the worms in the stool, or by finding the ova microscopically. Three important round worms may occur in the bowel: (1) The *round worm* resembles the common earth worm in size and color. It is a parasite of children, but also affects dogs and cats from which the infection may be acquired. (2) The *pin worm* or *thread worm* is a common parasite of the rectum and colon, occurring principally in young children. It is only $\frac{1}{2}$ inch long, often much shorter, and looks like a moving piece of white thread in the stools, but it is passed in large numbers, and causes intense itching of the skin around the anus. For the laboratory detection of pin worms a 2 inch strip of Scotch tape is placed with the adhesive side out over the rounded end of a small test tube. The tube is rocked to and fro in the perianal folds, and the tape picks up the fecal débris containing the worms. The tape is then removed from the tube, placed with the sticky side down on a glass slide and sent to the laboratory.

(3) The *hookworm* (Ankylostoma duodenale) is a very important parasite in tropical and subtropical countries on account of the severe and debilitating anemia which it causes. The worms themselves are seldom seen in the feces, and a diagnosis is made by finding the ova under the microscope.

The finding of the *ameba of dysentery* (Amœba histolytica) is a matter for the pathologist or the trained laboratory technician, but in this quest the nurse has one important duty to perform. The ameba is recognized microscopically by its peculiar motility, and this motility is soon lost when the specimen of stool is allowed to become cold. The nurse must, therefore, see to it that immediately after the stool is passed the receptacle containing it is wrapped up and sent to the laboratory. The pathologist should be notified that the specimen is on its way to the laboratory, so that he may arrange for its immediate examination.

Chapter

13

DISEASES OF THE LIVER AND GALLBLADDER

Structure and Function.—The liver, tucked under the ribs below the diaphragm on the right side of the abdomen, is the largest organ in the body. It is singularly simple in structure, being composed of columns of cells all apparently absolutely identical, and yet it is remarkably complex in function. The lungs have a single function, respiration, and the kidneys have a single function, excretion, but the liver has half-a-dozen functions. These may be divided into three main groups:

1. *Metabolism of Food.*—The foodstuffs brought to the liver from the intestine by the portal vein are altered so as to be more suitable for use by the tissues or are stored as in a bank so as to be paid out on demand. It is the proteins which chiefly undergo further preparation, and the waste product urea, which is one of the main constituents of the urine, is formed in the liver, so that in advanced liver disease the urea in the urine is greatly diminished. The sugar brought from the bowel in the form of glucose is stored in the liver as *glycogen*, and is restored to the blood as glucose when the demand arises.

2. *Production of Bile.*—The red blood corpuscles have a relatively short life, probably about a month, at the end of which time they are destroyed and the red pigment or hemoglobin which they contain is discharged from the body. It is first converted into a green pigment, known as bile pigment, and this is excreted by the liver in the bile. Throughout the entire liver there is a vast network of fine *bile canals*, and the columns of liver cells intervene between blood capillaries on one side and bile capillaries on the other, so that the bile pigment has to traverse these cells in order to pass from the blood into the bile. The liver cells add two other substances to the bile, namely, bile salts and cholesterol, the importance of which will be referred to presently. The bile is conducted from the liver by the *hepatic duct*, which is joined by the *cystic duct* from the *gallbladder*; the tube formed by the union of the hepatic and cystic ducts is called the *common bile duct*, which opens into the duodenum about 3 inches from the pylorus at the point where the duct from the pancreas also opens. The bile from the liver does not go straight into the duodenum, but passes back along the cystic duct into the gallbladder, where it is concentrated by absorption of water, stored, and sent down into the common duct and duodenum when a meal, particularly a meal rich in fat, is taken. For the bile, or rather the bile salts which it contains, is necessary for the proper digestion of fat. The bile does not act on the fat directly, but activates the ferment from the pancreas whose function it is to digest the fat. The reason for the bile and the pancreatic juice both entering the bowel at the same spot is

thus apparent. It is also evident that if the bile is prevented from entering the duodenum by the presence of a gall stone in the common duct the fats of the food will not be digested, an omission which can easily be recognized by the pale fatty color of the stools.

3. *Detoxifying and Antibacterial Function.*—Large numbers of bacteria pass with the foodstuffs from the intestine into the portal vein and thus reach the liver, where they are destroyed. Toxic substances which may pass from the bowel to the liver are likewise neutralized.

It is probable that the liver has a number of other functions, but as these have no direct bearing on its behavior in disease they will not be discussed here. In actual disease of the liver it is wonderful how little the normal functions may be interfered with unless the involvement is extremely widespread. One reason for this is that the liver has great reserve power, so that only a small part of it is sufficient to do the work of the whole organ. Moreover the liver has a great capacity for regeneration; large areas may be destroyed, but new liver cells are formed which take the place of those which are lost. These facts make the diagnosis of liver disease sometimes a matter of great difficulty.

HEPATITIS AND CIRRHOSIS

These two diseases may be considered together, because they seem to represent two phases of a single process. Hepatitis, as the word signifies, is an inflammation of the liver, whilst cirrhosis is a fibrosis which may represent the end stage of inflammation. The facts of the case are not nearly so simple and well-defined as the above statement might indicate. The word hepatitis indicates inflammation, but the actual change is cellular necrosis rather than inflammation in the ordinary sense of the word. Alcoholism may lead to necrosis and cirrhosis of the liver. The damage is probably produced as the result of dietary deficiency, partly because the chronic alcoholic loses appetite on account of the gastritis produced by the alcohol and partly because the alcohol itself can take the place of food but without protecting the liver cells against injurious influences in the way in which food does. In some native races such as the African Bantu in whom there is gross deficiency in the various protective food substances, cirrhosis of the liver is very prevalent. It is not possible to say, however, if the ordinary cases of cirrhosis which are seen in such a country as our own are due to food deficiency. It seems probable that the commonest cause of acute hepatitis is infection by a virus (virus hepatitis), but complete recovery without cirrhosis is usual in such cases. The cause of the great majority of cases of cirrhosis is still quite obscure.

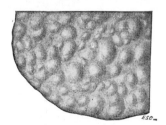

FIG. 63.—Cirrhosis of liver (hob-nail).

In cirrhosis of the liver the organ assumes a highly characteristic appearance. Although it may be enlarged in the early stages, as the disease develops it becomes smaller and smaller. At the same time the surface becomes nodular due to extensive scarring by fibrous tissue. In this way

the surface of the liver becomes covered with little knobs of tissue, so that it is sometimes called the "hob-nailed" liver (Fig. 63). The consistence of the liver becomes very firm and when it is cut with a knife it may feel almost leathery. This is due to the great increase of fibrous tissue.

Symptoms.—The most important effect of cirrhosis of the liver is obstruction to the portal vein. The pathways by which the blood passes through the liver are distorted and obliterated by the scarring and tissue destruction, so that blood is dammed back and collects in the portal vein and its branches. The portal vein collects blood from the stomach and intestines, from the peritoneum, and from the spleen. All of these organs therefore suffer in cirrhosis. The mucous membrane of the stomach is continually congested with blood so that the patient suffers from *dyspepsia*. The veins in the stomach and to an even greater extent those at the lower end of the esophagus become dilated to such an extent that rupture may occur. *Hemorrhage from the stomach and esophagus* is thus a common symptom, and the hemorrhage may be so profuse as to prove fatal. Back pressure in the veins of the peritoneum causes the blood plasma to pass out into the peritoneal cavity where it may accumulate in great amount, a condition known as *ascites*. This fluid causes so much distention and discomfort that it may have to be drawn off, but after each removal it tends to recur. *Enlargement of the spleen* is common on account of the blood which is continually dammed back in that organ. *Jaundice* may develop in the late stages owing to interference with the excretion of bile, which accumulates in the blood and tinges the skin, the whites of the eyes, and the tissues in general a yellowish or green color.

CHOLECYSTITIS

Structure and Function of the Gallbladder.—Cholecystitis means inflammation of the gallbladder (*chole*, bile), but before it can be studied intelligently it is necessary to consider briefly the structure and function of that organ. The gallbladder is a small muscular bag with a normal capacity of about 3 ounces, situated on the undersurface of the liver with its tip projecting beyond the free margin of that organ so that when the gallbladder is much distended it can be palpated by the physician. Bile continually flows into the gallbladder from the liver along the cystic duct, but the bile is only expelled by the gallbladder at intervals when a meal containing fat enters the duodenum. The liver produces twenty times the amount of bile which the gallbladder contains, so that a large amount of water must be absorbed from the bile during its stay in the gallbladder. This is easy to understand when we examine the structure of the mucous membrane, for it is thrown into a series of exquisitely delicate folds filled with capillaries, an arrangement which greatly increases the absorbing surface. As a result of the absorption of water there is marked concentration of the bile. One of the early signs of gallbladder disease is loss of this concentrating power. The *Graham visualization test* of gallbladder function is really a test of this power; an inorganic iodine compound is given which is excreted by the liver in the bile and is opaque to roentgen rays when concentrated sufficiently. This substance fills the gallbladder and is

seen in the roentgen-ray film when the gallbladder is concentrating normally. If this power is lost as the result of disease, the test substance is not concentrated sufficiently to be seen by the roentgen rays, so that the outline of the gallbladder remains invisible. The gallbladder has the same nerve supply as the stomach, so that the symptoms of gallbladder disease are usually referred to the stomach which seems to cry aloud in sympathy.

The chief *cause* of cholecystitis appears to be obstruction to the cystic duct, which connects the gallbladder with the common bile duct. The obstruction may be due to a gall stone or to inflammation of the wall of the duct, which closes off its already narrow lumen. The process appears to be chemical rather than bacterial in origin, and is caused by the action of the bile salts on the wall of the gallbladder. The inflammation may be acute or chronic. Acute cholecystitis is comparatively uncommon, but chronic cholecystitis, often associated with gall stones, is very frequent and is commonly referred to as gallbladder disease. The description which follows refers only to the chronic form.

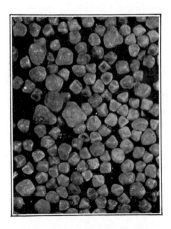

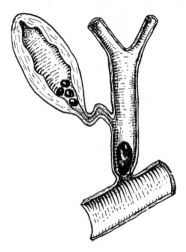

Fig. 64.—Gall stones.

Fig. 65.—Large stone obstructing the common bile duct; small stones in the gallbladder.

Lesions.—The lesions are the result of low-grade inflammation which goes on for months or it may be years. The wall becomes thickened and the cavity is often dilated owing to obstruction of the narrow neck of the gallbladder by which it opens into the cystic duct. The most significant change is seen when the gallbladder is opened and studied with a hand lens, for the beautifully delicate folds of mucous membrane are either greatly thickened or flattened out. As a result of this change absorption is seriously interfered with or completely suppressed, so that the gallbladder does not visualize in the Graham test. Gall stones may or may not be present; the longer the inflammation has lasted, the more likely it is to be complicated by stones.

Gall stones or biliary calculi (Fig. 64) are usually formed in the gallbladder itself, but may originate in the bile passages in the liver. They consist of bile pigment, cholesterol, and calcium, all of which substances are derived from the bile. The most important *cause* is infection of the gallbladder, which allows substances normally in solution in the bile to be precipitated in solid form. Pregnancy, the female sex, and obesity are accessory factors, so that those who are "fair, fat, and forty" are candidates for gall stones. In pregnancy the blood cholesterol is raised, an increased amount passes through into the bile, and the tendency to precipitation is thus increased. The number varies from one to several hundreds, and they may be large or small. It is little dogs that make the most noise, and the same is true of gall stones, for it is the little stones which are apt to pass along the cystic and common bile ducts causing the extreme pain of biliary colic. The stone may become lodged or impacted at the lower end of the common bile duct, causing the bile to accumulate on the proximal side of the obstruction and produce marked distention of the common bile duct and hepatic ducts (Fig. 65). The gallbladder may also become distended, but it is probable that the chronic cholecystitis which usually accompanies the presence of gall stones has resulted in such thickening and contraction of the gallbladder that it is incapable of distention.

The Basis of Symptoms.—Cholecystitis and calculi are frequently associated, so that the symptoms will be considered together. The *symptoms of chronic cholecystitis* are for the most part referable to the stomach, *i.e.*, indigestion, nausea, belching of gas, and a feeling of fulness and bloating. These symptoms are aggravated by fatty foods, (fried foods, etc.). Food containing much fat causes the gallbladder to contract and empty itself, and if the wall is inflamed this may cause much discomfort. *Dyspepsia* suggesting disease of the stomach is more often due to cholecystitis than to ulcer of the stomach or duodenum. The stomach suffers because it has the same nerve supply as the gallbladder, and irritation of one branch of the nerve is reflected in the other branch causing spasm of the pylorus with accompanying retention of food, a *feeling of bloating*, and *belching of gas*.

The *symptoms of gall stones* are in part those of the chronic cholecystitis which accompanies the condition, in part those of biliary colic, and in part those of obstruction. A gallbladder may contain numerous stones without any symptoms on the part of the patient. *Biliary colic* or gall stone colic is the result of the passage of a stone along the cystic duct. The patient is suddenly seized with pain of the most excruciating character, which starts under the ribs on the right side and passes up to the right shoulder. The pain is due to distention of the duct which is abundantly supplied with nerves. The agony endures during the slow passage of the stone along the narrow cystic duct, which to the patient seems endless, becomes eased when it enters the wider common duct, and ceases entirely when it passes into the duodenum. The patient may be mildly jaundiced after the attack. *Obstructive symptoms* occur in those cases in which the stone becomes *impacted* at the lower end of the common bile duct and fails to pass through the narrow opening into the duodenum. It may remain in this situation for many months. The bile is prevented from passing freely into the duodenum, and accumulates in the liver and finally in the blood, giving rise

to the symptoms of *jaundice*. The skin and the whites of the eyes become colored an intense green, bile escapes from the blood into the urine which it renders green, and the stools are *clay colored*, owing to the presence of fat which has not been digested because of the absence of bile in the duodenum. The irritation of the stone in the common duct causes inflammation and periodic attacks of fever. *Duodenal drainage* by means of a stomach tube passed into the duodenum followed by the administration of some solution, *e.g.*, magnesium sulfate, which will cause the discharge of bile from the gallbladder into the duodenum, may be useful in diagnosis. In cholecystitis pus cells may be present in the fluid obtained by the tube, and the presence of crystals suggests the possibility of gall stones.

Principles of Treatment.—The patient with gall-bladder disease must pay careful attention to his diet, particularly avoiding fats and foods fried in fat, substances which stimulate the gallbladder wall to contract with resulting reflex spasm of the pylorus. If diet fails to alleviate the symptoms, removal of the gallbladder (cholecystectomy) may be necessary. Stones in the gallbladder causing symptoms may require operation; they can never be dissolved by the various quack remedies sold for that purpose. This is equally true for stone in the common duct. The acute pain of biliary colic may demand morphine for its relief.

<h3 style="text-align:center">JAUNDICE</h3>

Jaundice or icterus is a coloration of the skin and sclerotics (whites of the eye) by bile pigment in the blood. The color varies from pale yellow to deep orange or even green. The pigment of the bile (bilirubin) is formed from broken down red blood cells by the reticulo-endothelial system (lymph nodes, spleen, etc.), and is excreted by the liver, passing first by the bile ducts to the gallbladder, and then along the common bile duct to the duodenum.

It is evident that there are three very different ways in which bilirubin may accumulate in excess in the blood and so give rise to jaundice.

1. If an excessive amount of blood is broken down, more bilirubin will be formed than can be excreted by the liver, so that it will remain in the blood. This is seen in extensive internal hemorrhage, when the wrong type of blood has been used for transfusion (the injected red cells becoming hemolyzed), and in the disease called congenital hemolytic jaundice in which the red corpuscles are abnormally fragile and easily hemolyzed. The type of jaundice caused by abnormal breaking down of red blood corpuscles (from whatever cause) is called *hemolytic jaundice,* so that the term is used in two senses. In this group bile does not appear in the urine.

2. If the liver is extensively diseased, as in hepatitis, it is unable to excrete the bilirubin brought to it, which therefore accumulates in the blood. The result is *catarrhal jaundice,* which is the commonest of the three varieties. Usually it clears up in a few days or weeks, but if the hepatitis is very severe the jaundice becomes extreme and the case may end fatally.

3. The liver may excrete the bile normally, but it may be unable to escape into the duodenum owing to some obstruction. The two common causes of obstruction are a gall stone lodged in the common bile duct, and carci-

noma of the head of the pancreas which blocks the opening of the duct into the duodenum.   Under these circumstances the bile is dammed back in the liver and is reabsorbed into the blood.   Such a condition is called *obstructive jaundice*.   The jaundice may become intense, and the urine is colored with bile.   As no bile reaches the intestine the stools are extremely pale and are described as clay-colored.   There is a marked tendency to hemorrhage, because absence of bile in the bowel prevents absorption of vitamin K, a substance which is necessary for the formation of prothrombin and normal clotting of the blood (see page 40).   This can be overcome by administering vitamin K and bile by mouth (through a duodenal tube), and when the prothrombin in the blood has returned to normal an operation for the removal of an impacted stone can be performed with safety.

Chapter

14

DISEASES OF THE PANCREAS

Structure and Function.—The pancreas, known in animals as the "sweet-bread," is an elongated flat organ which crosses the left side of the abdomen behind the stomach. It is the most powerful digestive gland in the body, and has been called the salivary gland of the abdomen, because, not only does it resemble the salivary glands in structure, but it pours its secretion into the digestive canal by a duct. The pancreatic duct opens into the duodenum at the same point as the common bile duct enters the bowel; indeed the two ducts usually have a common opening, the importance of which fact will soon become evident. The pancreas produces three powerful *digestive ferments*, one for the digestion of proteins, one for carbohydrates, and one for fats.

The pancreas is really a double organ. It produces an *external secretion*, the pancreatic juice, which is poured into the duodenum by the pancreatic duct, but it also produces an *internal secretion* which never enters the pancreatic duct, but is absorbed directly into the blood that passes through the pancreas. Were it to do so it would immediately be destroyed by the pancreatic ferments. This internal secretion had long been suspected, but it was only when Banting and Best, in 1921, hit upon a method of eliminating the pancreatic enzymes of the animals with which they were working that they succeeded in obtaining a solution of the internal secretion. This secretion, as all the world knows, is *insulin*, so named because it is produced by little groups or islands of specialized cells in the pancreas known as the *islets of Langerhans* (*insula*, an island). The function of insulin is to regulate carbohydrate metabolism; when insufficient insulin is produced, diabetes develops.

The three chief diseases of the pancreas are acute hemorrhagic pancreatitis, cancer, and diabetes mellitus.

ACUTE HEMORRHAGIC PANCREATITIS

The pancreas produces a powerful digestive ferment, *trypsin*, but as long as this remains in the duct it does no harm to the pancreas itself. Should the duct become blocked, however, the dammed-up secretion may rupture the finer branches of the duct and leak into the surrounding pancreatic tissue which it will proceed to digest. If bile, particularly infected bile, should enter the pancreatic duct, it may render the trypsin sufficiently active to enable it to digest the wall of the duct and thus the pancreatic tissue. The fact that the pancreatic and bile ducts frequently unite before entering the duodenum facilitates the passage

12

into the duodenum, especially when the common opening is blocked by a gall stone. The pancreatic tissue is then broken down by the activated trypsin, *i.e.*, it becomes necrosed, bloodvessels are destroyed, and extensive hemorrhage rapidly occurs into the pancreas. The pancreatic ferments are now free to escape into the abdominal cavity, where the fat-splitting ferment acts on the abundant yellow fat in the peritoneum and on the surface of the pancreas, producing little white patches of *fat necrosis*. When the surgeon opens the abdomen and sees these tell-tale white patches he is at once able to make a correct diagnosis even before the deep-seated pancreas has been exposed.

The Basis of Symptoms.—The disease is one of the acute abdominal accidents. The terrific *pain* which is the outstanding symptom usually comes on after a heavy meal when abundant bile is pouring out of the gall-bladder. The suddenness of the onset, the illimitable agony which accompanies it, and the high mortality dependent upon it render it the most formidable of catastrophies. The pain, more terrible than that of perforated gastric ulcer, causes the sufferer to remain motionless, whereas in gall-stone colic he changes his position every minute, seeking the relief which does not come. There is a marked condition of *shock*, and the face assumes a peculiar slate-blue color which is very characteristic.

Treatment.—The treatment consists in attacking the gallbladder, not the pancreas. There is usually an associated cholecystitis, and infected bile is much more irritating to the pancreas than normal bile. If the gall-bladder can be drained sufficiently early in the disease so that no more infected bile will enter the pancreas, the patient has at least a chance of recovery.

CANCER OF THE PANCREAS

Carcinoma of the pancreas usually occurs at the end which is in contact with the duodenum, the part known as the head of the pancreas. This position of the tumor is responsible for the characteristic symptoms of the disease, for it presses on and blocks both the pancreatic and common bile ducts. Owing to pressure on the pancreatic duct the pancreatic juice is prevented from entering the duodenum, so that digestion is interfered with. The patient therefore becomes extremely wasted, and much of the food in the stools passes out unchanged. The stools are clay-colored, due to the presence of undigested fat. Pressure on the bile duct leads to a gradually deepening jaundice, for the bile is unable to escape. This jaundice is painless, in contrast with the pain which accompanies jaundice due to obstruction of the duct by gall stones. A few cases of early cancer of the pancreas have been treated by removal of the whole pancreas, but the results of this procedure in the few cases which have been so treated have not been too encouraging. The patient develops a mild diabetes and of course no longer has available the pancreatic digestive enzymes. Occasionally, when cancer involves the head of the pancreas and produces a complete obstruction of the bile ducts, the jaundice becomes so troublesome from itching that surgical treatment will produce relief by joining the gall-bladder to the small intestine, thus by-passing the obstruction.

DIABETES MELLITUS

Diabetes means a "running through"; mellitus means "sweet" (literally honeyed). Diabetes mellitus is thus a condition in which there is an excessive outpouring of urine containing sugar. The word diabetes is also used for another disease, diabetes insipidus, in which the amount of urine is greatly increased but contains no sugar. As the latter condition is rare, diabetes mellitus is usually known simply as diabetes. The fact that the urine is increased and contains sugar might suggest that this was a disease of the kidneys. This is not so, for the kidneys are perfectly normal. It is a disorder of carbohydrate metabolism as a result of which the sugar of the food is not burnt by the tissues and converted into energy. The cause of the disorder is a deficient supply of insulin, and the lesion responsible is to be sought in the islets of Langerhans in the pancreas.

It might be thought that everything is known about diabetes that can be known. As a matter of fact the reverse is the case. We do not know the essential *cause* of diabetes, *i.e.*, the factor which damages the islets of Langerhans. The lesions in the islets are the reverse of striking, and may indeed be difficult to detect. The cells of the islets are of two kinds known as alpha and beta. The alpha cells have granules which stain red, the beta cells have blue-staining granules which are believed to be the source of insulin. In diabetes there is first loss of the granules of the beta cells, and later these cells disappear. Eventually it may be difficult to find any islets.

We do know, however, that insulin in some way serves as a spark which enables the glucose carried to the tissue cells, particularly the muscles, to unite with the oxygen there and be burnt with the production of energy. It also enables the glucose carried from the intestine to the liver to be converted into glycogen. When insulin is lacking it is evident that glucose will neither be changed into glycogen in the liver nor be burnt up by the muscles, so that it will accumulate in the blood in large amounts. When the blood reaches the kidneys the glucose will flow out into the urine. A diagnosis of diabetes can be made by testing either the urine or the blood for sugar, remembering that some is always present in the blood. The normal blood sugar is about 0.1 per cent, but in diabetes it may reach 0.4 per cent or higher.

There is an even greater danger than the failure to burn carbohydrates, namely, a failure to burn fats. For the proper combustion of fat a certain proportion of carbohydrates must be burnt at the same time. In the carburetor of an automobile the correct mixture must be present, else the engine will "smoke" and will miss fire. So also in the tissues if the correct fat-glucose mixture is not present it will "smoke" during combustion, the smoke representing toxic acid substances which are the result of incomplete combustion of the fat. These are known as *ketone bodies*, and the clinical condition is *acidosis* or *ketosis*. We may say, then, that diabetes is initially a derangement of carbohydrate metabolism, but that this leads to a perverted fat metabolism which if unchecked will result in death.

The Basis of Symptoms.—The chief signs and symptoms of diabetes are polyuria (excessive urination), glycosuria (sugar in the urine), high

blood sugar, excessive thirst and hunger, and marked weakness and loss of weight. Another group of symptoms due to the incomplete combustion of fats are manifestations of acidosis, *e.g.*, air hunger, coma, and ketone bodies in the urine. Still other accompaniments of the disease are itching, boils, gall stones, arteriosclerosis, and gangrene of the limbs. Nowadays as the result of insulin treatment most patients do not die of diabetes but of complications and infections.

The *glycosuria* is due to the excess sugar in the blood flowing out in the urine. As much as 1 pound of sugar a day may be excreted in the urine if a patient with marked diabetes eats all the sugar and starch he wants. The large amount of sugar dissolved in the urine *raises the specific gravity* or density so that it becomes 1.030 or 1.040 in place of the normal of around 1.020. The *high blood sugar* is the natural result of the sugar not being burnt up and not being converted into glycogen. Sugar acts on the kidney as a diuretic or stimulant to secretion, hence the *polyuria*. On account of the large amount of water the urine is characteristically pale in color. The tissues are dehydrated by the excessive loss of water in the urine and this causes great *thirst*. As the tissues are not able to use the sugar there is *hunger, weakness*, and *loss of weight*. The chief cause of the loss of weight, however, is the fact that the tissue protein is converted into sugar; the diabetic is unable to use the sugar in his blood, and so has to draw on his protein reserves for nourishment and fuel. *Itching* is probably due to sugar in the tissues, and the sugar is also responsible for *boils* and *carbuncles,* as it forms an excellent culture medium for bacteria. A carbuncle may be so severe as to prove fatal. The chief danger to life is from *acidosis* caused by incomplete burning of the fats. Ketone bodies appear in the blood and urine, and the presence in the urine of *diacetic acid* and *acetone* is always a danger signal. The onset of acidosis is indicated by the deep sighing respiration known as *air hunger*, and sometimes followed by drowsiness and later unconsciousness, a condition of *diabetic coma*, due to the action of the ketone bodies on the brain. For some reason which is at present unknown the blood cholesterol is raised; the cholesterol in the bile is accordingly increased, and this explains the frequency of *gall stones*. High blood cholesterol appears to favor the development of *arteriosclerosis*, and the consequent narrowing of the vessels of the limbs together with the devitalization of the tissues by the sugar stored in them tends to result in *diabetic gangrene*.

Principles of Treatment.—In the treatment of diabetes consideration must be given to: (1) The regulation of the patient's diet, habits, and life so as to minimize the effect of the imperfect carbohydrate metabolism and to throw as little strain as possible on the laboring pancreas; (2) the use of insulin, should that be necessary; (3) the prevention and treatment of complications, of which diabetic coma is the most serious.

The treatment adopted will vary with the severity of the case. Diabetics may be divided into mild, moderate, and severe groups. In a *mild* case the urine can be made sugar-free by omitting a few of the commoner carbohydrates without any serious curtailment of the diet as a whole. The disease is of *moderate* grade when the patient has to be on a carefully balanced diet in order to remain sugar-free. In a *severe* case insulin is needed in addition to a balanced diet if the patient is to remain sugar-free

and at the same time fit for work. Such a patient could also be kept sugar-free in the days before insulin, but only as a half-starved invalid whose miserable life was a burden to himself and to his family. Insulin has not only increased the span of life, especially in young children in whom there is great danger of coma, but it has added enormously to the happiness, comfort and usefulness of the great army of diabetics, of whom there are at least 1,000,000 in the United States alone. In addition to regular or crystalline insulin there have been developed modifications of this hormone by the addition of protamine and zinc or globin to provide a compound, which, when injected, will slowly liberate insulin over periods up to twenty-four hours or slightly longer. This has helped to provide a better degree of control of the diabetes than was possible with the shorter-acting regular insulin. Insulin is not a cure for diabetes, but it serves to give the over-taxed islets of Langerhans a much needed rest, and as a result of such rest they may regain to some extent the power of attending to the metabolic carbohydrate needs. The necessity for getting the urine sugar-free can hardly be overemphasized. If even a slight glycosuria is continually present, the tolerance to carbohydrates will steadily diminish, *i.e.*, the diabetes will increase in severity. On the other hand, even one sugar-free day will increase the tolerance so that the amount of carbohydrates can be increased without sugar appearing in the urine.

Once upon a time the treatment of diabetes consisted in cutting down the carbohydrates (sugars and starches) until the urine became sugar-free, at the same time maintaining the patient's strength with proteins and fats. The treatment was successful (in keeping the urine sugar-free), but the patient died (of acidosis and diabetic coma). In the absence of insulin an excessive amount of fat is broken down from the body stores to produce ketone bodies which are formed in excess of their excretion or utilization by the muscles, and this accounts for the development of ketosis and subsequent acidosis. Insulin has changed all this. It is now possible to kindle the carbohydrate fire with insulin, and the fats which are added to the fire are consumed completely and harmlessly. The supply of fuel for energy and heat is thus adequate and the body no longer needs to call on its own proteins and convert them into sugar for this purpose. It was this call in the past which made of the diabetic a half-starved wretch; now he is well nourished as well as reasonably vigorous.

It is beyond the scope of this book as well as far beyond the power of the author to go into detail about the constituents and proportions of a balanced diabetic diet or the dosage of insulin. The principle is to calculate a diet which will contain about 1 gram of protein per kilo of body weight with enough carbohydrate and fat to make up the necessary caloric value. This amount of protein is enough to maintain nutrition unimpaired. The proportion of carbohydrate to fat must be sufficient to insure that the fat is properly burnt, else it will "smoke" with the formation of ketone bodies. Normally the carbohydrates of the diet are from three to five times in excess of the fat, and the modern idea in the treatment of diabetes is to approach as closely as possible to a normal diet, even if insulin is needed to attain this ideal. The amount of exercise taken bears a relation both to the diet and the insulin required. A workingman needs more calories and

therefore more carbohydrates than a professor, but he needs less insulin, as the muscles in action use up more sugar than when they are at rest. The dose of insulin is that sufficient to keep the urine just sugar-free. As the pancreas becomes rested and recovers to some extent, the dose of insulin can be gradually decreased, until finally it may be omitted altogether. The patient must learn the very simple procedure of testing his own urine for sugar, so that he may detect at the earliest possible moment any reappearance of the glycosuria. After the preliminary analysis and check-up, for which hospital treatment is usually necessary, the patient will administer his own insulin. It is unfortunate that insulin has to be given by hypodermic injection. This is necessary because when given by mouth it is at once destroyed by the enzymes of the stomach and pancreas.

Many of the *complications of diabetes* can be prevented or at least nipped in the bud. *Coma* may be precipitated by indiscretions in diet, especially the excessive use of fats when the carbohydrates are low, exhaustion, mental excitement, infections, general anesthesia, indeed anything which upsets the metabolic balance and leads to acidosis. The early or warning symptoms are loss of appetite, nausea, vomiting, headache, and listlessness, followed later by the deep breathing of air hunger, drowsiness, and coma. The breath has a sweetish smell like that of new-mown hay, due to the presence of acetone. This and other ketone bodies are found in the urine, imparting to it a similar odor. The *acidosis* can be overcome by providing a bright carbohydrate flame in which the fat will burn, and this is most readily accomplished by the simultaneous injection of glucose solution intravenously and insulin hypodermically. Diabetic coma when at all advanced must be considered in the same light as a surgical emergency and demands the same prompt measures. Dehydration is the most dangerous feature in diabetic coma, being caused by paralysis and dilatation of the small bloodvessels, through whose walls there is a great loss of fluid and salt. Death may occur from dehydration alone, even though there are no ketone bodies in the urine. A valuable method of treatment is therefore to give large amounts of saline solution. Skin infections leading to *boils, carbuncles,* and *bed-sores* can be prevented to some extent by scrupulous attention to the skin. Gangrene of the feet and toes must be guarded against by avoidance of skin infection and injury. In the care of the feet attention may be directed to the following points. Wash the feet each night with soap and water. Do not use hot-water bottles or electric pads. Tight shoes must be avoided. Toe nails should be cut straight across, but corns and calluses should not be cut. "Athlete's foot" must be avoided at all costs, but strong antiseptics and patent remedies for "athlete's foot" are equally dangerous. Gangrene is one of the most frequent causes of death, now that insulin has conquered the previously dreaded acidosis and coma. *Arteriosclerosis,* which is the chief cause of gangrene and which attacks the arteries of the heart (coronaries) and legs, develops at an early age in diabetics, especially when they are kept, as used to be common, on a high-fat, low-carbohydrate diet; high blood fat (cholesterol) definitely predisposes to arteriosclerosis. The higher the proportion of carbohydrate in the diet, the less is the risk of arteriosclerosis and gangrene.

A complication which has developed since the introduction of insulin is *hypoglycemia* or insulin shock. If too large a dose of insulin is given or if the blood sugar happens to be low when an apparently safe dose of insulin is taken, the level of the blood sugar is forced to dangerously low levels (hypoglycemia), and the patient develops sudden nervousness, weakness, sweating, muscular incoördination, fainting, and even coma. Strange that coma may be the result both of too much and too little insulin! These alarming symptoms can at once be alleviated by the administration of glucose solution or even by eating some milk chocolate.

It is of great interest to note that in rare instances an apparently normal person may suffer from attacks of *spontaneous hypoglycemia* when he has gone without food for some time. Such a person is a victim of *hyperinsulinism*, or too great production of insulin by the pancreas, usually due to an innocent tumor (adenoma) of the islets of Langerhans which can be removed surgically. Such an individual presents the same picture as a diabetic suffering from insulin shock. One man of my acquaintance was arrested several times by the police for supposed intoxication, until finally an analysis of the blood showed that the essential trouble was a low blood sugar

Chapter

15

THE GENITO-URINARY SYSTEM

Structure and Function.—The urinary system is designed to remove waste products from the blood, particularly those containing nitrogen, *e.g.*, urea. Excretion is accomplished by means of a filtering mechanism in the *kidneys*, that removes water and solid material from the blood in the form of urine which passes from each kidney in the corresponding *ureter* to the *bladder* (Fig. 66), and thence in the *urethra* to the exterior. The

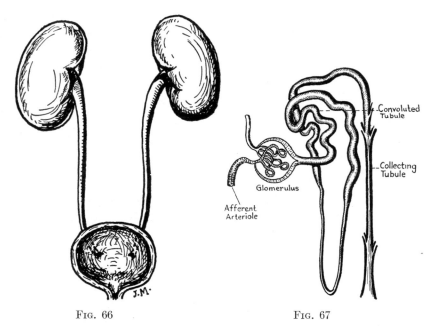

FIG. 66   FIG. 67

FIG. 66.—Kidneys, ureters, bladder, and commencement of urethra.
FIG. 67.—One of the kidney nephrons.

urinary bladder differs from the gallbladder in that it is merely a reservoir and does not absorb or concentrate the fluid which it contains. Such absorption and concentration does, however, go on in the kidney itself to a marked degree, and one of the early signs of renal disease is loss of this concentrating power.

(188)

The filtering mechanism is a very beautiful one. Each kidney is composed of some 2,000,000 units or *nephrons,* all of which are minute filters (Fig. 67). The nephron is a complex tube, partly coiled and partly straight, the upper end of which is formed by a spherical structure, the *glomerulus,* whilst the lower end opens into the chamber or *pelvis* of the kidney from which the water passes to the bladder. In the glomerulus, which is the actual filter, a small artery, the *afferent arteriole* of the glomerulus, breaks up into a little cluster of capillary loops that project like a bunch of grapes into the dilated upper end of the tubule. As the blood passes through the loops, water and solids in solution escape through the walls of the capillaries into the *convoluted tubule,* where much of the water is reabsorbed so that the urine becomes concentrated. It then passes into the *collecting tubules* and finally into the pelvis of the kidney.

The process of filtration or secretion of urine depends on the pressure under which the blood is forced through the glomerular capillaries. If the blood-pressure falls markedly the secretion of urine diminishes or stops. If a large number of glomeruli are eliminated as the result of nephritis or Bright's disease, the remainder have to do the extra work, and this is accomplished by means of a rise in the blood-pressure, so that high blood-pressure or hypertension is one of the important signs of advanced Bright's disease. There is a close reciprocal relationship between these two conditions, for not only may Bright's disease cause hypertension, but hypertension may cause one form of Bright's disease. This will be made clear a little later. Although water, urea, and salts pass from the blood through the walls of the glomerular capillaries into the tubules, the albumin and sugar of the blood plasma are not allowed to escape. The presence of albumin in the urine indicates inflammation of the glomeruli, whilst the presence of sugar is nearly always, though not invariably, due to the raised blood sugar characteristic of diabetes.

It is evident that in the formation of the urine there are two opposite factors at work, glomerular filtration and tubular absorption. Were it not for the absorption in the tubules, the body would soon be drained of its fluid, for only one-eightieth part of the fluid which passes through the glomeruli appears as urine. The normal amount passed is about 1000 cc. a day, but this will vary with the amount of water drunk, the amount lost in perspiration, etc.

One of the most important features of the urine is its specific gravity or density, which depends on the amount of solids in solution and indicates the concentration of the urine. In health this varies between 1.015 and 1.025, the specific gravity of distilled water being taken as 1.000. The gravity is high in diabetes because the urine contains so much sugar in solution; it is low in advanced Bright's disease because the kidney has lost its concentrating power owing to degeneration of great numbers of the tubules. In the latter disease it is fixed as well as low, and the normal variation of about 9 points in twenty-four hours is lost.

NEPHRITIS: BRIGHT'S DISEASE

Over a hundred years ago Richard Bright, of Guy's Hospital, London, recognized that the combination of edema of the face and ankles and

albumin in the urine was usually associated with a lesion of the kidneys which from that day to this has been known as Bright's disease. It is an inflammatory disease of the kidney, a nephritis, involving particularly the kidney filter, and as the filtration of the urine is dependent on blood-pressure, disturbance of the blood-pressure is one of the major symptoms.

The *cause* of the condition is bacterial infection; generally, perhaps invariably, streptococcal in type. The evidence in support of this view is the fact that an acute attack of the disease is usually preceded by a streptococcal infection such as tonsillitis, septic sore throat, occasionally even scarlet fever. The difficulty is that no streptococci are found either in the kidneys or in the urine. It may be that streptococcal toxins produced in the throat are carried to the kidneys by the blood. The course of the disease is chronic with so-called exacerbations, but it is probable that the exacerbations represent fresh onslaughts of toxins or bacteria on the already damaged kidneys.

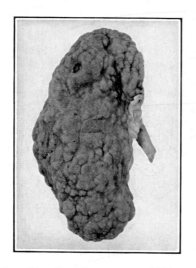

Fig. 68.—Granular contracted kidney.

Lesions.—The lesions vary much with the stage of the disease. Both kidneys are always affected. At first the kidneys are swollen and congested owing to the acute inflammation, but as time goes on they become small, shrunken, and present a characteristically granular surface. The kidney of chronic or advanced Bright's disease is therefore known as the *granular contracted kidney* (Fig. 68).

The *microscopic appearance* provides the key both to the gross change and to many of the symptoms. The brunt of the attack falls on the glomeruli, so that the condition is known as glomerulonephritis. At the first attack large numbers of glomeruli are involved. The capillary loops are inflamed, many of them are permanently blocked, and the permeability of the remainder is so much increased that the albumin of the blood plasma is able to pass through the capillary walls into the tubules and thus appears in the urine. With each attack an increasing number of glomeruli are irretrievably injured, their capillaries are closed off, and as the tubule is of little use without its glomerulus, the entire nephron atrophies and finally disappears. It is on account of this wholesale destruction that the kidney diminishes so greatly in size. The remaining nephrons have to carry on as best they can, and they hypertrophy in response to the added burden, this increase in size accounting for the little granules which project on the surface between the depressed atrophic areas. Finally, the strain becomes too great and the kidneys are forced to give up their losing fight.

The *hypertensive kidney, i.e.,* the condition of the kidney which may develop in the course of arterial hypertension or high blood-pressure, is

so similar in appearance to the kidney in the end stage of glomerulonephritis that it may be impossible to distinguish between the two at postmortem examination. The reason for this is that essential hypertension is accompanied by a great thickening of the walls of the small arteries with narrowing of the lumen, so that so little blood can reach the glomeruli through the afferent arterioles that they become ischemic and collapse. The entire nephron atrophies, and as this is taking place everywhere throughout the kidney, the result is a granular contracted kidney. Various names are given to the kidney of hypertension, such as the *arteriosclerotic kidney* (because the change in the bloodvessels is a form of arteriosclerosis) and *nephrosclerosis* (because the kidney becomes scarred or sclerotic).

The Basis of Symptoms.—The symptoms of nephritis are so multiform and their interpretation so difficult that large treatises have been written on this disease alone. In the space at our disposal we shall merely focus attention on the glomerular lesion and on the symptoms which may be attributed to it. Bright's disease may be acute or chronic, but the chronic stage may be marked by acute attacks. An acute attack, especially that which follows scarlet fever, may clear up completely and never progress to the chronic stage. On the other hand, repeated attacks so mild as hardly to be noticeable by the patient may lead to the inexorable and relentless downfall of the kidney which characterizes the chronic stage of the disease. Before this is reached the patient may or may not show symptoms of a subacute stage. The subacute stage is characterized by marked edema and is therefore known as *wet nephritis*; in the chronic stage the edema disappears so that it is called *dry nephritis*. The end picture is dry nephritis with little or no albumin in the urine, a very different affair from the conception of Bright's disease as a condition marked by albuminuria and edema with which we started. Some of the principal clinical features will now be considered in brief detail.

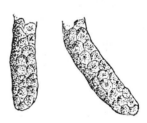

FIG. 69.—Urinary casts.

The main *urinary changes* are the presence of albumin, casts, and blood, and alteration in the specific gravity: (1) *Albuminuria* is due to the increased permeability of the glomerular capillaries caused by the acute inflammation. It is therefore marked in the acute stage, which is a matter of a few weeks' duration. In the subacute or wet stage the damaged glomeruli still allow a certain amount of blood to pass through them, so that albumin still pours out from the blood into the urine. In the dry chronic stage the affected glomeruli have become completely closed off, no blood can traverse them, and only a trace of albumin may appear in the urine. (2) *Casts* are moulds of the tubules which may be present in the urine in large numbers (Fig. 69). They consist of coagulated albumin and blood cells. (3) *Red blood corpuscles* in the urine indicate glomerular inflammation so acute that the capillaries give way or at least allow the escape of blood cells through their walls. They are therefore characteristic of the early or acute stage and of exacerbations. (4) In the late chronic

stage the *specific gravity* of the urine is *low* and *fixed, i.e.,* it does not show the normal variation of 9 or 10 points in the course of twenty-four hours. This is the result of loss of the concentrating power of the kidney, which in turn is due to the wholesale disappearance of the renal tubules. *Loss of concentrating power* as indicated by low fixed specific gravity is one of the most important signs of failure of renal function. This fact should emphasize to the nurse, on whom the duty of estimating the specific gravity of the urine often falls, the great necessity of accuracy in the performance of this simple test.

Edema may be present in both the acute and subacute stage of nephritis, but the explanation is different in the two cases. In the acute stage there are streptococcal toxins circulating in the blood which act on the capillaries in general as well as on those of the kidney. There is, therefore, a widespread increase in capillary permeability with resulting general edema, especially in the face and ankles, indicated by puffiness under the eyes and swelling of the ankles. General edema is also marked in the subacute stage as indicated by the name wet nephritis. Not only are the face and legs affected, but large amounts of watery fluid may accumulate in the pleural and peritoneal cavities, so that the patient becomes in truth waterlogged. Here the explanation is quite different. The fault lies not in the walls of the vessels but in the blood itself. Two more or less equal but opposite forces are always at work in the fine capillaries: (1) *Blood-pressure* which tries to force the fluid part of the blood out through the vessel wall into the tissues. (2) The *osmotic pressure of the blood proteins* which hold the fluid back within the vessels. The amount of blood proteins is seriously diminished by the great outpouring of albumin in the urine which characterizes wet nephritis, the osmotic pressure falls, and edema develops. In the dry or chronic stage, as the name indicates, the edema disappears because albumin is no longer poured in large amount into the urine.

Hypertension is one of the important manifestations of the later stages of Bright's disease, for it rather than the disease in the kidneys may be the cause of death. High blood-pressure may be the result of glomerulonephritis or pyelonephritis (see below); this form is called *secondary* hypertension. Or it may have no apparent cause, and is then called *primary* or *essential* hypertension. This is the form which is associated with the hypertensive contracted kidney; the hypertension appears to be the cause of the renal condition, but this is not certain, and the reverse may prove to be the case. Experimental work on animals has shown that when the blood supply to the kidneys is gradually reduced (ischemia) by narrowing the renal arteries, hypertension results. It is evident, therefore, that the kidney is able under certain conditions to produce a substance, which has been named renin, that has the power of raising the blood-pressure permanently. This is probably the mechanism of the hypertension of glomerulonephritis and pyelonephritis. It is not yet certain if essential hypertension is also renal in origin. The high blood-pressure is dangerous to the patient in two ways: (1) It may throw such a strain on the heart that the patient dies of heart failure rather than renal failure. (2) A blood-vessel may burst in the brain as a result of the high pressure causing death from cerebral hemorrhage.

Blood chemistry changes indicate the gradual failure of the kidneys to function, known to the physician as renal insufficiency. They are of great value in the difficult task of making a prognosis, of forecasting the probable length of time that the patient has to live. Two of the important waste products which pass from the blood into the urine are *urea* and *creatinine*. These are non-protein nitrogenous substances, known briefly as N.P.N. As the kidneys cease to function these substances accumulate in the blood in ever-increasing amount, and chemical examination of the blood will show the exact degree of retention of these nitrogenous substances. The normal blood urea is 12 to 20 mg. per 100 cc. of blood and the blood creatinine is 1.5 to 2 mg. In the late stages of nephritis, the urea may go to 100 mg. and the creatinine to 5 mg. Sometimes the urea may reach 200 mg. and the creatinine 13 to 15 mg. These figures indicate that the end is very near.

Uremia is the condition which results from renal insufficiency, and is the usual cause of death in the chronic stage of Bright's disease. Uremia is due to an accumulation of poisonous substances in the blood, although the exact nature of these poisons has not yet been determined. The blood urea and creatinine are very high, but the poisoning is not due to the presence of these nitrogenous substances. The symptoms are mainly cerebral, first headache, restlessness and vomiting, then muscular twitchings, convulsions and drowsiness, finally coma and death. The patient may be short of breath, and the respirations develop the peculiar and ominous Cheyne-Stokes character, *i.e.*, the breathing increases in depth up to a certain point and then decreases until finally all respiration ceases for half a minute or so, when it begins again as before.

It will be observed that no mention has been made of *backache* as a symptom of Bright's disease. In the acute stage, which is seldom seen, there may be some aching in the loins, but in chronic nephritis, which forms the great bulk of the cases, pain in the back is *not* a symptom. The numerous patent medicines advertised in the daily press as a sure cure for the backache which is supposed to spell Bright's disease are of no more value than a glass of water from the tap.

Principles of Treatment.—As the function of the kidneys is to excrete waste products, the matter of diet is of chief importance in the treatment of nephritis. The substances excreted such as urea, uric acid and creatinine are nitrogenous in character, and as nitrogen only occurs in proteins, chief attention has to be paid to the proteins in the food. Everything will depend, however, on the stage of the disease. *Acute nephritis* is an acute inflammation and as every acutely inflamed organ must be rested as much as possible, the diet, particularly the proteins, must be cut down to the irreducible minimum in this stage. Complete rest in bed is also essential. It is seldom, however, that the fully-fledged picture of acute nephritis presents itself for treatment. The disease is usually seen in the subacute and chronic stage.

In *subacute nephritis* there is marked generalized edema caused by the low level of the proteins whose constant outflow into the urine is indicated by the massive albuminuria. In this stage it would be folly to reduce the proteins in the food, for that would be the measure best calculated to in-

tensify the edema. There is no renal insufficiency in this stage, so that an adequate diet can be given. The salt in the food should be limited in wet nephritis, as an excess of chlorides in the tissues tends to accentuate the edema. Thyroid extract may prove of benefit. The accumulation of fluid may be so great that it has to be drawn off both from the tissues and from the large serous cavities by mechanical means. In *chronic nephritis* renal insufficiency develops, and again the kidney must be relieved of the strain of excreting nitrogen, so that the proteins in the food must once more be reduced. At any moment *uremia* may complicate the picture, and treatment then must be prompt and vigorous. Active purgation is found to be of benefit, the skin must be made to perspire by hot baths and packs, and about 500 cc. of blood may be withdrawn from a vein. All of these measures serve to relieve the kidneys. The withdrawal of cerebrospinal fluid by means of lumbar puncture will reduce the pressure on the brain and sometimes bring the patient out of a state of coma.

PYELONEPHRITIS

The word pyelonephritis means inflammation of the kidney and the renal pelvis. This inflammation is quite different from that of glomerulonephritis, for it is a suppuration. It is therefore caused by pyogenic bacteria, particularly Bacillus coli, streptococci and staphylococci. The colon bacilli ascend from the bladder in inflammatory conditions of the bladder, which are especially apt to occur in women and children. In men it is a common complication of enlarged prostate. The pyogenic cocci reach the kidney by the blood stream.

The kidneys are seldom equally affected, and often only one is involved. Numerous small abscesses are scattered throughout the kidney. These abscesses may open into the renal pelvis, so that one of the most characteristic symptoms is the presence of a large amount of pus in the urine, a condition called *pyuria*. The progress of the disease varies, and it may end in two very different ways:

1. The suppuration may extend, more and more renal tissue is destroyed, the small abscesses fuse and form large ones which communicate with the renal pelvis. The clinical picture is one of septic infection, and if the patient lives long enough one or both kidneys may become converted into large bags of pus. As so much kidney tissue is destroyed the patient will show symptoms of renal failure and will die of uremia, if he has not already died of septic infection.

2. In another group of cases the inflammatory process is much less violent, and in many of the inflamed areas healing occurs followed by scar formation. The infection continues in other areas, until these also become scarred. In this way the kidney is gradually destroyed, but it is now a mass of scar tissue instead of a bag of pus. The scar tissue contracts, so that the kidney becomes shrunken in size with a granular surface. In other words, it presents a picture of granular contracted kidney very similar to that of chronic glomerulonephritis. If both kidneys are involved the patient will again show evidence of renal failure and will die of uremia.

Hypertension is an invariable symptom of chronic Bright's disease. In a certain number of cases it develops in the chronic stage of pyelonephritis. Even though only one kidney is involved there may still be hypertension. This suggested the possibility of curing the hypertension by removing the diseased kidney. This has been done on a number of occasions, but the results have been disappointing. Although there is temporary benefit, sooner or later, and usually sooner, there is a return of the hypertension. There is also the danger that the remaining kidney may be affected, and then the last state of the patient will be worse than the first.

TUBERCULOSIS OF THE KIDNEY

Tuberculosis of the kidney is always secondary to tuberculosis elsewhere, usually in the lung or the lymphatic glands of the chest. The primary focus may be small and quiet, giving rise to no symptoms. The tubercle bacilli are carried by the blood to the kidney, where they are arrested. At first and often for a long time only one kidney is involved. The lesions are similar to those of tuberculosis of the lung, *i.e.*, gradual breaking down of tissue, discharge of the débris into the ureter, and formation of a series of cavities which finally coalesce and destroy the kidney (Fig. 70).

The *spread* of the disease is of great importance. The infection involves the ureter, producing thickening of the wall and narrowing of the lumen which may be so great that the lumen becomes completely blocked and the kidney is cut off from the bladder. The bacilli are carried by the urine down into the bladder, so that tuberculous ulcers are formed in that organ. The infection in the male may spread to the prostate gland situated in the floor of the bladder. Finally the other kidney may be involved either by upward spread from the bladder or from the original source in the lung.

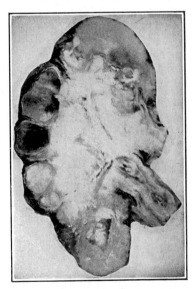

FIG. 70.—Tuberculous kidney, showing cavity formation.

The Basis of Symptoms.—It is a curious fact that the early symptoms of tuberculosis of the kidney are referable not to that organ but to the bladder. These symptoms are *painful* and *frequent urination*, and are explained by the tuberculous lesions in the bladder. The ulcers can be seen by means of a cystoscope passed into the bladder. In this way an early diagnosis can be made of which kidney is affected, because the urine from each ureter can be collected separately by means of the cystoscope. The urine contains pus, blood, and tubercle bacilli. The *pus* and *blood* come from the breaking-

down area in the kidney. In exceptional cases they may disappear after a time; this is due to the ureter becoming so completely blocked that the only urine which enters the bladder is from the sound kidney. The *tubercle bacilli* may be so scanty that they cannot be detected by the microscope. In such a case the urine is injected into a guinea-pig; if bacilli are present the animal will develop tuberculosis in the course of a few weeks. When the other kidney becomes seriously involved, symptoms of renal insufficiency will begin to make their appearance, and the development of uremia will finally ring down the curtain.

Treatment.—The treatment of renal tuberculosis is in part surgical, in part medical. The renal lesion will not heal of itself, because the kidney is an organ which cannot be put at rest. At the earliest moment that the diagnosis can be made the diseased kidney must be removed, else there is danger of spread of the disease to the other kidney. The bladder lesions will usually clear up spontaneously when the stream of bacilli from the kidney is cut off. Medical treatment in the form of rest, etc., is also advisable with a view to clearing up the original source of infection, lest the remaining kidney be involved at some later date.

URINARY CALCULUS

A urinary calculus is a stone which forms in the urinary tract. The common site of formation of the stone is the kidney, but it may form in the bladder. Stone in the kidney originates in the renal pelvis (Fig. 71),

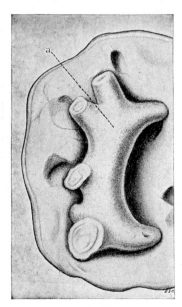 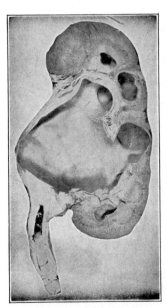

Fig. 71   Fig. 72

Fig. 71.—Stone in the kidney (*a*).

Fig. 72.—Hydronephrosis showing stone at upper end of ureter.

the chamber into which the urine is poured and from which the ureter collects it and conducts it to the bladder. Stone in the bladder may begin in the bladder, but more frequently it starts as a kidney stone and passes down into the bladder where it continues to grow.

The *causes* of stone can be guessed at, but not with certainty. *Infection* is an important factor, probably the most important in the case of stone in the bladder. In the kidney in addition to infection a *high concentration of crystalline salts* in the urine probably plays a part, for a urinary stone is composed of such inorganic materials as uric acid, oxalates, and calcium phosphate. Some stones consist entirely of one or other of these materials, but usually there is a mixture of two or more. *Diet* may be a factor in some cases, for stone is very common in countries such as India where a large proportion of the population lives on a vitamin-poor diet. Vitamin A is perhaps the most important of the vitamins in this respect. Recently it has come to be recognized that a small *tumor of the parathyroid glands* may be the cause of stone formation. These glands, which are four in number and lie in contact with the thyroid gland in the neck, are important regulators of calcium metabolism. When they become overactive, owing to the development of an innocent tumor, too much calcium phosphate is removed from the bones, carried by the blood to the kidneys, and deposited there.

The *effect on the kidney* is partly due to pressure, partly to blockage of the ureter. Pressure on the kidney due to a stone in the renal pelvis causes gradual destruction of that organ. Infection is always superadded and intensifies the destruction. The stone tends to block the upper opening of the ureter. Sometimes it passes down the ureter and blocks the lower end. In either case the urine accumulates behind the obstruction and produces great dilatation of the renal pelvis, a condition known as *hydronephrosis* (Fig. 72).

If severe infection with pyogenic organisms occurs, the fluid in the dilated pelvis will be pus instead of watery urine, and the condition is then called *pyonephrosis*. Pyonephrosis may also occur without the presence of a stone. The gradual accumulation of pus or watery urine leads to pressure on and destruction of the kidney. In time the kidney will cease to function and becomes useless to the patient. The *effect on the bladder* is similar. The combined irritation of the stone in the bladder and the infection which accompanies it causes inflammation of the bladder wall or *cystitis*. In addition the stone blocks the exit from the bladder (the urethra), and leads to dilatation not only of the bladder but also of both ureters and the pelvis of both kidneys, a condition of double hydronephrosis. This is much more dangerous than stone in the kidney, because the patient is threatened by renal failure owing to involvement of *both kidneys*.

The Basis of Symptoms.—The symptoms of urinary calculus are pain, the passage of pus and blood in the urine, and evidence of renal failure. The *pain* will be felt in the region of the kidney when the stone is in the renal pelvis. When it is in the bladder the chief pain is felt on urination owing to contraction of the bladder on the stone. If the stone in the kidney is small it may pass down the ureter causing *renal colic*. This is an agonizing pain felt along the line of the ureter, similar in nature and cause to the

13

extreme pain of biliary colic. The *pus* and *blood* in the urine are due to the irritation of the stone in the kidney and bladder, and the inflammation which results from that irritation. *Renal failure* may develop if there is a stone in both kidneys or if the outlet from the bladder is obstructed. It is due to the extensive destruction of renal tissue which occurs, and which may be caused as much by the accompanying inflammation as by the back-pressure of the accumulating urine.

Principles of Treatment.—The treatment of stone in the kidney is removal by surgical operation. Quack medicines, no matter what the claims of their purveyors, are powerless to dissolve a stone. In the early stages the stone can be removed through an incision in the renal pelvis. If the stone is allowed to become too large, it may be necessary to remove the kidney itself. If a parathyroid tumor is present this also will have to be removed to prevent the recurrence of the stone. A stone in the bladder can be crushed by means of an instrument passed along the urethra, and the fragments are then washed out without the bladder having to be opened. The temporary pain of renal colic must be treated by morphine.

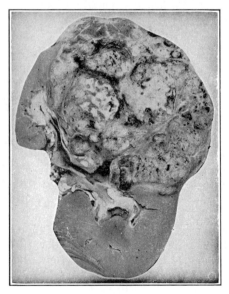
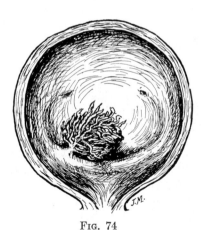

Fig. 73   Fig. 74

Fig. 73.—Hypernephroma.

Fig. 74.—Carcinoma of bladder, villous type.

TUMORS OF THE URINARY TRACT

Hypernephroma.—The only common tumor of the kidney is hypernephroma. This is a malignant tumor, a form of carcinoma, which gradually destroys the kidney and causes great enlargement of the organ (Fig. 73). The tumor invades the bloodvessels, so that secondary tumors are formed in the lungs, bones, and other organs. Sometimes the first indication of the

presence of a hypernephroma is the occurrence of a fracture due to weakening of the bone caused by the metastasis.

Symptom.—The chief symptom of hypernephroma is *blood in the urine*. In the early and sometimes in the late stages there is no pain in the region of the kidney. The presence of blood in the urine should always send the patient to his doctor.

Treatment.—The treatment is removal of the kidney containing the tumor. This is often successful if secondary growths have not occurred.

Carcinoma of the Bladder.—Carcinoma is the chief tumor of the bladder and is often of a low grade of malignancy, but it may be highly malignant. The tumor usually projects into the bladder in a papillary form. Sometimes it assumes a villous type, the growth consisting of delicate fern-like processes which unfold like a piece of seaweed when the bladder is filled with water and viewed with the cystoscope (Fig. 74). Each of these processes contains a thin-walled bloodvessel, which is readily injured when the bladder contracts during urination, so that hemorrhage is common.

Symptom.—The outstanding symptom is therefore *blood in the urine*, usually unaccompanied by pain (painless hematuria).

Treatment.—The treatment consists in opening the bladder and treating the tumor either by radium or by surgical removal. If an early diagnosis is made with the aid of the cystoscope, an instrument passed into the bladder by means of which a view of the interior can be obtained, the prognosis is good in very many cases.

THE PROSTATE

HYPERTROPHY OF THE PROSTATE

The prostate is a gland about the size of a horse chestnut situated at the neck of the bladder in the male and surrounding the urethra. It really belongs to the male reproductive system, but when diseased it produces symptoms associated with the urinary system on account of its position at the outlet of the bladder. Enlargement of the prostate is very common in men over sixty years of age, but fortunately it only produces symptoms in about 8 per cent of these cases. The disease is hardly ever seen in early life. The cause of the enlargement is probably some disturbance of the hormones from the sex glands which is likely to occur as the period of reproductive activity declines. It is comparable to the condition of the breast known as chronic mastitis which is described in the next chapter.

The *effects* of the prostatic enlargement are obstruction to the outflow of urine and an inability to empty the bladder completely. The *residual urine* retained in the bladder tends to undergo decomposition and becomes infected. The two great dangers which threaten the man suffering from enlargement of the prostate are (1) *urinary retention* with back-pressure on the ureters and kidneys, and (2) *infection* which ascends from the bladder to the kidneys. The results will be distention of the bladder, cystitis, dilatation of the ureters, hydronephrosis, and pyonephrosis (Fig. 75). Death is due either to sepsis or to renal failure.

Treatment.—Treatment has entirely changed the outlook for the man in declining years whose last days used to be made pitiable by prostatic enlargement. The enlarged gland can be removed by various surgical measures. One of these days it may be possible to control the enlargement by the use of hormones and thus render operation unnecessary.

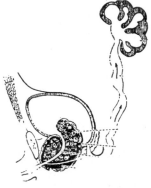

CANCER OF THE PROSTATE

Carcinoma of the prostate is unfortunately quite common. The prostate becomes enlarged and very firm, causing symptoms of urinary obstruction. The tumor infiltrates the surrounding structures early and extensively, and on that account surgical treatment is far from satisfactory. The bloodvessels are also invaded at an early date, and secondary growths are formed in various organs, particularly the bones. When an elderly man is found to be suffering from a tumor of bone, the prostate should always be examined. From what has been said it is evident that the prognosis in cancer of the prostate is very unfavorable.

FIG. 75.—Enlargement of prostate, the enlarged part projecting into the bladder and obstructing the urethra. The ureter and renal pelvis are dilated. (Joll and Leadley's Aids to Surgery; courtesy of Baillière, Tyndall & Cox.)

New light and new hope has been shed on the subject of carcinoma of the prostate by the demonstration that the male hormone of the testicle exerts an important influence on the growth of the prostate. Castration (removal of both testicles) before puberty prevents development of the prostate, and castration in adult life causes regression of the normal gland. These facts have been applied to the problem of the control of cancer of the prostate with remarkable results, for castration leads to marked shrinking of the tumor and great relief of the severe bone pains caused by metastases in the skeleton, particularly the spine. The administration of stilbestrol, the synthetic form of the female sex hormone, also affords marked relief, probably because of interference with the male hormone. This form of therapy is more widely used than is castration. Sometimes the two are combined.

A valuable means of determining the improvement produced by these methods of treatment is afforded by estimating the acid phosphatase in the blood. Phosphatase is an enzyme produced by the prostate, and the amount is greatly increased when cancer of the prostate develops, and especially when secondary tumors are formed in the bones. Under these circumstances there is a marked rise in the level of the blood phosphatase, a rise which disappears if the treatment is successful. The word success is used in only a relative sense, for it is not claimed that cancer of the prostate can be cured by these means.

TESTIS AND EPIDIDYMIS

The epididymis is the convoluted excretory duct of the testis, and although it lies separate from though attached to the testis, it may be considered with the latter in connection with disease.

Epididymitis.—By far the commonest cause of inflammation of the epididymis is the gonococcus, which extends from the male urethra during an acute attack of gonorrhea. The epididymis becomes enlarged, hard and tender. Minute abscesses are formed, but there is no extensive breaking down of tissue such as might be expected. The inflammation is acute and subsides quickly, but often leaves fibrous scars which obliterate the seminiferous tubules. When the condition is bilateral, complete sterility may result.

Orchitis.—The two common causes of inflammation of the testis (orchitis) are injury and mumps. Traumatic orchitis is caused by a blow, which is followed by an acute inflammatory edema of the organ. Mumps orchitis is usually unilateral, and is rarely seen before the age of puberty, being commonest in young men. It may follow or may precede the enlargement of the parotid gland which is characteristic of mumps.

Tuberculosis.—Tuberculosis usually starts in the lower pole of the epididymis. Tuberculous nodules are formed throughout that organ, and caseation may occur later with ulceration through the skin. Infection may spread to the testis and along the spermatic cord which is felt to be thickened and nodular. If the disease is progressive there may be successive involvement of the prostate, the other epididymis, the bladder, and finally the kidneys.

Tumors.—Tumors of the testis are fairly common. There are two principal groups named seminoma and teratoma. The *seminoma* appears to arise from the seminiferous tubules of the testis, whereas the *teratoma* is believed to arise from a primitive germ cell. Both of these tumors are highly malignant and tend to spread along the blood stream. Other rare tumors are found in the testis, but these do not need to be considered here.

THE URINE

Examination of the urine or urinalysis serves to show the presence of disease in the kidneys and bladder. It will also indicate the presence of diabetes, although this disease is not connected in any way with disorder of renal function. In a complete urinalysis the following points are noted: color, reaction, specific gravity, a chemical examination for albumin and sugar, and a microscopic examination for blood, pus, and casts.

Color.—The normal color of the urine is yellow or amber. The intensity of the color depends on the amount of water the urine contains. If the patient is drinking a large amount of water, the urine is dilute and pale. On the other hand if much water is lost by perspiration in hot weather or as the result of fever, the urine becomes highly colored. In diabetes there is a marked increase in the output of water, so that the urine is correspondingly pale. The same is true of chronic nephritis, where the kidneys lose their normal power of concentrating the urine. A smoky red or brown

color is usually due to the presence of large amounts of blood. Bile gives the urine a greenish-brown color; when a tube of such urine is shaken vigorously, the foam which appears on the surface is bright yellow instead of the normal white color. If the patient has been taking "gin pills," the urine is colored bright green. Normal urine is perfectly clear. Turbidity may be caused by the presence of blood or pus. On the other hand a normal urine may become turbid on standing owing to a deposit of phosphates or urates. Microscopic examination at once serves to distinguish between these conditions.

Reaction.—Although the blood is alkaline in reaction, the normal reaction of the urine is acid. This is readily shown by dropping a small piece of colored litmus paper into the urine. Blue litmus paper is turned red if the reaction is acid; red paper is turned blue if it is alkaline. In infections of the bladder the reaction tends to be alkaline owing to the action of bacteria. It is important for the nurse to remember that if the specimen of urine is forgotten and allowed to stand for many hours in a warm room, the normal acid reaction may be [changed to an alkaline one owing to the action of contaminating bacteria. The urine should therefore be fresh and sent at once to the laboratory. Decomposing urine has a characteristic ammoniacal smell (to be noticed in some urinals) owing to the production of ammonia from the urea in the urine.

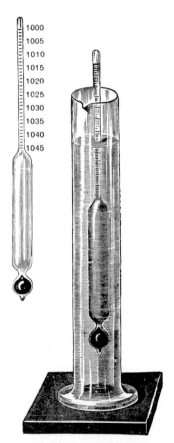

FIG. 76.—Urinometer.

Specific Gravity.—The specific gravity or concentration of the urine depends on the amount of solids (waste products of the tissues) held in solution. When the urine is secreted by the glomeruli it is of low concentration, but during its passage along the convoluted tubules a large amount of water is absorbed; this normal process is known as the concentrating power of the kidney. Extensive kidney disease, particularly chronic nephritis, results in destruction of large numbers of the renal tubules, with corresponding interference with the concentrating power. This loss of the normal concentrating power of the kidneys is one of the most valuable pieces of evidence of the presence of chronic Bright's disease. For this reason the estimation of the specific gravity of the urine is a procedure of the greatest importance, a fact which must be realized by the nurse who is often entrusted with the performance of the test.

The specific gravity is estimated by means of the urinometer (Fig. 76). This is a glass bulb with a graduated stem like a thermometer at one end,

and at the other end a mercury weight to keep the stem floating upright in the urine. It must not be allowed to touch the sides of the glass container. The *exact* level of the fluid is read against the graduated stem of the urinometer. This should be done in a good light, and the eyes must be on a level with that of the fluid.

The specific gravity of pure water is 1.000. The specific gravity of normal urine varies from 1.010 to 1.025, but it may be even higher as the result of loss of water through profuse perspiration, diarrhea, etc. In health there should be a variation of at least 10 points in the course of twenty-four hours, the first specimen in the morning being always the most concentrated. A low *fixed* specific gravity indicates chronic Bright's disease. A high gravity (1.030 to 1.040) suggests the presence of sugar, *i.e.,* diabetes.

Albumin.—When albumin is present in the urine (albuminuria) it comes from the blood, and is an indication of inflammation in the urinary tract as a result of which the permeability of the bloodvessels is increased. Two simple tests may be used, the heat and the salicylsulphonic acid tests. In the heat test a test-tube of urine is held by the bottom, and the upper part heated in the flame of a Bunsen burner. The appearance of a cloud in the upper part of the fluid (readily seen by contrast with the clear lower part) indicates either albumin or phosphates. The addition of a little dilute acetic acid dispels the cloud if it is due to phosphates, which are of no significance. In the salicylsulphonic acid test 3 cc. of a 3 per cent solution of this substance are added to 1 cc. of urine. This will produce varying amounts of turbidity depending on the amount of protein present in the urine.

Albuminuria is usually due to acute or chronic Bright's disease. The albumin may be present in very large amount, or there may be only a faint trace. As both blood and pus contain albumin, urine in which these substances are present will give a reaction for albumin. The commonest cause of albuminuria in the female is contamination with vaginal mucus, and so a positive test should always be confirmed on a catheter specimen of urine. If albumin is found in a urine it is essential to examine the deposit microscopically.

Sugar.—In nearly all cases the presence of sugar in the urine (glycosuria) indicates diabetes mellitus. The rare exceptions need not be discussed here. The kidneys are perfectly normal, but the blood sugar is so high that some of it leaks out into the urine. As the sugar is dissolved in the urine, the specific gravity is considerably above normal, *i.e.,* 1.040 or higher.

Sugar is tested for by means of Benedict's solution, which contains copper sulphate and is therefore blue in color. Five drops of urine are added to 5 cc. (a large teaspoonful) of the solution and boiled for one minute. If sugar is present the blue color changes to yellow or red.

Diacetic Acid and Acetone.—In the discussion of diabetes reference was made to the presence in the urine of diacetic acid and acetone, known as ketone bodies and indicative of acidosis, that grave complication of diabetes. When sugar is found in the urine it is therefore essential to test for the presence of ketone bodies. This is done by means of the nitroprusside test, known as Rotera's test. A few drops of a solution of sodium

nitroprusside are added to the urine and then a small quantity of ammonia is run onto the surface. A purple ring indicates the presence of ketone bodies.

In diabetes the ketone bodies may be present in large amount, particularly in severe acidosis with impending diabetic coma. Small amounts may appear in the urine in children after a general anesthetic, in fevers in children, and in the vomiting of pregnancy.

Blood.—If there is much blood in the urine it imparts to it a dark brown or smoky character. If the quantity is small there may be no naked eye change and microscopic examination for red cells is necessary. Two methods may be used in the microscopic examination of urinary deposits: (1) The specimen may be allowed to stand for a few hours in a conical glass or in a large test-tube; the deposit which collects at the bottom can then be removed by means of a pipette. (2) If the specimen has to be examined immediately it must be centrifuged, by which means the solid particles (blood cells, pus, casts, etc.) are rapidly drawn to the bottom of the tube. In examining for red blood cells the second method should be used, for when blood is allowed to remain in urine for some time many of the red cells become dissolved (hemolyzed).

Blood in the urine (hematuria) with rare exceptions indicates disease of the kidney, ureter, or bladder. The disease may be inflammation (acute or chronic nephritis), tuberculosis, stone, or tumor. Painless hematuria without any other symptoms suggests a malignant tumor of the kidney or bladder. When associated with pain it suggests a stone in the kidney or bladder, or tuberculosis of these organs.

Pus.—Pus in the urine (pyuria) gives a cloudy or turbid appearance. Microscopically large numbers of pus cells (polymorphonuclear leucocytes) are readily recognized. Pus in the urine may be caused by suppuration in the kidney (Bright's disease is non-suppurative), inflammation of the bladder (cystitis), tuberculosis or stone in the kidney or bladder. In the male, pus may come from the urethra, and in the female from the vagina. If pus is found in female urine, a second specimen should be obtained from the bladder by means of a catheter.

When tuberculosis of the kidney is suspected a search must be made for *tubercle bacilli*. These may be found in the centrifuged deposit. If not, a guinea-pig may be inoculated with a small quantity of urine or a culture made on special media. In both of these cases, unfortunately, several weeks must elapse before a definite result can be obtained.

Casts.—A urinary cast is a cast or mould of the renal tubules due to a collection in them of precipitated albumin. Red and white blood cells and epithelial cells from the lining of the kidney are often incorporated with the cast. Casts, which are oblong in shape, tend to disappear when the urine has been kept for some time; the specimen should therefore be fresh. The importance of casts is that they form an important feature of the urinary findings in Bright's disease. A few casts, spoken of in the report as "an occasional cast," may however be present in the absence of Bright's disease. When the urine is found to contain albumin it must always be examined for casts.

Crystals of various kinds are often found in the urine, but as they are of no special pathological significance they will not be described here.

Renal Function Tests.—In a sense every examination of the urine, except for sugar, is a test for renal function. But there may be pus or blood in the urine caused by a small tuberculous lesion or a stone in the renal pelvis without any real interference with the function of the kidney. There is a special group of tests known as functional renal tests which are designed to measure the excreting and concentrating power of the kidney. It is in Bright's disease that these essential functions of the kidney are interfered with or lost. Blood chemistry tests showing whether the waste substances (urea, creatinine, etc.) which the kidney should deal with are being normally excreted or retained in the blood, also afford valuable insight into the state of renal function. There is a multitude of renal function tests, but three of the simplest are the urine concentration test, the water test, and the dye test.

The urine concentration test is a test of the kidney's power to concentrate waste products removed from the blood. On the evening before the test the patient takes supper without fluid of any kind. He empties the bladder at bedtime, discarding the specimen. Next morning the bladder is again emptied and the urine saved in a bottle marked No. 1. An hour later a second specimen is collected and labelled No. 2. The specific gravity of both specimens is now taken with great care. If the specific gravity of either specimen is 1.025 or over, there is no serious impairment of renal function.

The dilution or *water test* also measures the concentrating power of the kidney. In the early morning, having emptied his bladder, the patient drinks 1000 cc. of water in the course of half an hour, but no more water during the day. The total amount of urine passed that day is measured and the specific gravity of each specimen passed is estimated. A normal person should excrete 1000 to 1200 cc. during the first four hours of the test. Some of the early specimens will have a specific gravity as low as 1.003. Later in the day the amount of urine decreases, and by the late afternoon the specimens will have a specific gravity as high as 1.025. When the function of the kidney is seriously impaired, as in chronic Bright's disease, the specific gravity may not go lower than 1.010, and as little as 400 cc. may be excreted in the first four hours. It will be noticed that in the urine concentration test attention is directed to how high the specific gravity goes, whilst in the water test we are interested in how low it goes. Both show *fixation of the specific gravity* to be one of the most valuable signs of serious impairment of renal function.

The dye test indicates the power of the kidney to excrete a dye injected into the blood stream. The dye employed is phenolsulphonephthalein, generally called P.S.P. for short. The patient drinks two glasses of water to promote active secretion of urine. Half an hour later he empties his bladder, and 1 cc. of the dye is injected into a vein. Specimens of urine are obtained in a quarter of an hour, half an hour, one hour, and two hours, and the amount of dye in each specimen is estimated. The average normal output of dye is 35 per cent in a quarter of an hour, 55 per cent in half an hour, 65 per cent in one hour, and 70 per cent in two hours. Less than

25 per cent in half an hour and 55 per cent in two hours indicates renal disease. In early disease the output of dye is merely delayed (this is why four specimens are taken), but in advanced disease the total amount is diminished. The dye test is an early indication of renal disease, but this is not necessarily Bright's disease. Urinary obstruction due to an enlarged prostate, etc., suppuration in the kidney, and congestion of the kidney due to heart failure, all interfere materially with the excretion of the dye.

An important use of the dye test is in the separate estimation of the function of the right and left kidneys. A catheter is passed into each ureter, so that the urine coming from each kidney together with the dye it contains is collected in a separate tube and labelled. In fifteen minutes each kidney should excrete 15 per cent of dye. The object of the test is to show *which* kidney is diseased in such a condition as renal tuberculosis, where one kidney has to be removed by the surgeon. From this the nurse will understand how vitally important it is that the tubes containing the urine from the two kidneys be correctly labelled. A mistake in the labelling may result in the healthy kidney being removed and may cost the patient his life. When the ureters are catheterized, even more important than the dye test is an examination for pus and blood.

Chapter

16

THE FEMALE REPRODUCTIVE SYSTEM

THE UTERUS

Structure and Function.—The reproductive system in woman consists
of four major parts (Fig. 77): (1) The *ovaries* where the ova or eggs are
produced; (2) the *Fallopian tubes* by which they are conducted to the uterus
and in which impregnation by the male element or spermatozoön occurs;
(3) the *uterus* or womb in which the impregnated ovum develops into an
embryo and then into a fetus; (4) the *vagina* or birth canal. The uterus is
divided into an upper part or *body* and a lower part or *cervix*. This distinction is important because the two parts are quite different in function
and in pathological behavior. The wall of the uterus is composed of involuntary muscle intermingled with fibrous tissue, and its cavity is lined
by a mucous membrane called the *endometrium*.

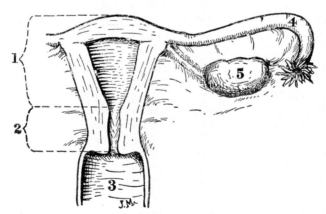

FIG. 77.—Female reproductive organs. 1, Body of uterus; 2, cervix; 3, vagina; 4, Fallopian tube; 5, ovary.

Every month the endometrium undergoes a change of the greatest
importance known as *menstruation* (*mensis*, a month), for every month
an ovum is discharged from one of the ovaries, and the endometrium shows
changes similar to those at the beginning of pregnancy in the expectation
that the ovum may be impregnated. When impregnation fails to occur the
prepared endometrium undergoes necrosis and is cast off, accompanied by

a discharge of blood lasting for several days. When the menstrual flow is excessive, it is known as *menorrhagia*; when there is bleeding between the menstrual periods it is known as *metrorrhagia*. Absence of menstrual bleeding is called *amenorrhea*. After menstruation has ceased the endometrium is reformed from the fragments that are left, only to be cast off again at the end of another month.

This strange cycle is directly dependent on a similar monthly cycle in the ovaries, the communication between the two organs being by chemical messengers or *hormones*. There are two of these hormones, each of which produces a different effect on the endometrium. In order to understand the origin of these hormones we must look a little more closely at what is going on in the ovary. Each ovary contains thousands of ova, but only one is discharged from the ovary every month. The chosen ovum undergoes a process of ripening. It lies in a little cavity, the *Graafian follicle*, containing a watery fluid and lined by specialized cells. The follicular fluid is the source of the first of the ovarian hormones, which is carried by the blood to the uterus where it acts on the endometrium and also to the kidneys by which it is excreted in the urine. It is known as *œstrin* or the female sex hormone. The follicle approaches the surface of the ovary, and at the very middle of the month, about the fourteenth day, the ovum is discharged into the end of the Fallopian tube (ovulation). The follicle at once undergoes a peculiar series of changes, as a result of which it is converted into a solid yellow body, the *corpus luteum*, which in turn produces a hormone of its own. This hormone is responsible for the changes in the endometrium designed to nourish the impregnated ovum when it reaches the uterus, so that in the absence of the corpus luteum pregnancy is impossible, for the fertilized ovum cannot be retained. When pregnancy occurs the corpus luteum becomes greatly enlarged (corpus luteum of pregnancy) and produces a correspondingly increased amount of hormone. The reason for this increase in size will be apparent presently. The corpus luteum hormone is called *progestin*, because it prepares the uterus for pregnancy (gestation). It will be seen presently that failure of the corpus luteum to develop will give rise to serious pathological changes.

Just as the endometrium is under the influence of the ovary, so the ovary is under the influence of the *pituitary gland*. The periodicity of the ovary is not inherent in itself, but is dependent on the pituitary which regulates it. Injections of pituitary extract will cause an immature female animal rapidly to become mature with development of Graafian follicles and production of the female sex hormone. The starting motor of the complex monthly menstrual cycle is undoubtedly the tiny pituitary gland lying on the floor of the skull and covered by the brain. The pituitary hormone which produces these effects has been called the pituitary sex hormone, the gonad (ovary) stimulating hormone, and *prolan*. The prolan is excreted from the blood into the urine.

To complicate matters still further it appears that another very powerful hormone is produced by the *placenta*. This structure is the organ of communication between the mother and fetus, being derived partly from the maternal endometrium, partly from the chorion, a membrane which covers the developing fetus (Fig. 78). The chorionic part of the placenta

contains large quantities of hormone. It used to be thought that this was produced by the pituitary and stored in the placenta, but the work of Collip has made it clear that the hormone is produced by the placenta itself. As it resembles the action of the sex hormone of the pituitary it is known as the *A-P-L* or *anterior pituitary-like principle*. It is absorbed into the blood stream, and is excreted in large quantities in the urine. It is carried by the blood to the ovaries and there stimulates the corpus luteum to develop into the corpus luteum of pregnancy. Its presence in the urine is the basis of the well-known Aschheim-Zondek test for pregnancy. In this test the patient's urine is injected into the ear vein of an immature female rabbit. If the woman is pregnant the A-P-L hormone in the urine will stimulate the rabbit's ovaries to such a degree that in the course of one hundred hours they become greatly enlarged, and present small red spots which are follicles into which hemorrhage has occurred. This test has other uses which will be referred to later.

It will make for clearness of thinking and serve to assist the memory if it be kept in mind that there are four hormones of interest to us in relation to the female sex cycle. These are œstrin and progestin from the ovary, prolan from the pituitary, and A-P-L from the placenta. Œstrin and progestin act on the endometrium, prolan and A-P-L act on the ovary and thus indirectly on the uterus.

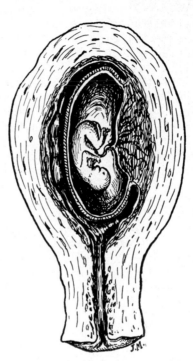

FIG. 78.—Pregnant uterus showing placenta and fetus.

It is well to recall that nearly all the remarkable facts which have just been described are of very recent discovery. The phenomenon of menstruation used to be a complete mystery, and no one dreamed that its regulator and starting motor was to be sought for in a little gland inside the skull. The whole story is one of the romances of medicine, a romance which has been brought to a rapid as well as a satisfactory conclusion.

ENDOMETRIAL HYPERPLASIA AND FUNCTIONAL HEMORRHAGE

At the time of the menopause or change of life a woman may begin to suffer from irregular uterine hemorrhage, which may take the form either of periodic bleeding or of prolonged and continuous bleeding. This irregu-

lar hemorrhage may occur at earlier age periods, and sometimes even in young women. The endometrium is markedly thickened. It used to be thought that this bleeding condition was due to some disease of the uterus, but we now know that the essential trouble lies not in the uterus but in the ovaries. For this reason the condition is called functional uterine hemorrhage, the associated thickening of the endometrium being endometrial hyperplasia.

We have already seen that two ovarian hormones act on the endometrium to produce normal menstruation, the one, œstrin, from the ripening follicles, the other, progestin, from the corpus luteum. It is apparently œstrin which is mainly responsible for menstruation, whilst progestin brings the process to a conclusion. The onset of pregnancy is marked by an immediate cessation of menstruation due to the continuous overproduction of progestin by the enlarged corpus luteum which persists during the entire duration of pregnancy. The corpus luteum is only formed after ovulation has occurred, i.e., when the ovum is discharged from the follicle. The basic trouble in functional uterine hemorrhage is failure of ovulation, with overproduction of œstrin and insufficient production of progestin. The A-P-L hormone of the placenta produces the opposite state of affairs, i.e., ovulation, suppression of œstrin and stimulation of progestin formation. For this reason many cases of functional uterine hemorrhage are being treated with A-P-L hormone. If this fails, the activity of the ovaries may have to be destroyed by radiation. Before the nature of the condition was understood the only effective treatment used to be removal of the uterus (hysterectomy). Owing to lack of the usual monthly destruction and removal of the endometrium, the lining of the uterus becomes greatly thickened (endometrial hyperplasia). This may have to be rectified by scraping of the uterus (curettage).

PUERPERAL SEPSIS

The normal uterus is remarkably resistant to infection, but in the puerperium, the period after childbirth, it is extremely liable to infection on account of the raw surface of the interior and the presence of blood clots and fragments of placenta. The danger of infection is much greater after an abortion than after delivery at full term, owing to the greater likelihood of fragments of placenta being retained and acting as a suitable culture medium for any bacteria which may be introduced. Secondary factors which predispose to infection are instrumental interference, exhaustion, and hemorrhage. In the vast majority of cases infection is introduced either by the examining hand or by an unsterilized instrument used to produce abortion. The less manual examination a woman receives during labor, the less likely is she to develop puerperal infection, for the hand is apt to carry microörganisms from the vagina up into the uterus. The commonest cause of fatal puerperal infection is Streptococcus hæmolyticus. This may come from the throat of the attending physician or nurse, so that the wearing of a mask is a valuable protective measure. In a small proportion of cases the hemolytic streptococci apparently come

from the throat of the patient, being carried to the uterus by the blood stream.

In the fatal cases the cavity of the uterus is lined by dirty, necrotic, breaking-down material swarming with streptococci which have also widely invaded the uterine wall and may in this way set up general peritonitis. Infection may reach the peritoneal cavity from the uterus by passing along the Fallopian tubes, with resulting fatal peritonitis. An equally great danger is infection of the large blood clots which occupy the gaping and torn vessels. These infected clots become broken down, converted into septic emboli, and carried by the blood stream throughtout the body causing septicemia and pyemia. In such cases the streptococci will readily be found in blood culture, and the clinical picture is that of acute blood poisoning. The patient is thus exposed to the double threat of septicemia and general peritonitis.

The above account is now largely of historic interest, because with modern chemotherapy the infection can be nipped in the bud. It is well, however, for the student to know something of the risks from infection which women used to run in giving birth to a child.

Penicillin and other antibiotics are so effective against puerperal sepsis that the fear of this complication of pregnancy no longer exists. This condition was one of the first infections in which the efficacy of sulfonamide therapy was demonstrated, but the sulfonamide drugs have now largely been replaced by penicillin and other antibiotics.

ENDOCERVICITIS

The uterus, as we have already seen, is divided into an upper part, the body, and a lower part, the neck or cervix. The changes characteristic of menstruation and pregnancy are confined to the endometrium of the body. As it is on this part of the uterus that the ovarian hormones act, this is naturally the part affected by such disorders as functional hemorrhage. Up to the present the cervix has seemed remarkably immune from disease. We have now to learn that it is the site of two common pathological conditions, namely, chronic inflammation and cancer.

Inflammation of the cervix, or rather the lining of the cervix, is known as endocervicitis. Its frequency is due partly to the structure of the mucous membrane of the cervix, partly to the fact that the lining of the cervix is not swept away every month as in the case of the uterine body, so that infection can lodge in it for long periods. The glands in the lining of the body of the uterus are comparatively simple and tubular, but those in the cervix are highly complex and branching like the streets in the native quarter of an oriental city, so that infecting organisms may lurk there for long periods, not only causing local inflammation but sallying forth and causing trouble at a distance. Two sets of organisms may give rise to chronic endocervicitis: (1) the ordinary pyogenic bacteria such as staphylococcus, streptococcus, and Bacillus coli, which tend to invade the tissue as the result of a tear during childbirth; (2) the gonococcus, the infection of the cervix occurring during an attack of gonorrhea.

Cervical erosion is the name given to the inflammatory lesion which follows injury to the cervix during delivery. When the cervix is examined by means of a speculum in the vaginal canal a red patch is observed which has an appearance of rawness or erosion. The underlying tissue is filled with inflammatory cells, and the bacteria responsible for the inflammation may keep it going for months or years.

The *chief symptom* of inflammation of the cervix is *leucorrhea*, a word which means white discharge. This discharge is a sticky glairy fluid which is poured out by the irritated cervical glands. Leucorrhea is one of the commonest of female disorders. The *chief danger* of cervical erosion is the possibility that cancer may develop later, *i. e.*, that the inflammatory lesion may prove to be a precancerous one. This matter will be referred to again in connection with cancer of the cervix.

FIBROIDS OF THE UTERUS

A fibroid of the uterus is an innocent tumor consisting essentially of involuntary muscle, but containing a varying amount of fibrous tissue. Pathologically, therefore, it is a myoma, but the old name of fibroid is universally used. It is an extremely common tumor, but very often it gives rise to no symptoms. One of its most striking characteristics is that it only develops during the period of reproductive activity. It never appears before puberty nor after the menopause, although naturally fibroids which are already present will persist after the change of life. This suggests very strongly that ovarian hormones play some part in stimulating the growth of the tumor. The tumors are frequently multiple. In size they vary from a pea to a child's head. They somewhat resemble the surrounding uterine muscle, from which they are separated by a definite capsule, but they are whiter and more dense. The tumor may grow towards the cavity of the uterus, pushing the mucous membrane in front of it, and is then known as a *submucous* fibroid (Fig. 79). Or it may grow outwards, projecting from the surface of the uterus and pushing the peritoneum in front of it; it is then called a *subperitoneal* fibroid, and may only be attached to the uterus by a narrow stalk or pedicle.

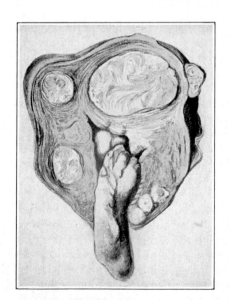

FIG. 79.—Fibroids of uterus; some tumors are in the muscular wall, and one hangs down in the cavity.

has o
cervi
impr(

Th
accou
tissue
and a
fetal t
be pr
pregn
aborti
Morec
30 per
of the
hydati
in the
The
very s(
it inva
the la:
early in
by the
ularly
second:
The
hemorr
weeks
should
theliom
firmed
Zondek
Hyda
"like h
mole is
in abou
ceases t
there is
not a n
the A-F
in the u
test rem
from the
developi
the mol
to form

Symptoms.—The symptoms are variable. Often there are none. A submucous fibroid is likely to cause *uterine hemorrhage*. This may take the form of excessive menstrual bleeding (*menorrhagia*) or bleeding between the periods (*metrorrhagia*). A large fibroid may cause *pelvic pain,* pressure on the rectum with *constipation,* or pressure on the veins from the leg with resulting *edema.* Occasionally the narrow pedicle of a subperitoneal fibroid may become twisted, causing a sudden attack of severe pain.

Principles of Treatment.—Frequently the symptoms are not sufficiently severe to demand any drastic form of treatment. If operation is necessary it may be possible to remove the tumor without the uterus, especially in the case of subperitoneal pedunculated fibroids. When, as is usually the case, the tumors are in the uterine wall and submucous in character, the uterus has to be removed together with the fibroids, an operation known as hysterectomy.

CANCER OF THE UTERUS

Cancer of the uterus is one of the commonest forms of cancer and this tumor grows from the cervix in 90 per cent of the cases (Fig. 80). The great susceptibility of the cervix compared with the body of the uterus is possibly related to the frequency with which the cervix is injured during childbirth, for at least 96 per cent of the cases are in women who have borne children.

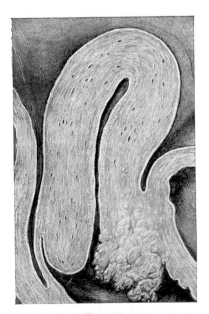

Fig. 80

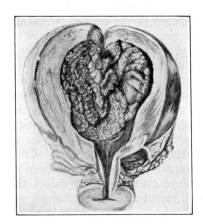

Fig. 81

Fig. 80.—Carcinoma of the cervix uteri. The tumor has destroyed one side of the cervix and is invading the bladder wall. (Schmitz, Surg., Gynec. and Obst.)

Fig. 81.—Carcinoma of body of uterus. The tumor projects into the uterine cavity, but does not involve the cervix.

14

The practical application of all this now becomes evident. Hydatidiform mole is an essentially innocent condition, which requires no more drastic treatment than clearing out the uterus. It always holds the threat, however, that it may develop into a chorionepithelioma. This tumor, although highly malignant, can be cured if the uterus is removed sufficiently early. The change from the benign mole to the malignant tumor is indicated by the continuance of the Aschheim-Zondek reaction in the urine after the mole has been removed.

THE FALLOPIAN TUBES

The Fallopian tubes are the ducts, one on each side, which lead from the ovaries to the uterus, along which the ovum passes, and in which fertilization of the ovum takes place. The inner end of the tube opens into the uterus and the outer end into the peritoneal cavity. Both ends are readily closed by inflammation, which is by far the commonest pathological condition to affect the tubes and which is called salpingitis.

SALPINGITIS

By far the most important cause of salpingitis is gonorrhea, which is responsible for at least 80 per cent of the cases. Pyogenic cocci, especially streptococci, cause 15 per cent. The remaining 5 per cent are tuberculous in nature. The effect on the tube depends largely on the virulence of the infection. The outer end usually becomes closed early, so that the peritoneal cavity is shielded from infection. If the inner end still remains open the condition is called a *pus tube*. When both ends are closed the tube becomes markedly distended with fluid. If the infection is virulent the inflammation will be purulent in type, the tube is filled with pus, and the condition is known as *pyosalpinx*. If the infection is mild the inflammation is more in the nature of a catarrh and the fluid is watery in type, a condition of *hydrosalpinx*.

The infection usually reaches the tubes from the uterus, so that salpingitis is usually bilateral. The distention of the tubes may be enormous, and they may resemble bananas. Adhesions to surrounding structures may be very dense, so that operative removal may be a matter of great difficulty. *Sterility* is an inevitable result if both tubes are closed, as the ovum is unable to pass along the obstructed tubes. In addition there is often pelvic pain, menstrual disturbances, and general invalidism.

Tuberculous salpingitis is very similar to the salpingitis produced by gonococci and other organisms except that the inflammation is not purulent. The tubes are thickened, and may be greatly distended with caseous tuberculous material. The infection reaches the tubes by the blood stream from some tuberculous focus elsewhere.

TUBAL PREGNANCY

Impregnation of the ovum takes place during its passage along the Fallopian tube, not in the uterus itself. If the fertilized ovum should

be entrapped in the folds and crevices of the mucous membrane of the tube, it will develop into an embryo in the tube instead of in the uterus, a condition known as tubal or *ectopic* pregnancy (Fig. 83). Chronic salpingitis causes thickening of the folds and deepening of the pockets between them, so that it acts as a strong predisposing cause of tubal pregnancy.

As the embryo grows in size it burrows deeper into the wall of the tube and causes increasing distention of the lumen. An accident is almost certain to happen by the end of the second month. The pregnancy may terminate in one of two ways, by tubal abortion or by tubal rupture. *Tubal abortion* is the usual course. There is hemorrhage into the placenta which has formed in the tube, with destruction of the embryo and distention of the tube with blood clot, a condition called *hematosalpinx*. This is accompanied by severe pain in the right or left groin, and a flow of blood from the uterus. These symptoms together with amenorrhea for two months will usually allow a correct diagnosis to be made.

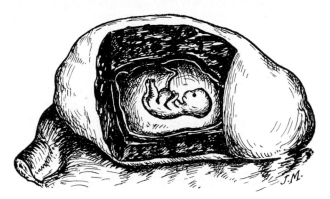

Fig. 83.—Tubal pregnancy.

The great danger of ectopic pregnancy is *tubal rupture*, which occurs in about 25 per cent of the cases. The wall of the tube ruptures, severe bleeding occurs into the abdominal cavity, and the patient may die of internal hemorrhage. It is on account of the danger of tubal rupture that the correct treatment of ectopic pregnancy is surgical removal of the tube.

THE OVARIES

The ovaries are two small flat organs, rather larger than a bean, which lie one on either side of the uterus, and are connected with it by the Fallopian tubes. Each ovary contains more than 100,000 Graafian follicles in which ova are formed, but only a small number of these may come to maturity. The chief pathological conditions affecting the ovaries are cysts and tumors.

CYSTS AND TUMORS OF THE OVARY

Ovarian cysts may be of two kinds, retention cysts and tumor cysts or cystadenomas. *Retention cysts* are of very common occurrence. They arise

from Graafian follicles which have never matured and discharged their ova on the surface, and are usually multiple but small in size, so that the ovary is only slightly enlarged. On account of their origin they are called *follicular cysts*. It used to be a common practice to remove such cystic ovaries under the belief that they were responsible for pelvic pain and other common female complaints, but this practice has been largely given up.

Cystadenomas are of very different character. Although they take the form of cysts, *i.e.*, cavities filled with fluid, they are really innocent tumors, and may accordingly grow to an enormous size. Before the days of modern surgery it was not unusual to see the entire abdomen filled with one of these great bags of fluid. The contents are sometimes watery, sometimes jelly-like. The cavity is often multiloculated so that the main cyst contains many smaller cysts. The lining is usually smooth, but may be covered by papillary processes; in the latter case there is a distinct danger that the tumor may become malignant. The papillary processes perforate the wall of the cyst, become scattered over the peritoneal cavity, and form there large secondary malignant masses. The irritation to the peritoneum leads to an outpouring of watery fluid, a condition of ascites.

As long as the cystadenoma is innocent, removal of the tumor will bring about cure. Even when it becomes malignant, removal may be successful if secondary growths have not been formed.

Dermoid cyst is a common form of ovarian tumor which takes a cystic form. It is a teratoma, a developmental tumor arising from an ovum and representing an attempt to form a new individual. It may, therefore, contain a variety of structures such as skin, hair, teeth, bone, brain tissue, etc. It is filled with yellow buttery material produced by the glands in the skin which it contains, and hair is a constant ingredient. Although this cystic tumor may attain a large size, it is essentially innocent in character.

Tumors of the ovary may be cystic or solid. The cystic tumors are the cystadenomas which have just been described. The solid tumors are nearly all malignant, for the most part carcinoma. Carcinoma of the ovary may be primary or secondary. *Secondary cancer* is much commoner than primary, being usually secondary to cancer of the stomach or large bowel. The tumor cells are carried from the stomach through the peritoneal cavity and are implanted on both ovaries so that the tumor is bilateral. *Primary cancer* is comparatively uncommon. It forms a large solid mass which replaces the ovary; tumor cells are often implanted on the second ovary, so that both ovaries must be removed, although only one may appear to be affected.

Chapter

17

THE BREAST

Structure and Function.—The breast resembles the uterine endometrium in many respects, for it changes markedly in structure in response to the needs of reproduction, it is played upon by influences from the ovary and pituitary, some of its commonest disorders are connected with disturbance of these influences, and it is a very common site of cancer. It varies markedly in microscopic appearance as well as in size at varying periods of life. At all periods, however, it consists partly of glandular tissue, for the breast is essentially a gland, and partly of fat.

In the *newborn*, both male and female, the breasts may be slightly swollen and contain milk (witch's milk), due to stimulation by the female sex hormone in the mother's blood. Up to puberty there is almost no glandular tissue in the breast, but at *puberty* under the influence of ovarian hormones there is rapid growth of glandular tissue in the female breasts, the outlines of which become rounded and full. It is, of course, during *pregnancy* and *lactation* that the glandular overgrowth is most marked, the stimulus being again due to ovarian and now also to placental hormones. At the *menopause* there is great atrophy of the glandular tissue.

It is evident that the breast is capable of great hypertrophy, and of correspondingly great involution in which there is an attempt to return to the former state. A similar but much smaller swing of the pendulum takes place during each menstrual cycle, the glandular tissue enlarging and then regressing. As a result of pathological conditions, *e.g.*, abnormal ovarian stimuli, there may be deviations from the normal. In the first place the hyperplasia and involution may be more localized to one part of the breast than another. In the second place, involution may be less complete than hyperplasia, as a result of which some of the gland spaces may remain dilated and become converted into cysts. These two results are often combined, so that localized areas of overgrowth are produced, which may be well or poorly demarcated from the surrounding breast and which contain cysts of varying size. There are only three common diseases of the breast, cystic hyperplasia, fibroadenoma, and carcinoma; the first two appear to be a direct outcome of the cyclic changes which have just been described.

CHRONIC MASTITIS.   CYSTIC HYPERPLASIA

This, which is the commonest lesion of the female breast, is generally called *chronic mastitis,* but this name was given when it was supposed to be a chronic inflammation of the breast and when the true nature of the

condition was not known. It usually occurs about the time of the meno-pause, but is by no means confined to that period of life, and a group of cases are seen in young unmarried women with menstrual evidence of disturbed ovarian function. Both in the young and in the elderly the hyperplasia is due to irregular and abnormal stimuli coming from the ovaries. As a result of these irregular stimuli a hyperplasia of the breast occurs which is patchy in character, affecting groups of the lobules into which the breast is divided. Cyst formation is a prominent feature. Each month the process is repeated, so that the lesion is gradually intensified.

The *clinical features* are characteristic. The woman, usually between the age of forty and fifty years, has commonly borne a number of children, and now complains either of *pain* or of a *lump in the breast*. The pain, as a rule, is worse at the menstrual period, and there is tenderness of the breast as well as pain. Both breasts are often involved and there may be several lumps in each breast. The lump may feel exactly like a tumor, especially if it contains one or more large cysts; these are so tense that they give the feeling of a solid mass.

Chronic mastitis is an innocent lesion, which can be treated by local removal. But it must be treated with respect for two reasons: in the first place, the doctor can never be certain before operation whether a lump in the breast is innocent or malignant, and in the second place lobular hyperplasia may act as a precancerous lesion, *i.e.*, it may develop later into cancer. The area affected may be very small and localized, so that the operation does not need to be a mutilating one. On the other hand it is advisable in an elderly woman, in whom the danger of cancer is greater and the importance of the breast less, to remove the entire breast.

FIBROADENOMA

This is an innocent tumor of the breast, occurring chiefly in young women, often originating at puberty and growing during the years of de-veloping sexual activity. It forms a firm, circumscribed, peculiarly movable mass with no attachment to the overlying skin or the underlying tissue. It is easily removed, and carries no threat of developing into cancer. As its name implies it is formed by an overgrowth both of fibrous and glandular tissue. Although we have spoken of the lesion as a tumor, it is really more of a localized and encapsulated form of cystic hyperplasia, although without cyst formation, and may be attributed to abnormal ovarian stimuli at the beginning of the reproductive period.

It is not wise to draw too close a parallel between lesions of the breast and those of the uterus, but it is allowable to compare lobular hyperplasia of the breast with endometrial hyperplasia and fibroadenoma of the breast with fibroids of the uterus.

CANCER OF THE BREAST

Carcinoma of the breast is one of the commonest forms of malignant disease. It usually occurs in the years before the menopause, but may

develop at the age of eighty or ninety years; it is rare before the age of thirty-five. It is rather commoner in those who have not borne children. Injury to the breast bears no relation to the development of cancer. Lobular hyperplasia, however, may act as a predisposing cause. Cancer of the breast is often called *scirrhous cancer*. The term means hard, and describes a common characteristic of breast cancer. Other forms of cancer also occur, but for convenience in this brief outline only the characteristics of scirrhous carcinoma will be described.

It usually begins in the upper and outer segment of the breast, and forms a hard nodule which can be best appreciated by the palm of the hand rather than the fingers. It may not be nearly so readily felt as a fibroadenoma. It is important to realize that no matter how small a lump in

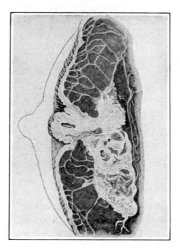

FIG. 84.—Cancer of the breast. The white mass is the tumor. The nipple is retracted. Dotted line shows normal outline of breast.

the breast may be it may still be cancer. I have seen a nodule of the breast no larger than a pea, but when it was removed it was found to be carcinoma. It is wise to regard every lump in the breast as malignant until it has been proved to be innocent. If the advanced signs are waited for, it is then too late. These advanced signs are fixation of the tumor to the overlying skin and to the chest wall, indrawing of the nipple (Fig. 84), dimpling of the skin, and enlargement of the lymph glands in the axilla (armpit) and in the neck.

The tumor in the patient may feel to be a circumscribed lump, but when it has been removed it will be found to blend with the surrounding breast. It cuts with the peculiar hard grittiness of an unripe pear, and the cut surface is concave instead of convex, as in the fibroadenoma.

Spread of the tumor occurs by infiltration, by the lymph stream, and by the blood stream. By *infiltration* the tumor cells spread throughout the breast, to the overlying skin, and to the underlying muscle (Fig. 85). This microscopic spread is very much wider than the tumor which can be seen

with the naked eye, so that the surgeon has to remove a wide area of skin and muscle as well as the entire breast itself. *Lymph spread* carries the tumor cells to the lymphatic glands in the axilla, so that the contents of the axilla have also to be dissected away lest any cancer be left from which a recurrence of the tumor may occur. Unfortunately lymph vessels may also carry tumor cells to lymphatic glands in the chest and in the neck. *Blood spread* carries the tumor to distant organs such as the brain, lungs, and bones.

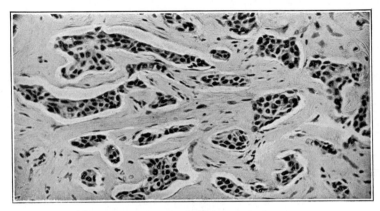

Fig. 85.—Microscopic picture of cancer cells infiltrating the breast.

Principles of Treatment.—The prognosis or outlook for the patient depends partly on the earliness of the diagnosis, partly on the thoroughness of the treatment. Statistics vary much in different clinics and in different countries, but it has been estimated that of patients treated efficiently and thoroughly, 50 per cent are alive and well after three years and 30 per cent after ten years. Of patients in whom the disease is confined to the breast without involvement of the lymph nodes, over 85 per cent are alive and well at the end of ten years.

The breast must be completely removed, together with a wide area of overlying skin, the underlying pectoral muscle and the lymphatic glands in the axilla. If the removal is not wide, there is every chance of a recurrence. In addition to operation, radiation is beginning to play a part of ever-increasing importance. The radiation may be in the form of radium or roentgen-rays, and it may be given before operation or after operation. In some cases radiation without operation has been employed. It is not possible to say at present what the ultimate place of radiation may be in the treatment of cancer of the breast. With increasing improvements in apparatus and in methods of application it appears probable that it will come to assume a position of commanding importance.

Chapter

18

THE DUCTLESS GLANDS

THE *ductless* or *endocrine glands* form the most interesting group of organs in the body. Ordinary glands, such as those concerned with digestion, pour their secretion into the mouth, stomach or intestine where they act upon the foodstuffs. The endocrine glands have no ducts, so that their secretions, instead of passing into one of the cavities of the body, are absorbed directly into the blood. But the difference between the two sets of glands is much greater than this, for the secretion of the ductless glands, known as hormones, governs some of the most fundamental metabolic processes of the body, and exert a far-reaching influence on the personality itself. This becomes evident when we remember that the sex glands belong to this group. Moreover, it is now known that subtle and but dimly understood relationships exist between the various endocrines. They may be compared to an orchestra in which, when on instrument is out of tune, a perfect ensemble is impossible. As has been remarked in a previous chapter, the leader of the glandular orchestra is the pituitary.

Large treatises have been written on the ductless glands, but in this place it will be possible to give brief consideration to only five members of the group, disturbance of the function of which is reflected in the symptoms of disease. These are the thyroid, parathyroids, adrenals, islets of Langerhans, and pituitary. Reference has already been made to disorders of the female sex glands. Speaking generally, the endocrine glands may show evidence of disorder in one of two ways: there may be *hyperactivity* associated with the production of an excess of hormone, or there may be *hypoactivity* associated with an insufficient production of hormone. Overproduction of hormone may be caused by the presence of a tumor, usually benign in character, but this is not necessarily the case. Hypoactivity is usually the result of destruction of the gland produced by disease.

THE THYROID GLAND

Structure and Function.—The thyroid gland is an organ of some size, shaped like a shield, which lies on either side of the neck in the region of the larynx or Adam's apple. It is composed entirely of a large number of spaces or *acini*, lined by low epithelial cells, and filled with jelly-like material known as *colloid*, which is richer in iodine than any other substance in the body (Fig. 86). Between the acini run thin-walled capillaries, into which the secretion of the epithelial cells is poured. But part of this secretion, when not actively needed by the body, passes into the acini and is

(223)

stored as colloid, which may be regarded as an emergency ration to be given up to the body on demand.

The chief *function* of the thyroid is to maintain a certain rate of metabolism, as evidenced by oxygen consumption and heat production, and to regulate this rate according to the needs of the body. This is done by means of its iodine-containing hormone, *thyroxin.* The effect of feeding thyroid gland or injecting thyroxin is to raise the rate of metabolism. Removal of the thyroid is followed not only by a loss of heat production, but also by poor physical, mental, and sexual development, most marked, of course, in the young. It would appear, therefore, that an adequate supply of thyroid secretion is necessary for the development of the young animal. Similarly an excess of secretion will accelerate development, as can be shown by the rapidity with which thyroxin brings about the change from a tadpole into a frog. Thyroid secretion appears to act as a general and necessary stimulant without which there can be no health or vigor of the body, no flash and speed of the mind. Someone with a turn for the picturesque has remarked that thyroxin converts the sluggish toad into the lively frog. The bearing of these observations will become very evident when diseases of the thyroid are considered.

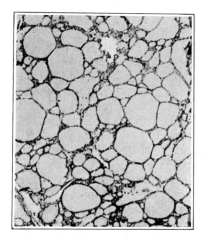

Fig. 86.—Microscopic picture of normal thyroid gland.

The activity of the thyroid is gauged by estimating the *basal metabolic rate,* the amount of metabolism in a person at complete physical and mental rest. This is actually done by determining the amount of oxygen consumed when a person is under these basal conditions. If during the test the person makes the slightest physical or mental exertion, the metabolic rate at once goes up, and the test is invalidated. Even the effort required to digest a meal is sufficient to spoil the test.

The thyroid takes iodine from the blood which flows through it and converts it into thyroxin, and gives it back to the blood or stores it as the case may be. If there is an insufficiency of iodine in the food or water, the thyroid finds itself in the same position as the Children of Israel when they were ordered by the Egyptians to make bricks without straw. But as the Israelites rose to the occasion by redoubling their efforts, so the thyroid responds by working overtime, and in doing so it becomes larger. This enlargement is known as *goiter.* It is evident that this enlargement is compensatory in character, being analogous to the enlargement of the heart when that organ is given too much work to do. It is not associated with symptoms of hyperthyroidism or overactivity of the thyroid. Other

forms of goiter, as we shall see, are of a different nature, and are accompanied by marked symptoms of hyperthyroidism.

The term goiter simply means an enlargement of the thyroid. As this enlargement may be due to more than one cause, it is obvious that the symptoms will vary correspondingly. Three forms of goiter may be recognized: these are simple goiter, adenomatous goiter, and exophthalmic goiter.

SIMPLE GOITER

This is by far the commonest form of goiter. It is known by a variety of names: *adolescent goiter*, because it so frequently occurs during the years of adolescence; *endemic goiter*, because it is prevalent in certain regions and peoples (*demos*, people); and *colloid goiter*, because it is characterized by an accumulation of colloid in the acini with corresponding dilatation of these spaces and consequent enlargement of the gland. The regions where goiter is endemic are the Alpine districts of Switzerland and the Himalayas where almost every thyroid gland is more or less enlarged, the region of the Great Lakes in North America, and the vally of the St. Lawrence. These areas have one thing in common: the soil is poor in iodine, so that the enlargement of the thyroid is compensatory in character, a work hypertrophy in order to perform the necessary amount of work with an inadequate supply of raw material. Animals as well as men living in these regions tend to suffer from this deficiency form of goiter. The occurrence of goiter during adolescence is due to a relative deficiency in iodine. The demands on the thyroid made by the girl at puberty blossoming out into womanhood are greater than those in later life, and it is for this reason that the enlargement is usually only temporary, the gland returning to its normal size when the period of stress is past.

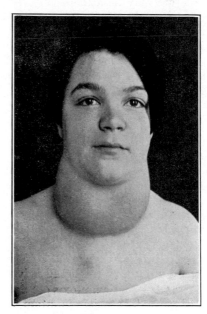

FIG. 87.—Simple goiter. (Eberts.)

The incidence of this form of goiter has been greatly diminished in certain endemic districts by the judicious use of iodine. In one part of Ohio a mass experiment was performed by giving the school children a small amount of iodized salt for one or two weeks twice a year (spring and fall), and this simple expedient was followed by an astonishing reduction in the incidence of goiter in the school community, a striking demonstration of

the value of the application of the results of scientific research in the laboratory to the needs of the people.

Lesions.—The lesions of simple goiter depend on the stage of the disease. During the early and more active stage of hyperplasia, the chief microscopic change is hyperplasia, an overgrowth of the glandular epithelium which will be more fully described in connection with exophthalmic goiter. When the demand for increased work is no longer felt the gland tends to return to its former state. Should the supply of iodine be much below normal, a stage of exhaustion follows the overactivity, and although the epithelial hyperplasia disappears, the acini become distended with colloid, and the thyroid may remain permanently enlarged. Such colloid goiters are met with at any period of adult life, and these are the goiters which are so prevalent in Switzerland and the hill districts of India.

Symptoms.—The symptoms of simple goiter, apparent from enlargement of the neck, are naturally few or absent, for the needs of the body are attended to by the work hypertrophy. Occasionally the hyperplasia may be carried too far, so that the girl may suffer from nervous irritability and other signs of hyperthyroidism. On the other hand, the return of the gland to a colloid state may be attended by symptoms of thyroid insufficiency. In the great majority of cases, however, the only evidence of disease (if it can be called such) is the enlargement of the neck (Fig. 87).

Treatment.—The treatment of simple goiter consists of providing an adequate supply of iodine, and regulating the life of the patient so that no undue strain is thrown on the organism during the critical period at which the goiter is likely to develop. From what has already been said it is evident that operation is the worst thing that could be done for such a patient.

NODULAR OR ADENOMATOUS GOITER

In adult life a rather different form of goiter may develop, again more common in goitrous districts. The thyroid is not only enlarged, but is also nodular, the nodules being called adenomas. These may be regarded as the result of repeated hyperplasia followed by involution, the process affecting some parts of the gland more than others so that a series of nodules tend to develop, some of considerable size. Microscopically, these nodules may show either hyperplasia or a resting colloid condition. With the passage of years they tend gradually to become larger.

Symptoms.—The symptoms of adenomatous goiter may be of two different varieties. The chief symptom is *pressure* of an adenoma upon surrounding structures, especially the trachea, causing difficulty in breathing. Or there may be so-called *toxic symptoms*, indications of hyperthyroidism, such as rapid pulse, tremors, nervousness, sweating, and an increased basal metabolic rate. In these cases there is evidently an overproduction of thyroxin by the adenomas, for these are the very symptoms produced by an injection of thyroxin or by an overdose of thyroid extract. Such a clinical condition is known as *toxic adenoma*, and is similar in many ways to that of exophthalmic goiter except that there is no exophthalmos. The main danger is the effect on the circulatory system. The blood-pressure

is raised, and the constant acceleration of the heart's action, which may last for years, gradually leads to cardiac exhaustion.

Treatment.—Treatment consists in removal of the part of the thyroid containing the adenomata. It is evident that this must not be delayed too long, else the heart may suffer irreparable damage.

EXOPHTHALMIC GOITER

This variety of goiter is also known as Graves' disease. It is by far the most serious form of the disease. It is characterized by hyperplasia of the gland and great overactivity of its function, but without any corresponding call on the part of the body for such overactivity. There is

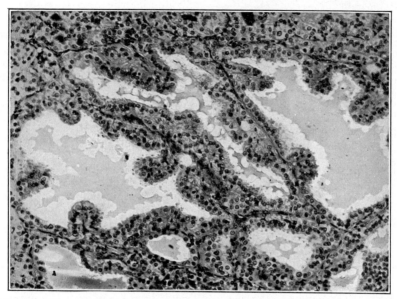

FIG. 88.—Thyroid of Graves' disease undergoing involution under iodine treatment. The papillary processes are being withdrawn from the enlarged acini, and the colloid is reappearing. Above and below there is still dense hyperplastic tissue. × 150. (Boyd, Textbook of Pathology.)

often a very definite history of nervous or psychic shock, or some terrifying experience, which is sometimes followed in the course of a few days by the development of the symptoms. This suggests that the disease is in some way connected with the nervous system. It seems probable that overstimulation of the thyroid by one of the hormones of the pituitary gland is the basis of the disease. This idea may ultimately lead to some satisfactory form of treatment.

Lesions.—The lesions are due to diffuse epithelial hyperplasia. The thyroid is diffusely enlarged, but not necessarily to a great degree, and presents no nodules. The cut surface has a dense, meaty appearance, in marked contrast to the translucency of the normal thyroid or the colloid

goiter. The microscopic appearance presents a great change in structure, for the normal colloid in the acini has disappeared and is replaced by numerous projections of epithelium from the lining of the acini (Fig. 88). It is, therefore, a picture of great glandular activity. The thyroxin which is normally stored in the colloid has gone, having been poured into the blood stream. The bloodvessels in the walls of the acini are widely dilated.

Symptoms.—The symptoms are those of extreme overactivity of the thyroid. The patient has a strained tense expression and is in a highly *nervous excitable condition.* The outstretched hands show a fine *tremor.* The pulse is very rapid (*tachycardia*) and *palpitation* is common, the *skin* is *moist*, and the patient is peculiarly *insensitive to cold*, owing to the heat produced by the excessive metabolism which is indicated by the *high metabolic rate*. It is as if some blast were blowing on the furnace of the body, fanning it to furious activity. The nitrogen of the tissues is consumed by this fire, so that the patient wastes away. A peculiar symptom which gives its name to the disease is *exophthalmos* or protrusion of the eyeballs. The staring eyes, the strained expression, and the enlargement of the neck give the patient so striking an appearance that in a severe case the diagnosis can be made at a glance (Fig. 89).

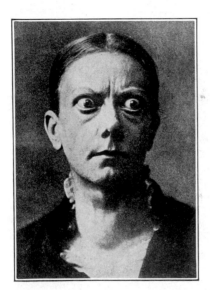

FIG. 89.—Characteristic appearance in Graves' disease. (Bramwell's Atlas of Clinical Medicine.)

Course.—The course of the disease varies. In some cases it is acute and fulminating, the patient being consumed by the inward fire and dying of exhaustion. More frequently the course is marked by exacerbations and remissions without any apparent cause; gradually the fire burns itself out, the thyroid becomes incapable of hyperplasia, and the final picture may be one of thyroid insufficiency or myxedema.

Treatment.—There are several methods of treatment of hyperthyroidism now available and the choice of treatment in an individual case depends upon several factors and must be decided upon in light of the severity of the disease, the patient's age, heart complications and other situations. Propylthiouracil or methylthiouracil will control the disease in many cases by reducing the amount of thyroxin liberated from the gland. Some cases may be controlled in this manner for periods of six to twelve months or longer, and subsequently they remain normal after one or more courses of such treatment. Or alternatively, after such preparation with this drug removal of the thyroid gland may be performed which will result in a cure

of the condition in a large majority of patients. Preparation for operation with iodine alone is not used very much at the present time, although many surgeons prefer to add iodine to the thiouracil drugs prior to operation. The introduction of radioactive iodine as a treatment measure in this condition offers another possibility. Here radioactive iodine is deposited in the active thyroid gland and emits radiation in diminishing amounts over a period of two weeks, during which time the active tissue is either destroyed or returned to normal functional state. This method of treatment requires the provision of very careful laboratory control of the administration of this potentially dangerous method of treatment, and is available only in a few centres.

CRETINISM AND MYXEDEMA

So far we have discussed overactivity of the thyroid as evidenced by symptoms of hyperthyroidism. An exactly opposite picture results from hypothyroidism, but the effect differs greatly, depending on whether the deficiency of thyroid secretion is due to absence of development of the gland during fetal life or to atrophy of an already developed thyroid in adult life. The former condition, which is congenital, is known as cretinism; the latter condition, which is acquired, is called myxedema.

Cretinism.—A cretin is an individual in whom the thyroid has failed to develop, so that a study of the disease serves to throw light on the functions of the gland. We have already seen that normal thyroid function is necessary for the proper development of the body and the mind. The cretin is a dwarf physically and mentally (Fig. 90). The mind, the skeleton, and the sexual organs do not develop. Like Peter Pan, the cretin never grows up, but he has none of Peter's vivacity, for the vitalizing influence of the thyroid is lacking. He is a sad, old child. Sir William Osler's pen picture of the cretin is a masterpiece: "No type of human transformation is more distressing to look at than an aggravated case of cretinism. The stunted stature, the semibestial aspect, the blubber lips, retroussé nose sunken at the root, the wide-open mouth, the lolling tongue, the small eyes half closed with swollen lids, the stolid

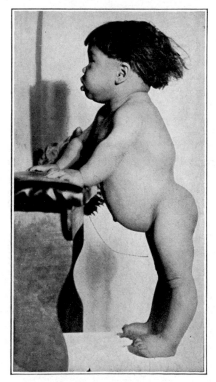

Fig. 90.—A cretin.

15

expressionless face, the squat figure, the muddy dry skin, combine to make the picture of what has been termed 'the pariah of Nature'."

Cretinism occurs in two forms, endemic and sporadic. *Endemic cretinism* is very common in the great regions of endemic goiter, the Alps and the Himalayas. The mother suffers from simple goiter, and the tragedy of cretinism can be prevented by giving the pregnant woman a sufficient supply of iodine. The *sporadic form* develops in non-endemic regions, and is fortunately a rare disease. The mother is not goitrous, but apparently something interferes with the development of the thyroid during fetal life.

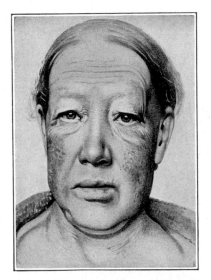

Fig.91.— Myxedema. (Bramwell's Atlas of Clinical Medicine.)

Treatment.—Treatment by means of thyroid extract may be effective if started early enough, but it must be kept up during the rest of the patient's life. If treatment is not commenced until a few years have passed it is useless to hope that the child may be restored to normal, for the critical period of brain development has been lost; "the moving finger writes, and, having writ, moves on."

Myxedema.—This is thyroid deficiency in the adult. Like other diseases of the thyroid, it is commoner in women, usually appearing about the age of forty years. The thyroid atrophies until only a remnant is left, but the cause of the atrophy is unknown. It is not commoner in the regions of endemic goiter than elsewhere.

Clinical Picture.—The clinical picture in an advanced case can be recognized at a glance, for it is the reverse of that of Graves' disease (Fig. 91). All the processes, both mental and physical, are slower, the fire burns low, the basal metabolism is much below normal. The patient is heavy, obese, intensely phlegmatic, and will sit for hours without moving. The face is broad, the features coarse like those of an Eskimo. The skin is rough, dry, and wrinkled, and the patient is very sensitive to cold. Premature baldness is common and the hair falls out of the outer third of the eyebrow. There is an infiltration of the skin with a mucus-like substance, giving an appearance of edema but not pitting on pressure. It is this infiltration which gives the disease its name, and which is responsible for the ironing away of all lines of expression in the face, so that most myxedema patients look more or less alike.

The above description applies to the full-blown case. Milder degrees of thyroid insufficiency are very much commoner, and are much more difficult to recognize. Increased sensitiveness to cold is always suggestive of the

condition, and the diagnosis can be confirmed by testing the basal metabolic rate.

Treatment.—Treatment consists in giving thyroid extract (thyroxin) by mouth. Few therapeutic results are more dramatic. The metabolic fire begins to burn again, the infiltration of the skin disappears, the normal lines and expression of the face return, the mind reawakens, the patient becomes indeed a new man, or rather a new woman. When health has been restored the dose of thyroxin is cut down to that amount which will just maintain the basal metabolic rate at a normal level, but the administration has to be continued during the remainder of the patient's life.

THE PARATHYROID GLANDS

Structure and Function.—In the wonderful volume of endocrine romance there are few more thrilling chapters than that dealing with the story of the parathyroids. For more than fifty years the presence of these four tiny glands, each no larger than a pea, has been known. They are situated in the neck, two on each side behind the thyroid, but their function was not even guessed at. Gradually it came to be suspected that they had something to do with the regulation of calcium metabolism, but it was not until Collip, in 1925, succeeded in preparing an extract of their active principle, which he called parathormone, that a flood of light was cast upon the subject.

By injecting the extract into animals it was found that an amazing mobilization of the calcium in the body was brought about. Normally the calcium in the food is absorbed from the bowel, carried by the blood to the bones, and stored in the skeleton which acts as the great reservoir of calcium in the body, just as the thyroid is the reservoir of iodine. Calcium is essential for tissue health and activity, but it must be supplied in minute and exactly correct amounts. In health this small amount is given up by the bones to the blood, and carried to the body in general and to the muscles in particular. When parathyroid extract is injected into an animal, the mobilization of calcium is enormously augmented, and the blood is flooded with calcium, which pours through the kidneys into the urine and is lost to the body. As a result of this loss the bones become decalcified, they lose their rigidity and are easily bent, they no longer cast a dense shadow in the roentgen-ray film, and cystic spaces develop in their substance.

Like the thyroid and other ductless glands the parathyroids may show disturbance in the direction either of underactivity or overactivity. In underactivity or *hypoparathyroidism* there is insufficient mobilization of calcium, and the tissues are starved of that element; in overactivity or *hyperparathyroidism* there is undue mobilization of calcium; the blood is flooded but the bones are depleted.

TETANY

The chief clinical mainfestation of hypoparathyroidism is tetany. This is a disorder marked by intermittent muscular contractions affecting par-

ticularly the hands and feet which are drawn into peculiar attitudes that are highly characteristic. These spasms are due to increased irritability of the muscles, which in turn is due to the low calcium content of the blood. The condition used to be common in the early days of the surgical treatment of goiter, when the great importance of leaving the parathyroids behind when the thyroid was removed was not properly recognized. Tetany may also occur in other disturbances of calcium metabolism such as rickets, but this aspect of the subject need not be entered into here. The disorder is at once relieved by the administration of parathyroid extract which ensures an adequate supply of calcium to the starved muscles.

PARATHYROID TUMORS

Hyperparathyroidism can be produced experimentally by the administration of parathyroid extract, but in human pathology it is the result of the growth of a parathyroid tumor. This is an innocent tumor, an adenoma, but the effect it produces on the body may be far from innocent. The adenoma may be no larger than a bean or it may be the size of a plum, but even a large tumor may not be detected by the physician because it is tucked away behind the thyroid. It is readily recognized, however, by the remarkable effects which it produces.

In 1891 the Viennese pathologist, von Recklinghausen, described a peculiar disorder of bones which is known as *osteitis fibrosa cystica* or von Recklinghausen's disease. In this condition the bones are softened

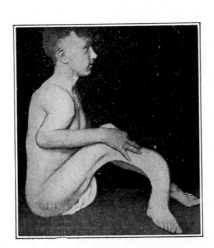

FIG. 92.—Osteitis fibrosa cystica. Showing marked bending of the arms and legs.

as the result of decalcification, and the softened bones, having lost their rigidity, become greatly deformed. The arms and legs are bent (Fig. 92), the pelvis is wedge-shaped, there is spinal curvature, and there is a loss of weight. Severe pains in the bones are a distressing feature. Only within the last few years has it been discovered that this long-recognized disease of bones is due to the presence of a hitherto unsuspected tumor of one of the parathyroids. A striking feature in many cases is the formation of cysts in the bones, readily seen in the roentgen-ray picture; these cysts may so weaken the bones that spontaneous fractures occur.

Two other points of importance are the condition of the blood and the condition of the kidneys. The *blood* is flooded with calcium from the bones, so that the normal blood calcium of 10 mg. per 100 cc. is raised, sometimes to 18 or even 20 mg. Other conditions associated with decalci-

fication, such as secondary tumors of bone, may cause the blood calcium to be raised, but there is an additional blood change which is even more characteristic of hyperparathyroidism, *i.e.*, lowered blood phosphorus. Calcium in bone is combined with phosphorus in the form of calcium phosphate, so that it might be supposed that the blood phosphorus would also be raised in the decalcification of hyperparathyroidism. But in this condition the permeability of the kidney for phosphorus is markedly lowered, so that more escapes into the urine than is poured into the blood from the bones, and the level of the blood phosphorus is accordingly lowered.

The *kidneys* may show a change of very great importance, namely, deposits of calcium. The calcium pouring from the blood into the urine may be partly arrested in the kidney, giving a shadow in the roentgen-ray film. Sometimes these deposits of calcium form a stone in the kidney, even though the changes in the bones may be comparatively slight. It is, therefore, desirable in every case of stone in the kidney to estimate the blood calcium and phosphorus in order to determine if a parathyroid tumor may be the underlying cause of the stone.

Treatment.—Treatment by removal of the tumor in the neck, even though this be so small that it cannot be felt, is followed by dramatic consequences. The blood calcium at once falls and the phosphorus rises to normal, the pains in the bones are relieved; in a remarkably short space of time the bones become recalcified, and the patient is converted from a chronic invalid to a robust individual.

THE ADRENALS

Structure and Function.—The adrenals are two little glands shaped like a cocked hat, one on either side of the spinal column situated just above the kidney. They are about the size of a flattened thimble. Each adrenal consists of two parts, an outer portion or *cortex* and an inner portion or *medulla*. These are not merely two parts; they are two different organs joined together as one, different in origin, in structure, in function, and in pathology.

The *cortex* is essential to life, for when removed on both sides in the animal, death occurs in a few days. For over a hundred years it has been known that patients with adrenal insufficiency often die from minor infections and stresses. We now know that it is the adrenal which enables the body to withstand the large variety of environmental stresses and strains to which it is subjected. The adrenal plays perhaps the largest single role in determining whether a person is sick or well. It is, however, the pituitary which controls the adrenal cortex, so that the pituitary still remains the master gland. More than twenty distinct steroids with varying degrees of physiological action have been isolated from the adrenal cortex. These may be divided into three groups which regulate three broad types of body activity, namely, salt or electrolyte balance, metabolism, and sex function. For those of weak memory or mentality, the three functions may be represented as the letter S: salt, sugar and sex.

(1) *The salt or electrolyte group* of hormones governs sodium and chloride retention and potassium excretion, and therefore the amount of fluid in the body. Administration of the hormone leads to edema and increase of body weight due to retention of sodium and chloride, and also fatigue and electrocardiographic changes due to depletion of potassium. It is essential to life. Deficiency of this group of hormones results in the picture of Addison's disease and leads to death.

(2) *The sugar or S group* convert amino acids into sugar instead of into protein, thus increasing blood sugar and the amount of glycogen in the liver. They cause the eosinophils of the blood to disappear. The best known example of this group is cortisone, the production of which is stimulated by the action of the pituitary hormone known as ACTH, the adrenocorticotropic hormone. Cortisone produces an immediate and dramatic beneficial response in rheumatic fever and rheumatoid arthritis, as well as in related diseases. It appears to provide the tissues with a buffer against the attacking irritant. It does not put out the fire nor does it repair the damage after the fire, but it does seem to provide the tissues with an asbestos suit.

(3) *The sex group* of hormones tend to masculinize the body and to build up amino acids and protein from nitrogen. When this hormone is metabolized the substances known as 17-ketosteroids are formed and excreted in the urine. The urine is examined for these steroids in cases of virilism where some disorder of the adrenal is suspected.

The *medulla* is derived from the sympathetic nervous system, and an extract made from the medulla, known as *adrenalin* or epinephrin, has a remarkable stimulating effect on that system. When injected into an animal or person it causes a marked rise in the blood-pressure, owing to contraction of the involuntary muscle in the walls of the arterioles, this contraction in turn being due to stimulation of the sympathetic nerves which supply this muscle. Adrenalin also converts the glycogen in the liver into sugar which is poured into the blood and at once carried to the voluntary muscles, allowing these to perform a markedly increased amount of work. It appears that under severe emotional stress such as rage or fear a marked excess of adrenalin is poured into the blood, thereby enabling the animal or person to perform feats of muscular exertion (attack, flight, etc.) of which he would not ordinarily be capable. This has been called the emergency function of the adrenals. It is much more difficult to say what the function of the adrenal medulla is under conditions of ordinary life.

ADDISON'S DISEASE

This is a condition of *chronic adrenal insufficiency*, which was described over a hundred years ago by Addison, of Guy's Hospital, London. It is of great historic interest, because Addison's description was the means of directing attention for the first time to the ductless glands, which had previously been structures of complete mystery. In the years which have intervened since this epoch-making contribution we have come to regard the endocrine glands as amongst the most important in the entire body.

Lesions.—The lesions responsible for the condition are those which destroy both adrenals. Of these, the commonest is chronic tuberculosis, the infection being carried by the blood from some focus in the lung or elsewhere. Sometimes there is merely atrophy of the adrenals for some unknown reason. In very rare cases there are tumors of both glands, either primary or secondary.

Symptoms.—The symptoms are multiform. The two most characteristic are a gradually progressive *weakness* and a remarkable *pigmentation of the skin.* This pigmentation varies from a light yellow to a deep brown, and in severe cases the patient may resemble a Hindu in appearance. It is most marked on the nipples, the genital region, and other places which are normally pigmented, as well as on exposed parts such as the face and hands. The *blood-pressure* is very low. There may be *gastro-intestinal symptoms,* such as nausea, vomiting, and diarrhea. Sometimes these occur in an acute and alarming form known as *crises,* in which abdominal pain is a prominent feature.

It appears probable that the muscular weakness and low blood-pressure are due to lesions of the cortex and the pigmentation to lesions of the medulla. Owing, however, to our lack of knowledge of the normal function of the adrenals, it is not possible to give a satisfactory pathological basis for the symptoms of Addison's disease.

Treatment.—Mild cases of Addison's disease may be treated by the addition of salt to the daily intake. However, in the more severe cases, the use of desoxycorticosterone, a synthetic compound which controls the salt and water metabolic disturbances of Addison's disease, will restore the patient to a normal state in many cases. This may be given by injection or by the implantation of pellets under the skin, from which the drug is slowly absorbed. Aqueous extract of adrenal cortex is also of use, particularly in acute episodes in the disease, but is more expensive as a maintenance treatment. Cortisone has been found to be satisfactory in the maintenance treatment of these cases. It has to be emphasized that these treatments are by no means a cure for the disease, but merely act as a replacement of the missing hormones.

CORTICAL TUMORS

Tumors of the adrenal cortex are rare, but as the symptoms they produce serve to throw some light on adrenal function, they deserve brief consideration. These tumors are malignant and may be regarded as carcinoma, spreading by the lymph and blood stream.

The clinical picture may be of one of two groups, known as the adrenogenital syndrome and Cushing's syndrome.

The adrenogenital syndrome is marked by premature sexual development in children with an intensification of maleness, a condition known as *virilism.* In boys, even when quite young, there is precocious development of the sex organs, growth of hair on the face (hirsutism) and great muscularity, so that the boy may present the picture vividly termed the infant hercules. In girls and women the uterus and ovaries atrophy, but the clitoris hypertrophies, hair appears on the face and upper lip, the voice

alic is unable to increase his stature, but his face becomes very large with a markedly projecting lower jaw, which serves to match the huge hands and feet. Curvature of the spine develops, and the patient with his bent back, enormous hands reaching to the knees, and protruding lower jaw, may present a gorilla-like picture in extreme cases. The overgrowth affects the connective tissue as well as the bones, and the skin becomes thick, coarse, and furrowed. The disease does not necessarily shorten life, for it is self-limited, and the tumor responsible for the condition not only stops growing but tends to undergo degeneration.

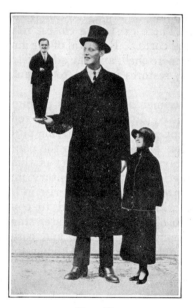

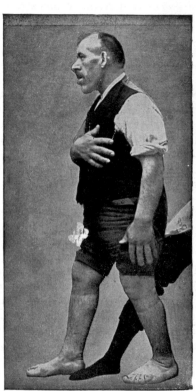

Fig. 93   Fig. 94

Fig. 93.—Effects of pituitary disease, showing a pituitary giant and dwarf; the woman is of normal height.

Fig. 94.—Acromegaly showing protruding lower jaw and large hands and feet. (Purves-Stewart, Diagnosis of Nervous Diseases, courtesy of Edward Arnold and Company.)

HYPOPITUITARISM

This is a much commoner condition than hyperpituitarism, but the clinical pictures produced are more varied and confusing, and a detailed consideration of their complexities would be out of place here. The most common form is *Fröhlich's syndrome*, which is a disturbance of genital development and fat (Fig. 95). It commonly develops about the time of puberty.

Lesions.—The lesions responsible for the condition are those which destroy both adrenals. Of these, the commonest is chronic tuberculosis, the infection being carried by the blood from some focus in the lung or elsewhere. Sometimes there is merely atrophy of the adrenals for some unknown reason. In very rare cases there are tumors of both glands, either primary or secondary.

Symptoms.—The symptoms are multiform. The two most characteristic are a gradually progressive *weakness* and a remarkable *pigmentation of the skin*. This pigmentation varies from a light yellow to a deep brown, and in severe cases the patient may resemble a Hindu in appearance. It is most marked on the nipples, the genital region, and other places which are normally pigmented, as well as on exposed parts such as the face and hands. The *blood-pressure* is very low. There may be *gastro-intestinal symptoms*, such as nausea, vomiting, and diarrhea. Sometimes these occur in an acute and alarming form known as *crises*, in which abdominal pain is a prominent feature.

It appears probable that the muscular weakness and low blood-pressure are due to lesions of the cortex and the pigmentation to lesions of the medulla. Owing, however, to our lack of knowledge of the normal function of the adrenals, it is not possible to give a satisfactory pathological basis for the symptoms of Addison's disease.

Treatment.—Mild cases of Addison's disease may be treated by the addition of salt to the daily intake. However, in the more severe cases, the use of desoxycorticosterone, a synthetic compound which controls the salt and water metabolic disturbances of Addison's disease, will restore the patient to a normal state in many cases. This may be given by injection or by the implantation of pellets under the skin, from which the drug is slowly absorbed. Aqueous extract of adrenal cortex is also of use, particularly in acute episodes in the disease, but is more expensive as a maintenance treatment. Cortisone has been found to be satisfactory in the maintenance treatment of these cases. It has to be emphasized that these treatments are by no means a cure for the disease, but merely act as a replacement of the missing hormones.

CORTICAL TUMORS

Tumors of the adrenal cortex are rare, but as the symptoms they produce serve to throw some light on adrenal function, they deserve brief consideration. These tumors are malignant and may be regarded as carcinoma, spreading by the lymph and blood stream.

The clinical picture may be of one of two groups, known as the adrenogenital syndrome and Cushing's syndrome.

The adrenogenital syndrome is marked by premature sexual development in children with an intensification of maleness, a condition known as *virilism*. In boys, even when quite young, there is precocious development of the sex organs, growth of hair on the face (hirsutism) and great muscularity, so that the boy may present the picture vividly termed the infant hercules. In girls and women the uterus and ovaries atrophy, but the clitoris hypertrophies, hair appears on the face and upper lip, the voice

becomes deep, and normal healthy interest in the opposite sex is lost. Men naturally show none of these changes. A puzzling feature is the frequent occurrence of *high blood pressure,* which is usually paroxysmal rather than constant. Removal of the tumor in women has been followed by a dramatic return to a normal sexual condition, the change including the voice, the abnormal hair, the blood-pressure, and the sex instincts.

In Cushing's syndrome there is a confusing array of symptoms, the only ones which we shall mention being painful adiposity confined to the face, neck and trunk; hirsutism in females and preadolescent males; sexual atrophy; and muscular weakness. The adiposity gives the face a peculiar round appearance to which the name of "full moon face" has been given. Although adrenal tumors are rare, Cushing's syndrome has suddenly become of importance, because when patients are given ACTH or cortisone for too long a period they tend to develop this peculiar appearance. It is in rheumatic fever, which is an acute relatively short-lived disease, that cortisone is of the greatest value, whereas in a long drawn-out disease like rheumatoid arthritis it would hardly be expected to give such satisfactory results.

THE PITUITARY GLAND

It is no exaggeration to say that in the light of modern knowledge the pituitary gland is the most remarkable organ in the human body. In size it is insignificant, being only slightly larger than a cherry stone, but its importance is indicated by the care with which it is protected from injury, for it lies in a little roofed-in chamber on the floor of the skull with the entire mass of the brain above it and the nasal cavity below. Its name indicates the relation which it bears to the nose, for the ancients, who were well aware of its existence, imagined that its function was to produce the "pituita" or nasal secretion. Others, more idealistic, considered it to be the seat of the soul. Modern materialistic medicine regards it as the master gland of the body, regulating and coördinating the action of the other endocrine glands, and exercising a profound influence on the growth of the body, on the development of sex, on the subsequent functioning of the sex organs, and on the mind of the individual.

Like the adrenals, the pituitary consists of two parts which may be regarded as two separate organs which happen to be united in one. These parts are the *anterior lobe,* which is formed by an upgrowth from the pharynx and is glandular in nature, and the *posterior lobe,* which is derived from a downgrowth from the base of the brain, remains connected with the brain by a narrow stalk, and is composed of nervous tissue.

The *anterior lobe* is the part which produces the various hormones that play such an important part in the development and functioning of the body. The principal hormones are as follows:

1. *The Growth Hormone.*—If the anterior pituitary is removed in an animal, growth is retarded to an extreme degree and the animal remains a dwarf. The human dwarf is usually an individual in whom the growth hormone of the pituitary has been lacking. When the dwarfed animal is given the growth hormone, it catches up with its normal brother and may

even surpass it in size, provided that the period of growth is not ended. Removal of the anterior lobe in a tadpole prevents its metamorphosis into a frog, but if an extract of the lobe is injected, normal development takes place.

2. *The Gonadotropic Hormone, i.e.,* the *Gonad-stimulating Hormone.*— This is necessary for the proper development of the reproductive organs, both male and female. It is on this hormone that the menstrual cycle in the female depends, for it stimulates the ovaries to monthly activity, and these in turn produce hormones which are responsible for the changes in the uterus that result in menstruation. One of the first signs of pituitary disease in the female is cessation of the menstrual function.

3. *The Thyrotropic Hormone.*—Injection of this hormone in an animal stimulates the thyroid to great activity, and produces both the symptoms and the thyroid lesions of exophthalmic goiter.

4. *The Lactogenic Hormone.*—When this is injected, it stimulates the production of milk in the female animal, and it is probably through the pituitary that the changes of pregnancy finally lead to lactation.

5. *The Adrenocorticotropic Hormone.*—There exists the closest relationship between the pituitary and the adrenal cortex. Removal of the anterior pituitary reduces the adrenal cortex to a mere shell, and the administration of this hormone, now known as ACTH, restores it again to normal and stimulates it to produce cortisone.

6. *The Diabetogenic Hormone.*—If experimental diabetes is produced in an animal by removal of the pancreas, the condition is relieved by removal of the pituitary. It would, therefore, appear that the anterior pituitary exercises an antagonistic effect on the islets of Langerhans in the pancreas.

The *posterior lobe* is much more of a mystery. An extract of this lobe when injected produces marked contraction of the involuntary muscle. This action is exerted on the arterioles, producing a marked rise in blood-pressure, and on the pregnant uterus which is stimulated to contract strongly. The latter action is utilized in obstetrics in the later stages of labor. This stimulating substance is known as pituitrin, and curiously enough it was discovered long before a single hormone was known to exist in the much more important anterior lobe.

Like the other endocrine glands, disturbance of the pituitary may manifest itself either by overactivity, *i.e.,* hyperpituitarism, or by underactivity, *i.e.,* hypopituitarism. The former is associated with and dependent on the presence of an adenoma or benign tumor of the anterior lobe. The latter is caused by destruction of the anterior lobe by disease.

HYPERPITUITARISM

This manifests itself by excessive growth, particularly of the skeleton, but the results depend on whether the disturbance develops during the period of skeletal growth or after it is completed. In the former case the result is *gigantism* (Fig. 93). Every giant has an overactive pituitary, and at autopsy an adenoma of the anterior pituitary will be found. If the adenoma develops after growth is completed the result is *acromegaly,* a name which signifies enlargement of the hands and feet (Fig. 94). The acromeg-

alic is unable to increase his stature, but his face becomes very large with a markedly projecting lower jaw, which serves to match the huge hands and feet. Curvature of the spine develops, and the patient with his bent back, enormous hands reaching to the knees, and protruding lower jaw, may present a gorilla-like picture in extreme cases. The overgrowth affects the connective tissue as well as the bones, and the skin becomes thick, coarse, and furrowed. The disease does not necessarily shorten life, for it is self-limited, and the tumor responsible for the condition not only stops growing but tends to undergo degeneration.

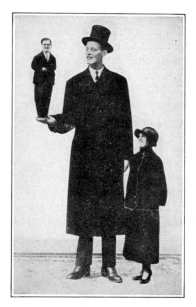

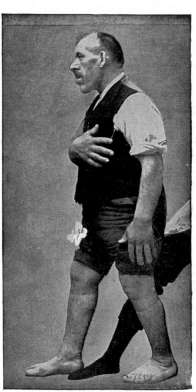

Fig. 93   Fig. 94

Fig. 93.—Effects of pituitary disease, showing a pituitary giant and dwarf; the woman is of normal height.

Fig. 94.—Acromegaly showing protruding lower jaw and large hands and feet. (Purves-Stewart, Diagnosis of Nervous Diseases, courtesy of Edward Arnold and Company.)

HYPOPITUITARISM

This is a much commoner condition than hyperpituitarism, but the clinical pictures produced are more varied and confusing, and a detailed consideration of their complexities would be out of place here. The most common form is *Fröhlich's syndrome*, which is a disturbance of genital development and fat (Fig. 95). It commonly develops about the time of puberty.

Depression of the sexual function is the earliest and most constant symptom. In the female there is absence of menstruation, and lack of libido in the male. The sexual organs remain undeveloped. The connective tissue of the skin atrophies, so that the skin is smooth and delicate like a child's, the reverse of the condition seen in acromegaly. Adiposity may be very marked or may be absent. When the condition develops in an adult male, deposits of fat in the breasts, hips, and buttocks give th figure a distinctly feminine cast. Mental dulness and lethargy are common. The syndrome or collection of clinical features is perfectly illustrated by the Fat Boy in Pickwick, with his round, chubby face, his fat body fairly bursting through his buttons, his slow mind, and his ability to drop asleep at a moment's notice.

A different form of hypopituitarism is *pituitary dwarfism* (Fig. 93). The patient is bright mentally, but remains small and undeveloped sexually. When he grows up he remains like a graceful and attractive child, a Peter Pan who never really grows up.

The common *cause* of hypopituitarism is an adenoma of the pituitary composed of undifferentiated cells which apparently have not the power of producing pituitary hormones. The cells do not stain well with the dyes used in microscopic work, so that the tumor is known as a *chromophobe adenoma*, in contrast to the *chromophil adenoma* responsible for hyperpituitarism which is composed of cells that stain intensely. The chromophobe adenoma is not only non-functioning, but it destroys the functioning cells which produce the hormones and thus lead to pituitary insufficiency. Other lesions may destroy the pituitary, but these are much rarer.

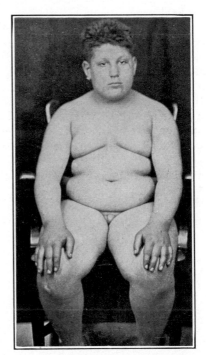

Fig. 95.—Frölich's syndrome showing adiposity and sexual underdevelopment. (Bell, Textbook of Pathology.)

THE ISLETS OF LANGERHANS

The islets of Langerhans are small groups of cells scattered through the pancreas, which really constitute one of the endocrine glands, for they pour their secretion or hormone into the blood and not into the intestine like the pancreatic cells proper. The hormone of the islets is known as insulin. Like the other endocrine glands, there may be underactivity or overactivity of the islets, *i.e.*, hypoinsulinism and hyperinsulinism. *Hypo-*

insulinism is the condition known as diabetes, which has already been studied in connection with the pancreas. It is relieved by the administration of insulin.

HYPERINSULINISM

Hyperinsulinism is caused by the presence of a tumor of the islets, which may be either a benign adenoma or a carcinoma of low malignancy. The symptoms, which are remarkable and highly distinctive, although only recently recognized, are due to a condition of hypoglycemia or lowering of the blood sugar (glucose). The normal blood sugar is about 1 per cent, but when an excess of insulin is produced the blood sugar may fall to low levels. When it reaches 0.5 per cent symptoms of hypoglycemia develop, which are similar to those caused by an overdose of insulin (insulin shock). The patient suffers from attacks of faintness of increasing severity, convulsions, and loss of consciousness. The tell-tale feature of these attacks is that they always occur when the patient has been fasting for some hours, the sugar absorbed from his last meal being exhausted. The attacks can be prevented by eating sugar, and even when the patient is unconscious the injection of glucose solution into the blood will at once revive him. As the tumor grows in size, the attacks increase in severity, and the only adequate treatment is removal of the tumor. Such removal is usually not difficult for the skilled surgeon, and is followed by brilliant and most satisfactory results.

Chapter

19

THE BLOOD AND LYMPHATIC GLANDS

THE BLOOD

Structure and Function.—The total volume of the blood is from 4000 to 8000 cc., depending on the size of the individual. The blood consists of a fluid part, the plasma, and a solid part, the blood cells. In this consideration of the diseases of the blood and the blood-forming organs we are concerned only with the blood cells. These are of two varieties, the red cells or erythrocytes (*erythros*, red), and the leucocytes or white cells (*leukos*, white). In addition there is a third element, the blood platelets, minute particles which cannot be regarded as cells. In the case both of the red and the white cells there may be too few cells or too many cells. A diminution in the number of cells is always a sign of disease. An increase in the number may be a manifestation of blood disease, or it may be a physiological response to a temporary demand from the body for more red or white cells; the leucocytosis of infection is an example of the latter condition.

The *erythrocytes* or red blood cells are globules filled with hemoglobin, which gives them their color, and possessing no nucleus. In health they number from 5,000,000 to 6,000,000 in the male, and from 4,500,000 to 5,000,000 in the female. They are formed in the bone-marrow. Some knowledge of this formation is necessary for an understanding of what happens in anemia, the commonest disease affecting the red blood cells. In the bone-marrow, in addition to the vessels through which the blood circulates, there is a series of lagoons or sinusoids in which red cells are formed and released into the blood stream as required. The endothelial cells lining the sinusoids give rise to large nucleated cells called *megaloblasts* (Fig. 96). These are the earliest blood cells, and they do not at first contain any hemoglobin, the coloring matter of the red cells which enables them to perform their sole function, the carrying of oxygen from the lungs to the tissues and the return of carbon dioxide from the tissues to the lungs. The megaloblasts multiply, and their daughter cells develop into *normoblasts*, *i.e.*, smaller cells which become filled with hemoglobin but still retain a nucleus. The last stage of development is the change from a normoblast into an *erythrocyte*, which is brought about by loss of the nucleus. The adult erythrocyte is the only cell in the body which does not possess a nucleus, and as a nucleus is essential to the life of a cell, it follows that the days of an erythrocyte are numbered. Their average duration of life is from one hundred to one hundred-twenty days. The megaloblast and the normoblast are primitive blood cells, and in health they are not allowed to escape from the sinusoids into the blood stream. When the stage of the

(241)

mature erythrocyte is reached the doors are opened, and the red corpuscles are launched on the blood stream, to perform their life-giving function of respiration. In conditions of anemia, particularly pernicious anemia, immature red cells escape from the bone-marrow into the blood stream, and are found when a blood count is made. They are readily recognized by the fact that they possess a nucleus, whereas the adult erythrocytes are non-nucleated.

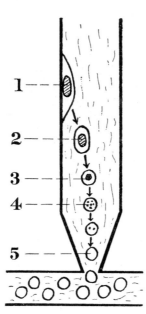

FIG. 96.—Steps in the formation of red blood cells. Immature cells in marrow sinusoids maturing and entering blood stream. 1, Endothelial cell; 2, megaloblast; 3, normoblast; 4, reticulocyte; 5, erythrocyte.

The *leucocytes* or white blood cells number from 6000 to 8000 per c.mm. of blood. Large numbers, however, are trapped in the unused capillaries, and as physical exertion causes great numbers of these capillaries to become opened up, the leucocyte count shows a corresponding rise after exercise. The white blood cells are not uniform in type like the erythrocytes, but are of three different kinds: the polymorphonuclear leucocyte, the lymphocyte, and the monocyte. The *polymorphonuclear* (*polyps*, many, *morphe*, form, and *nucleus*) is a cell whose nucleus may have various forms, in comparison with the spherical nucleus of the lymphocyte and monocyte. It is further characterized by the presence of fine granules in the cytoplasm. In one variety the granules are large and stain bright red with eosin, a red dye used for staining blood films; this is known as the *eosinophil*. The polymorphonuclears constitute about 70 per cent of the leucocytes, but this figure varies considerably. The eosinophils form only 2 per cent of the total leucocyte count. Both types of cells are formed in the sinusoids of the bone-marrow, in very much the same way as the erythrocytes are formed, *i.e.*, they go through two immature stages before the adult form is reached. These stages are the myeloblast and the myelocyte. Granules appear for the first time in the myelocyte, and these cells are present in large numbers in the marrow, but do not enter the blood stream under normal conditions. Some of the myelocytes are eosinophil myelocytes. Both forms are found in the blood in large numbers in the disease known as leukemia. The *function* of the polymorphonuclears is defense of the body against bacteria by means of phagocytosis, a process which has already been studied in connection with inflammation. The number in the blood is enormously increased in acute infections, owing to the depots in the bone-marrow pouring their reserve into the blood stream, and at the same time speeding

up the rate of production. The function of the eosinophils is not known.

The *lymphocytes* form about 20 per cent of the total leucocyte count. They are rather small, uninteresting-looking cells, with very little cytoplasm around the spherical nucleus. Large numbers of lymphocytes appear at a focus of chronic inflammation, some being derived from the blood, others from the tissues. Though they arrive on the field of battle, they appear merely to play the part of interested spectators, for they have no phagocytic power. This appearance is deceptive, however, for the lymphocytes are an important source of the immune bodies which play so important a part in the defense of the body against bacterial infection. The lymphocytes are produced in the lymphoid tissue, mainly the lymph glands and spleen.

The *monocytes* or large mononuclears, on the other hand, are actively phagocytic, and play an important part in the inflammatory process. In acute inflammation they form the second line of defense, arriving later than the polymorphonuclears and serving the useful purpose of scavengers. They are formed in the bone-marrow and constitute about 8 per cent of the total leucocytes.

In a blood examination the leucocytes may be examined in two ways: (1) Leucocyte count; (2) differential count. The object of the *leucocyte count* is to estimate the total number of leucocytes, and to determine if there is a leucocytosis or increase in the number. This extremely useful procedure is quite simple and takes only a few minutes. In a *differential count* several hundred leucocytes are examined, note being taken whether each cell is a polymorphonuclear, eosinophil, lymphocyte, or monocyte. In this way the percentage of the various cells is determined. Such a procedure is much more laborious and time-consuming, and in most diseases gives information of little value. In selected cases, however, it may prove of great use. It is essential in the leukemias.

BLOOD TRANSFUSION

The novelist speaks of the life blood ebbing away. The phrase is hardly an exaggeration, for, as we have seen in Chapter 1, it is the blood which carries to the innumerable cells of the body their requisites for life, namely, food and oxygen. Without sufficient blood the cells are both starved and asphyxiated. As a severe loss of blood is so injurious, it is natural that the injection of blood from another person should be correspondingly beneficial. When this injection is made into a vein it is called transfusion of blood.

The chief value of blood transfusion is replacement of blood after a severe, acute hemorrhage, when it is truly a life-saving procedure. It is also useful for combating shock following surgical operations, especially those associated with much loss of blood, as in operations on the brain. Repeated small transfusions are sometimes used in the treatment of chronic anemias with a low red cell count and in severe infections.

Unfortunately it is not possible to use the blood of all and sundry for the purpose of transfusion. The red blood cells and serum of each individual are perfectly adapted to one another, but the cells of one person

may not be adapted to the serum of another; they may be incompatible. The gravest accidents may follow transfusion of an incompatible blood. It is this fact which has for centuries retarded the use of so obvious a procedure as blood transfusion.

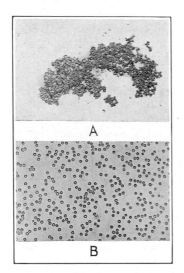

FIG. 97.—Blood grouping. *A*, Incompatible bloods. *B*, Compatible bloods.

When two bloods are incompatible the red cells of the injected blood from the donor are clumped together or agglutinated by the serum of the patient, the recipient, owing to the presence of agglutinins in the serum of the latter (Fig. 97). The basis of the incompatibility lies in the fact that in human blood the red cells contain either no antigens or one or both of two antigens, known as A and B, which may produce agglutination, whilst the serum contains corresponding antibodies or agglutinins known as beta or Anti B and alpha or Anti A. Under natural conditions an antigen and its corresponding agglutinin cannot be present simultaneously in the same blood. If, however, blood containing antigen A or B is introduced by transfusion into a person whose blood contains the corresponding antibody, agglutination occurs. Moreover, solution as well as agglutination of the transfused red cells may occur. This solution of red cells or hemolysis is the real danger of blood transfusion.

Depending on the presence of the two antigens the blood of all persons can be divided into four great groups known as O, A, B, and AB. Group O contains no antigen, group A contains A antigen, group B contains B antigen, and group AB contains both A and B antigens. As group O contains no antigen, it does not react with the blood of other groups, even though they contain agglutinins. Persons belonging to this group are therefore called universal donors because their blood is compatible with that of any of the four groups. Fortunately this is the largest group, comprising over 40 per cent of persons. A person in any one group may receive blood from anyone in the same group.

The specific antigens and agglutinins (antibodies) are governed by hereditary factors and are transmitted from parent to child, a fact which is sometimes made use of in cases of disputed parentage. An agglutinin in the blood of a child must also be present in at least one of the parents. If the blood group of one parent and the child is known, in certain cases the group of the other parent can be determined.

The suitability of a donor is determined by two methods known as *grouping* (or typing) and *matching* (or cross-matching). The blood group to which an individual belongs can be decided by testing his red cells

against serum from both a known Group A (which contains Anti B agglutinins) and a known Group B (which contains Anti A agglutinins) and noting if any agglutination occurs. The blood group to which an individual belongs can be decided by testing his red cells against serum from both a known Group A (which contains Anti B agglutinins) and a known Group B (which contains Anti A agglutinins) and noting if any agglutination occurs.

Cells agglutinated by serum from a known:		Individual belongs
Group A	Group B	to
No	No	Group O
No	Yes	Group A
Yes	No	Group B
Yes	Yes	Group AB

When this has been done both the cells and serum of the prospective donor should be cross matched against the serum and cells of the patient, even though both belong to the same group, because each group contains subgroups which are not shown by the usual method of grouping. If the same donor is to be used after an interval of time for a second transfusion, the two bloods should be matched again even though they belong to suitable groups, for agglutinins may develop in the patient's blood as the result of the first transfusion with alarming and even fatal results.

Reference has just been made to the subject of what is called intragroup incompatibility. An important example of this incompatibility is afforded by the antigen known as the *Rh factor*, so-called because it was first discovered in the blood of the rhesus monkey. About 85 per cent of persons possess this factor or antigen, so that they are said to be Rh positive, whilst 15 per cent lack the factor and are Rh negative. Anti-Rh agglutinins are not normally present in human serum, but may be formed in Rh negative persons following transfusion by Rh positive blood. If a second transfusion is given, using the same donor, it is evident that there will be a transfusion reaction owing to combination of the antigen with the corresponding agglutinin.

The Rh factor may prove a menace in another and more subtle way. It has been found that a Rh positive father can transmit the factor to the fetus. If the mother is Rh negative, anti-Rh agglutinins may be formed in her blood in response to the presence of the Rh factor in the fetus. There is now a twofold danger. (1) If the mother is transfused because of excessive blood loss at delivery, and the donor (probably the husband) happens to be Rh positive, there will be a transfusion accident, even though the two bloods belong to the same general group (intra-group incompatibility). (2) The maternal anti-Rh agglutinins may reach the fetal blood through the placenta and cause a slow continuous hemolysis of that blood. The result of this intra-uterine hemolysis of fetal blood is a severe and often fatal hemolytic anemia known as *erythroblastosis fetalis*. The reason for this name is that the most striking feature of the blood, apart from the anemia, is the presence of great numbers of nucleated red cells or erythroblasts.

16

These are immature red cells turned out in feverish haste by the bone marrow of the fetus in an effort to compensate for the progressive destruction of red blood cells.

In testing for incompatibility the criterion is the presence or absence of agglutination of the red cells in the test-tube, but it is hemolysis rather than agglutination which is the great danger in *transfusion reactions*. If the bloods of the donor and recipient are incompatible there may be immediate signs of shock as evidenced by restlessness, pallor, shortness of breath, feeble rapid pulse and fall in blood pressure. Or there may be a more delayed type of reaction, marked by chills, fever, pain in the back, jaundice and the presence of hemoglobin in the urine. These delayed symptoms are all due to breaking down of the red blood cells. About 40 per cent of the patients showing these symptoms of hemolysis make a complete recovery. In the remaining 60 per cent symptoms of renal failure develop in the course of a week, there is complete suppression of urine, and the patient dies in convulsions or coma. From a consideration of these facts it is evident how extremely important it is to prevent transfusion reactions, and how necessary are the preliminary laboratory tests to determine the question of blood incompatibility. It is essential that blood for cross matching be correctly and adequately labelled so that there can be no doubt about the identity of the person from whom it was collected. For many purposes, particularly in the treatment of shock, *blood plasma* can be used instead of whole blood. As the plasma contains no red cells, the question of incompatibility does not arise and the dangers of using unsuitable blood are thus avoided. Plasma has a great advantage over whole blood in that it can be dried, and can be kept in the dry form for an indefinite period, but unfortunately it may contain a virus which will cause jaundice.

It has already been pointed out that diseases of the blood may affect either the red cells or the leucocytes, and that the change may be either an increase or a decrease in the number of these cells. By far the commonest disease is *anemia*, a diminution in the number of the red cells. An increase of these cells is known as *polycythemia*, a rare condition. A permanent increase in the number of the leucocytes is called *leukemia*, in contrast to the temporary increase of leucocytosis in response to a bacterial infection. A marked decrease of the leucocytes is known as *leucopenia*, of which the most serious variety is *agranulocytosis* or diminution in the number of granular cells, *i.e.*, the polymorphonuclears. Anemia may be of two types, nutritional anemia and secondary anemia. Nutritional anemia can again be divided into two types, pernicious anemia and idiopathic hypochromic anemia. By nutritional anemia is meant a condition of bloodlessness due to some defect in the supply of substances necessary for the proper building up of the red blood corpuscles.

PERNICIOUS ANEMIA

The form of anemia known as pernicious provides one of the romances of modern medicine. Known for more than a hundred years since Addison, of Guy's Hospital, London, first described it, the disease has merited its grim appellation on account of its slow but remorseless progress to a fatal

conclusion. Every form of treatment was tried, but all without avail. Now the patient merely visits the butcher and buys a pound of liver!

The all-important discovery of the therapeutic effect of liver was made as the result of painstaking scientific research, but, as often happens, that research was not directed initially against the problem of pernicious anemia. George Whipple, of the University of Rochester Medical School, produced chronic anemia in dogs by repeated bleeding, and then determined which articles of diet brought the blood back to normal most quickly. The most effective substance was found to be liver, but the anemia was of the so-called secondary type and bore no resemblance to pernicious anemia. In spite of this fact Minot and Murphy, of Boston, tried liver therapy on a series of pernicious anemia patients—and it worked. For this work Whipple, Minot, and Murphy received the Nobel prize in 1934.

Pernicious anemia is now classed among the nutritional anemias. This does not necessarily mean that it is due to some defect in the diet; the defect is rather in the mechanism which converts certain elements of the diet into substances necessary for proper blood formation. The end-result, however, is the same as if the defect was primarily in the food. We have seen that erythrocytes are formed in the bone-marrow from normoblasts, and that these in turn are formed from the more primitive megaloblasts. A continuous evolution is going on in normal marrow, primitive nucleated blood cells being converted into adult non-nucleated erythrocytes, which are then liberated into the circulation. It would appear that for this process to continue, a stimulating substance which has been called the antianemic principle is necessary. If this principle is missing the primitive red blood cells fail for the most part to develop into erythrocytes and accumulate in great numbers in the marrow. Only a few erythrocytes reach the blood stream, so that a condition of bloodlessness or anemia develops which tends to be steadily progressive. Some of the primitive red cells, especially megaloblasts, escape into the blood, but for the most part they crowd the bone-marrow, where, of course, they are of no use to the patient. In biology as well as in economics it is evident that there may be the paradox of poverty in the midst of plenty.

Experiments have shown that the stimulating or antianemic principle is more abundant in the liver than in any other organ, so that feeding the patient on liver or injecting liver extract containing the principle is the best way to stimulate the marrow to normal activity. But the principle is not formed in the liver. It is produced in the normal stomach just as insulin is produced in the pancreas, although the primary function both of the stomach and the pancreas is digestion. In pernicious anemia the stomach has lost the power to produce the antianemic principle. This loss may be associated in some way with loss of the power to form hydrochloric acid, but many persons have no gastric hydrochloric acid and yet do not suffer from pernicious anemia. The disease may be treated by the administration of an extract of an animal's stomach, but it is much more convenient to use liver, seeing that the principle is stored in large amounts in that organ.

The Blood Picture. The red blood corpuscles are greatly diminished in number, so that a condition of extreme anemia may exist. Instead of

the normal 5,000,000 red cells per c.mm. the number may fall to 1,000,000 or even less. The hemoglobin or coloring matter of the red cells is also diminished but not to a corresponding degree, so that each red cell is more highly colored than normal and is said to be *hyperchromic*. Pernicious anemia is, therefore, a hyperchromic anemia, in comparison with the great majority of anemias which are hypochromic in type (Fig. 98). In several other respects the red cells are far from normal. Some are very small (*microcytes*), but the average size is larger than normal and these large cells are known as *macrocytes*. This is a highly characteristic feature of the blood picture, so that pernicious anemia is called a *macrocytic anemia*. The average diameter of normal red cells is 7.5 microns, but in this disease it may be 8 or 8.5 microns, and individual macrocytes may be 12 microns in diameter. From the standpoint of diagnosis this is the most important

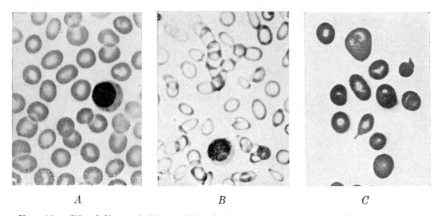

A   B   C

Fig. 98.—Blood films. *A*, Normal blood; *B*, hypochromic anemia; *C*, hyperchromic, macrocytic pernicious anemia. (Nicholson.)

single feature of the blood picture. Primitive red cells, sometimes normoblasts but usually megaloblasts, may be found in the blood. Normal erythrocytes are perfectly rounded and are all of the same size. In pernicious anemia many of the red cells are misshapen and distorted (*poikilocytosis*), and they vary much in size (*anisocytosis*).

Reference must now be made to one of the most important features of the blood picture, the presence of *reticulocytes*. These are primitive red cells which have lost their nucleus, but in which a fine network or reticulum is present in the cytoplasm. Normally about 1 per cent of the red cells are reticulocytes, but in pernicious anemia there may be 5 per cent. The great importance of reticulocytes, however, lies in their relation to liver therapy. If a patient with severe anemia is given liver diet there will be a marked rise in the number of reticulocytes, a sure indication that the treatment is proving of benefit. If there is no increase in the reticulocytes it is a strong indication that the case is not one of pernicious anemia.

The Basis of Symptoms.—The disease, which usually develops in middle life, is marked by a *progressive anemia*, and the development of a blood

picture which has already been described. The basis of the anemia is the inability of the immature red cells to develop into mature erythrocytes, so that they remain locked up in the bone-marrow and are unable to enter the blood stream. This lack of maturation is due to the absence of the normal antianemic principle, which in turn is caused by lack of the intrinsic factor in the stomach. One of the most characteristic features of the disease is the *absence of the normal hydrochloric acid* of the stomach. Unless this is absent, a diagnosis of pernicious anemia must not be made. The alteration in the gastric juice is responsible for digestive disturbances which may be severe. There may be marked *loss of appetite* which may amount to aversion for food, and in severe cases there may be dyspepsia, nausea, and even vomiting. The *tongue* is often characteristically *sore*, smooth, and of a glazed appearance.

Every patient with severe anemia is *pale* and suffers from *shortness of breath and palpitation*. The shortness of breath (*dyspnea*) is due to the fact that there are not enough red blood cells to carry oxygen from the lungs to the tissues. Just as dyspnea may result from disease of the heart or the lungs, equally so it may result from disease of the red blood cells.

There is one more group of symptoms which must be mentioned, those pointing to disease of the nervous system. Common symptoms of pernicious anemia are *numbness, tingling*, and a *feeling of pins and needles in the arms and legs*, particularly the hands and feet. In more severe cases there may be *unsteadiness in walking* or other indications of changes in the spinal cord. Very definite degenerative lesions are often found in the cord at autopsy. The exact cause of these changes is still uncertain, but it is apparently due to some deficiency similar to, but not necessarily identical with, that which is responsible for the changes in the bone-marrow. Treatment with large doses of liver serves to arrest these changes, and may relieve the symptoms either partially or completely. Treatment of severe nervous symptoms, however, is much less satisfactory than treatment of the blood condition.

Principles of Treatment.—As has been described above, the principle of treatment of pernicious anemia is the administration of liver. This can be done most effectively by the intramuscular injection of liver extract. Liver extract by mouth may also be used, but it is important to make sure that adequate dosage is provided. It is much better to use the intramuscular extract.

It has been shown that the substance known as Vitamin B_{12} is as effective as liver extract in the treatment of pernicious anemia and this may well be the essential material which is required for blood production. However, this material is not very effective by mouth and should only be used by injection. Fortunately liver extract or Vitamin B_{12} will prevent and in some cases improve the changes in the nervous system which accompany pernicious anemia.

Pernicious anemia resembles other deficiency diseases such as myxedema and diabetes in that the administration of the deficient substance must be continued for the rest of the patient's life, for the fundamental gastric defect is never restored to normal. That, however, is a small price to pay

for one of the greatest gifts, one of the most notable triumphs, of medical science. "Peace hath her victories no less renowned than war."

PRIMARY HYPOCHROMIC ANEMIA

Pernicious anemia is a hyperchromic as well as a macrocytic anemia, that is to say, each red blood cell contains rather more hemoglobin than normal. Though the total amount of hemoglobin in the blood is diminished, the total number of red cells is decreased to an even greater extent. In hypochromic anemia conditions are reversed, and the hemoglobin is diminished to a greater degree than the red cells, so that each erythrocyte has a pale, washed-out appearance. Again in contrast to pernicious anemia, this is a microcytic anemia, the average diameter of the red cells being smaller than normal.

In spite of these facts, the *clinical picture* resembles in many respects that of pernicious anemia. There are the same digestive disturbances, loss of appetite, absence of hydrochloric acid, glazed tongue, and numbness and tingling in the arms and legs. One important difference is that the finger nails are brittle and easily broken, and are turned up at the edges so that they become "spoon-shaped." The disease is much commoner than pernicious anemia, being essentially a disease of middle-aged women, often following pregnancy.

Like pernicious anemia this form of anemia is a deficiency disease, but in this case it is a *deficiency in iron*, which is an essential ingredient of hemoglobin. Several factors combine to produce this deficiency. During pregnancy there is a great depletion in the store of maternal iron which is needed for the formation of the red blood cells of the baby. The absence of hydrochloric acid and the gastric disturbance probably interfere with the digestion and absorption of the iron in the food. Finally, the marked distaste for food is apt to lead the patient to adopt a diet of slops which is greatly deficient in iron. An exact determination by examination of the blood of the type of anemia is of the highest importance, because the administration of large amounts of iron in hypochromic anemia is followed by as dramatic an improvement as is produced in pernicious anemia by the administration of liver.

SECONDARY ANEMIA

The so-called secondary anemias form rather a heterogeneous group in which the blood is of the hypochromic type. The hemoglobin is diminished to a greater degree than the number of red cells, so that each erythrocyte is correspondingly poor in coloring matter. The cause of the anemia is defective formation of hemoglobin, and this occurs as the result of all sorts of acute and chronic infection, Bright's disease, cancer, etc. Secondary anemia is, therefore, a complication or accompaniment of many other diseases. The same type of anemia develops as the result of hemorrhage, which may be acute and profuse, as in the vomiting of blood due to gastric ulcer, or chronic and almost unnoticed, as in the continued bleeding from piles. In the treatment of secondary anemia, iron is again the most valuable therapeutic agent.

HEMOPHILIA

Several blood conditions are apt to be complicated by a tendency to hemorrhage, either from a mucous membrane such as that of the mouth or from the injured skin. Purpura and leukemia are examples of bleeding diseases. Although rare, one of the best-known members of the group is hemophilia, "the bleeding disease," on account of its peculiarly hereditary character, and the fact that a number of famous examples have occurred among the royal houses of Europe. It is the most hereditary of hereditary diseases, and repeats itself from generation to generation. It is a perfect example of what is known as sex-linked heredity, for it is a disease of the males but is transmitted only by the females of the family, a striking demonstration of the adage that the female of the species is more deadly than the male.

The bleeding tendency may show itself in early childhood, as in the famous case of the Tsarevitch, whose illness is associated with the name of Rasputin. A simple injury such as the extraction of a tooth or a cut to a finger may prove fatal, owing to the uncontrollable hemorrhage which may follow it. The blood is unable to clot as normal blood should, the opening in the torn vessel remains unplugged, and the blood drains away slowly but remorselessly. The cause of the loss of clotting power has long been a mystery, but this has been solved recently. The fault is found to lie in the blood platelets. These minute bodies are necessary for normal blood coagulation; indeed it is they which start the process. In another bleeding disease known as purpura there is an extreme diminution in the normal number of platelets, so that the blood is unable to clot. In hemophilia their number is normal, but they are abnormally stable. When blood is shed, the blood platelets are disintegrated and liberate a substance which starts the whole complex mechanism of coagulation. If the platelets are not sufficiently fragile to be broken up, this activating substance will not be liberated and clotting will not occur. This lack of the normal platelet fragility, a defect which is transmitted from mother to son, is the real secret of the hemophilic mystery.

PURPURA

Purpura is a condition in which there are hemorrhages in the skin and mucous membranes. The tendency to bleeding is connected in some way with a marked fall in the number of blood platelets.

Two forms of the disease can be recognized, a *primary* form in which no cause for the fall in blood platelets can be discovered, and a *secondary* form in which it is possible to demonstrate some definite cause for the fall.

The primary form is known as *purpura hemorrhagica*. The platelets fall from 250,000 (normal) to below 60,000, and may indeed disappear completely. There are small and large hemorrhages in the skin, and bleeding from the mucous membranes of the nose, mouth, stomach, intestines, and uterus; blood appears in the urine. When a tourniquet is applied to the arm petechial hemorrhages develop below the tourniquet.

Acute cases may end fatally in a few weeks. In chronic cases removal of the spleen (splenectomy) may produce great benefit.

Secondary purpura may be caused by replacement of the bone-marrow by secondary carcinoma. The reason for this is that the cells which produce the platelets in the marrow are destroyed by the cancer. In septicemia and in infectious fevers there may be purpuric hemorrhages, owing to damage to the capillary walls by the bacterial toxins. Secondary purpura is seldom so severe as the primary form.

LEUKEMIA

Leukemia is the very antithesis of anemia, for it is an excess of the white blood cells, whereas anemia is a diminution of the red blood cells. It must be distinguished from leucocytosis which is also an increase in the number of leucocytes, but this increase is temporary and serves the definite object of combating infection, whilst leukemia is permanent and purposeless. In this respect leukemia may be regarded as a tumor growth of the white blood cells, or rather of the tissues which form these cells. It also resembles a malignant tumor in that it progresses inevitably to a fatal conclusion.

There are two main forms of white blood cells, the polymorphonuclears which belong to the granular series of leucocytes and are formed from myelocytes in the bone-marrow, and the lymphocytes which are formed in the lymphatic glands. It is evident that there must be two forms of leukemia, one involving the polymorphonuclears and the myelocytes which form them, called *myelogenous leukemia*, and the other involving the lymphocytes, called *lymphatic leukemia*. In the first the essential lesion is in the bone-marrow, in the second it is in the lymphatic glands. In both forms there is a tremendous increase in the total number of leucocytes, which commonly reach 100,000 and sometimes even 500,000 instead of the normal, 6000 or 8000. In both forms there is a progressive anemia, owing to infiltration and replacement of the bone-marrow by enormous numbers of white cells, just as any organ may be infiltrated by cancer cells with destruction of its function.

The *blood picture* in the two forms is so different that they can usually be distinguished at a glance. In myelogenous leukemia the teeming multitudes of leucocytes represent all the types of granular cells, *i.e.*, polymorphonuclears, eosinophils, and, much more important, the myelocytes and eosinophil myelocytes which give the disease its name (Fig. 99). In lymphatic leukemia the picture is uniform in place of varied, for the white cells are all of one type, *i.e.*, lymphocytes (Fig. 99).

The Basis of Symptoms.—A patient suffering from leukemia presents two entirely different groups of symptoms: The first are those of *anemia*, *e.g.*, weakness, dyspnea, palpitation, etc.; the second are due to infiltration and enlargement of the organs. In addition there is often a marked tendency to hemorrhage, as shown by bleeding from the gums, the uterus, etc. Extraction of a tooth may be followed by prolonged bleeding. In myelogenous leukemia the *spleen* is usually much *enlarged*, and sometimes it may be so huge that it fills the greater part of the abdominal cavity, producing a feeling of dragging and great weight. The liver and other

organs may be enlarged to a lesser degree owing to accumulation of white cells within their substance. In the lymphatic form the chief organs enlarged are the *lymphatic glands,* in which the lymphocytes are formed. Not only the superficial glands are enlarged such as those in the neck, axilla, and groin, but also the deep glands in the thorax and abdomen, and these may produce symptoms by pressure on neighboring structures.

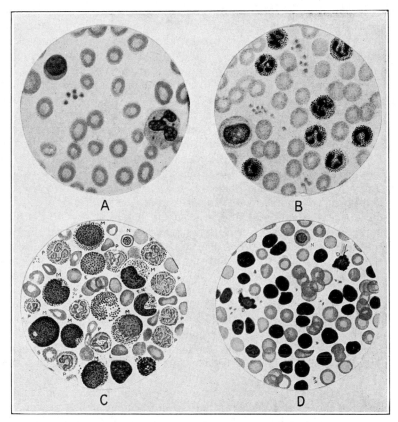

Fig. 99.—*A,* Normal blood film, showing polymorphonuclear (right) and lymphocyte (left). *B,* Leucocytosis. *C,* Myelogenous leukemia, showing numerous large myelocytes and smaller polymorphonuclears. *D,* Lymphatic leukemia; all the white cells are lymphocytes.

Principles of Treatment.—Leukemia in both its forms is a progressive condition which will eventually take the life of the patient. Sometimes it runs an acute course of a few weeks, particularly in children, but usually it is a matter of several years. The best means of holding the disease in check is by periodic courses of *roentgen-ray treatment.* The radiation at first produces a dramatic change in the blood picture, reducing the leucocytes from 100,000 to normal in a remarkably short time, but in the course of years it gradually loses this power,

It is doubtful whether radiation treatment produces any definite prolongation of life, but in most cases of chronic leukemia it will produce improvement in symptoms. Urethane is a drug which has been of value in the treatment of chronic myeloid leukemia, but again it is temporary in its effect.

AGRANULOCYTIC ANGINA

This is a disease in which an ulcerative or even gangrenous condition of the mouth (*stomatitis*) is associated with a remarkable drop in the number of leucocytes (*leucopenia*). The word angina in this sense means an acute inflammation of the throat. Agranulocytosis indicates a diminution in the number of granular leucocytes (polymorphonuclears) as distinguished from the lymphocytes. It is of special interest to those who are attending the sick, because doctors, dentists and nurses are frequently the sufferers.

Two groups of cases can be distinguished: (1) those occurring in persons who have been taking too much of some of the pain-killing drugs, particularly amidopyrine; (2) cases in which no obvious cause can be discovered. The two factors, diminished leucocyte count and severe mouth infections, probably assist one another. Disappearance of the leucocytes, which are the natural defenders of the body against infection, facilitates the spread of infection in the mouth. On the other hand a severe mouth infection with production of bacterial toxins is known in some cases to depress the production of leucocytes. Certain persons are peculiarly susceptible to the action of amidopyrine and other drugs, and respond by a marked lowering of the leucocyte count. Unfortunately the victim, on account of the pain of the mouth lesions, may continue to take even larger doses of the drug, and such cases cannot fail to go on to a fatal termination, as the leucocytes fall almost to the vanishing point.

The disease often begins with the extraction of teeth. It is marked by fever, increasing weakness and fatigue, sore mouth and sore throat. There may be extensive destruction of the gums and even the jaw, so that the teeth may fall out. Some cases are very acute, death occurring in a week or two.

It is important to discontinue the use of any dangerous drugs which the patient may have been taking. The use of penicillin has prevented the occurrence of serious infections in these cases, so that the patient's bone-marrow will have a better chance of recovery from the damage done by the toxic drug. Repeated transfusions of fresh blood may be of help also in the treatment.

THE LYMPHATIC GLANDS

LYMPHOSARCOMA

This is a malignant tumor of the lymphoid tissue, so that it is characterized by enlargement of the lymphatic glands, both superficial and deep, the lymphoid tissue in the throat and intestine, and sometimes the spleen. It presents a clinical picture very similar to lymphatic leukemia, but the lymphoid cells which multiply and cause such great enlargement of the

lymphatic glands do not escape into the blood. Treatment with roentgen rays is remarkably effective for a time, the masses of enlarged glands melting away like snow before the sun, but eventually this power is lost, and the patient is killed by the pressure of huge masses in the chest and abdomen.

HODGKIN'S DISEASE

The clinical picture of Hodgkin's disease is very similar to that of lymphosarcoma, being marked by the development of large glandular masses in the neck, axilla, groin, thorax, and abdomen (Fig. 100). Enlargement of

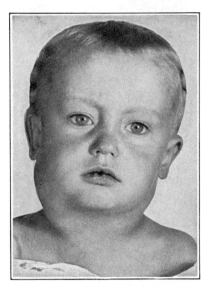

Fig. 100.—Hodgkin's disease, showing enlarged glands in the neck.

the spleen is more frequent and more marked than in lymphosarcoma. The microscopic picture is quite different from that of lymphosarcoma and suggests an infection rather than a tumor. In lymphosarcoma the cells are all of the same type, all lymphocytes. In Hodgkin's disease, on the other hand, the cells are extremely varied, resembling the picture seen in an inflammatory condition such as tuberculosis. In spite of this fact the disease has the same progressively fatal character as lymphosarcoma, although the progress may be arrested for a time by means of radiation.

TUBERCULOSIS OF THE LYMPHATIC GLANDS

Tuberculosis used to be one of the commonest causes of glandular enlargement in the neck, but improvement in the milk supply has greatly diminished the number of these cases. Glands in the neck are infected from the mouth and throat, the bronchial glands are infected from the

lungs, the abdominal glands from the bowel. The enlarged glands are at first firm, but when caseation occurs they undergo softening and break

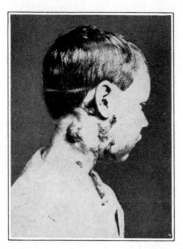

Fɪɢ. 101.—Tuberculous glands of the neck, showing sinuses and scars.

down, and the softened material is discharged on the surface if the glands are in a superficial position. Sinuses are formed which connect the softened glands with the skin of the neck. These persist for a long time, but eventually they heal, leaving deep scars which cause considerable deformity (Fig. 101). In many cases the glands heal without undergoing softening and sinus formation, especially if the patient is placed under the best hygienic conditions.

Chapter

20

THE NERVOUS SYSTEM

Structure and Function.—The nervous system is divided into a central part consisting of the brain and spinal cord, and a peripheral part consisting of the nerves carrying motor messages from the brain and cord to the muscles and those carrying sensory messages from the skin and other parts of the body to the cord and brain. In this place only the central nervous system will be considered.

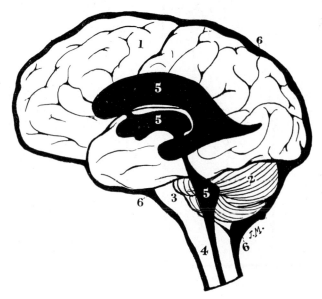

Fig. 102.—Brain and cerebrospinal fluid. 1, Cerebrum; 2, cerebellum; 3, pons; 4, medulla; 5, ventricles; 6, subarachnoid space.

The brain is made up of the cerebrum consisting of the right and left cerebral hemispheres, the brain stem which connects the cerebrum with the spinal cord, and the cerebellum or little brain (Fig. 102). The *cerebrum* initiates motor impulses which pass to the muscles, receives sensory impulses from the periphery, and is the seat of thought and reason. The *brain stem* is composed from above downwards of the midbrain, the pons, and the medulla which is continued into the spinal cord. Through the brain stem pass the innumerable motor and sensory nerves, and it also

(257)

houses the groups of nerve cells from which arise the cranial nerves that pass to the eye, ear, face, mouth, etc. The *cerebellum* is concerned principally with coördination and equilibrium, so that cerebellar disease is marked by incoördination and loss of equilibrium (ataxia).

The *spinal cord* is traversed by all the nerves going to and coming from the body. Those passing to the arm leave the cord in the upper or cervical region, whilst those passing to the leg leave in the lower or lumbar region. The motor fibers from the brain end around nerve cells in the gray matter which occupies the center of the cord, and from these motor cells a second set of fibers carries the motor messages to the muscles. The upper relay is called the *upper motor neurone* and is injured in cerebral hemorrhage; the lower relay is called the *lower motor neurone* and is injured in infantile paralysis. Complete paralysis may be produced by destruction of either neurone, and by injury to the nerve cell or the nerve fiber which arises from it.

The central nervous system is composed of neurones and neuroglia (Fig. 103). The *neurones* consist of nerve cells and the nerve fibers which arise from them and pass sometimes for a long distance through the brain and cord. The word *neuroglia* means nerve glue, and the neuroglia cells and fibers which occupy the spaces between the neurones used to be regarded merely as so much packing. There can be no doubt that the neuroglia has much more important functions to perform than that of sawdust, but what these functions are is at present uncertain. From the standpoint of disease the neuroglia is of importance, because it is from this structure that most brain tumors arise.

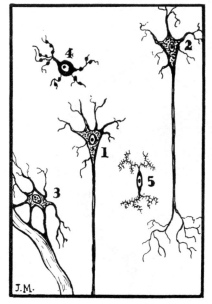

Fig. 103.—Nerve cells and neuroglia. 1 and 2, nerve cells; 3, 4, and 5, various types of neuroglial cells.

The nerve cells which send out motor impulses along nerve fibers and those which receive sensory impulses along corresponding fibers are situated in the *gray matter* of the brain which is spread for the most part as a thin layer over the surface to form the cerebral cortex. These cells are collected in groups known as *centers* or nuclei. The various centers are linked by bundles of fibers known as association fibers. In the performance of an action many centers are associated, and when this is repeated many times the nervous impulse appears to flow along the corresponding *association paths* with increasing ease; the resistance to their passage seems to be diminished. Some such mechanism may form the physical basis of *habit*.

Every act, indeed every thought, serves to make these paths more open and easily traversed. Every smallest stroke of virtue or of vice leaves its never so little scar. Nothing we ever do is, in strict scientific literalness, wiped out.

The brain and spinal cord are enclosed in two bony cases which are continuous with one another, namely, the skull and the spinal column. They are, therefore, unable to expand when they become swollen with blood or as the result of inflammation, and the increased tension causes headache, that commonest of symptoms. And yet there is an ingenious mechanism which serves to take up some of the temporary increases of pressure which may occur inside the skull. This mechanism is the *cerebrospinal fluid*, which bathes the brain and in which it is suspended as in a water-bath. This fluid not only covers the brain but also passes down the spinal canal outside the spinal cord. There is far more spare space in the canal than in the cranial cavity, so that when the brain becomes swollen the fluid flows out

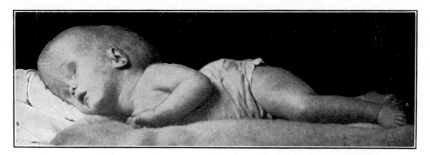

Fig. 104.—Hydrocephalus, showing extreme enlargement of the head.

into the spinal canal and thus provides a much needed safety-valve. The fluid is produced in a series of cavities in the interior of the brain which are known as the *cerebral ventricles* (Fig. 102). From these it escapes by one or two tiny openings to reach the exterior of the brain. Should these become blocked the fluid accumulates and distends the ventricles, pressing the brain against the skull with serious results, a condition of *hydrocephalus* or water on the brain (Fig. 104). In an advanced case of hydrocephalus the cranium is fearfully enlarged, dome-shaped, and surmounts the little wizened face like an enormous turban. In the end the head becomes a great bag of water, and all the mental faculties are completely lost. Such a state of affairs is only possible in a young child, in whom the various bones of the skull have not yet fused.

The spinal fluid can be withdrawn by the simple procedure of *lumbar puncture*; a hollow needle is passed into the spinal canal between two contiguous vertebræ in the lumbar region, below the point where the spinal cord ends, and the fluid which escapes is collected. This procedure is of great value in two ways: (1) It is a simple means of lowering a dangerously high intracranial pressure, which may be threatening the life of the patient by injuring the vital centers; (2) it is a valuable means of diagnosis in diseases of the nervous system, for the fluid is a mirror in which are reflected

many of the changes which may be affecting the brain and spinal cord.

One structure still remains to be described, the membrane or rather membranes which cover the brain and cord, just as the pleura covers the lungs and the peritoneum the abdominal organs. These membranes are known as the meninges, of which there are three, the dura mater, the arachnoid mater, and the pia mater. The *dura* is a tough membrane which lies in the cranial cavity and the spinal canal. The *pia* clothes the brain and cord like a glove, and the *arachnoid* like a mitt; there is, therefore, a space between these membranes, and that space, known as the *subarachnoid space*, is occupied by the cerebrospinal fluid. Fortunately this space extends a good deal lower than the termination of the spinal cord, so that in lumbar puncture a needle can be inserted into the space without danger of damaging the cord.

CEREBRAL HEMORRHAGE

With advancing years the arteries in the brain tend to degenerate and become brittle. If at the same time the blood-pressure is raised, there is danger of one of the brittle arteries bursting. When this happens the person is said to have a stroke or *apoplexy*. The effect will naturally depend on the site of the hemorrhage and also on the extent. The most common position is unfortunately that part of the brain where the motor nerves to the body are gathered together into a comparatively small space before passing down the spinal cord. The hemorrhage destroys these nerves, the motor impulses are cut off from the muscles, and the side of the body (face, arm, and leg) supplied by the side of the brain affected is paralyzed, a condition known as *hemiplegia*. Should the patient survive, the paralyzed arm and leg gradually become flexed and assume the characteristic appearance shown in Figure 105. As the motor nerves from one side of the brain cross to the opposite side before passing down the cord, it follows that hemorrhage on the right side of the brain will be followed by a left-sided hemiplegia, and *vice versa*. The speech center in right-handed persons is on the left side of the brain, so that hemorrhage on the left side will destroy the nerve fibers which go to the organs of speech, producing a condition of speechlessness or *aphasia* in addition to a right-sided hemiplegia.

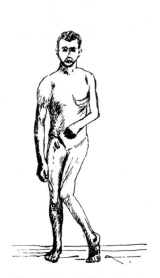

FIG. 105.—Old hemiplegia due to cerebral hemorrhage.

Apoplexy almost never produces sudden death, because the part of the brain in which it occurs contains no vital centers. Sudden death is nearly always due to sudden heart failure. But if the hemorrhage is large and close to the ventricles it may rupture into those cavities in the course of a day or two, a complication which is sure to prove fatal. On the other hand, if the hemorrhage is small the amount of damage to the brain is correspond-

ingly limited, and only the arm or the leg may be affected. The blood is gradually absorbed, and the patient may make a good recovery, with only a slight disability in the affected limb. Of course, there is always the danger of another hemorrhage later, a danger which hangs suspended over his head like the sword of Damocles but may never fall. The cerebral faculties are not necessarily interfered with. Pasteur did some of his best work after a stroke of apoplexy.

Fracture of the Skull.—This may be considered in connection with cerebral hemorrhage, because the essential danger of this condition is laceration of the surface of the brain with accompanying hemorrhage. The fracture may involve the upper part of the skull or *vault*, or the *base* of the skull. The latter is by far the more serious, and is apt to prove fatal if not properly treated. The fracture itself is of little moment, although it may open into the ear or nose, causing bleeding from those organs. There is nearly always an accompanying laceration of the base of the brain with rapidly developing edema of that struc-

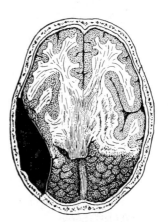

ture. Some of the most important vital nerve centers essential for life, those for the heart and for respiration, are situated in this part of the brain, and the increasing pressure on these centers caused by the edema may prove fatal. At the same time there is an accumulation of cerebrospinal fluid in this region which still further increases the pressure. It is evident that the most urgent need is to reduce the pressure inside the skull before the vital centers become paralyzed, and this is done most readily and effectively by repeated lumbar puncture and withdrawal of large amounts of spinal fluid. Since this method of treatment has been introduced, the mortality in cases of fracture of the base of the skull has been greatly reduced. Lumbar puncture also serves as a means

Fig. 106.—Extradural hemorrhage. A dark blood clot lies between the skull and the brain.

of diagnosis, for the fluid is found to contain blood when the skull has been fractured and the brain torn.

Hemorrhage inside the skull may come not from the brain but from the vessels in the meninges, the blood accumulating between the brain and the skull. There are two entirely different types of meningeal hemorrhage, known as extradural and subarachnoid hemorrhage.

Extradural Hemorrhage.—Extradural hemorrhage (Fig. 106) is a condition in which blood is poured out between the skull and the dura mater. It is commonly called *middle meningeal hemorrhage*, because the bleeding occurs from the middle meningeal artery. This artery lies in contact with the inside surface of the skull in the region of the temple, and is liable to be torn by a fracture of the skull in this region. The condition is readily diagnosed because the patient is first stunned by the blow to the skull; he then recovers consciousness and appears to be all right for a few hours—

17

this is known as the "lucid interval"; at the end of that time he becomes dull, drowsy, and finally loses consciousness again owing to the increasing pressure of the blood which is accumulating between the skull and the brain outside the dura mater. The condition *must* be diagnosed, for by immediate operation the collection of blood can be removed, the bleeding vessel tied, and the life of the patient saved. There is no blood in the cerebrospinal fluid at lumbar puncture, because the thick dura mater intervenes between the bleeding vessel and the cerebrospinal fluid.

Subarachnoid Hemorrhage. — Subarachnoid hemorrhage is hemorrhage into the subarachnoid space between the arachnoid and the pia mater. As the cerebrospinal fluid is contained in this space, blood in large amount will be found in the fluid at lumbar picture. Such hemorrhage occurs when the surface of the brain is torn by a fracture of the skull, or it may be due to rupture of an aneurism of one of the arteries which lie beneath the arachnoid at the base of the brain. The latter variety is known as *spontaneous* subarachnoid hemorrhage, and produces a clinical picture which is easily mistaken for ordinary cerebral hemorrhage. The condition, which is not uncommon in young people, usually proves fatal.

ABSCESS OF THE BRAIN

The microörganisms which cause abscess of the brain may come from a focus of infection in the skull or may be carried by the blood stream from a distance. By far the commonest local source is the middle ear or mastoid, which is so often the site of suppuration. The infection spreads inwards and causes abscess formation in the adjacent part of the brain. Another source of danger is infection in the frontal and other air sinuses which communicate with the nose. Here the abscess is likely to be in the frontal part of the brain. If the infecting organisms come from a distance, the most common source is an abscess or other septic process in the lung. Indeed, one of the dangers of abscess of the lung is the formation of a secondary abscess in the brain.

Symptoms. — The symptoms of abscess of the brain are apt to be very misleading. It might be imagined that a collection of pus in so delicate a piece of mechanism as the brain would cause a violent disturbance, but the reverse is the case. Many parts of the brain are what are called *silent areas*, that is to say, a lesion of that part produces no characteristic symptoms, and this is particularly true of those parts in which an abscess is likely to occur. Moreover, the inflammation is usually of a quiet rather than a violent character. For these reasons the abscess may give rise neither to "localizing symptoms" nor even to those indicating infection. The clinical picture will rather be that of gradually increasing intracranial pressure, which may suggest a tumor instead of an abscess. Suspicion, however, will be aroused by the coëxistence of middle-ear and mastoid infection, inflammation in the frontal sinus, or lung abscess.

Remarkably good results may follow the opening of a brain abscess, providing that the operation is performed by a surgeon who knows what he is doing, but there is always danger of the infection reaching the meninges with the production of a fatal meningitis. This complication may now be avoided by the use of antibiotics.

MENINGITIS

We have already seen that the brain and spinal cord are covered by membranes or meninges, inflammation of which constitutes the condition known as meningitis. This inflammation is confined to the pia and arachnoid, which are in intimate contact with the brain, and which contain between them the cerebrospinal fluid. Many organisms may cause meningitis, but the common ones are the meningococcus, streptococcus, pneumococcus, and tubercle bacillus. These cause, respectively, *meningococcal meningitis*, *streptococcal meningitis*, *pneumococcal meningitis*, and *tuberculous meningitis*, of which the first and the last are the most frequent. The first three organisms are pyogenic or pus-forming bacteria, so that the diseases they produce are acute and violent in type; the tubercle bacillus is less violent in action, yet it is the most fatal of the four types.

The streptococcus and pneumococcus reach the meninges from the middle ear or the frontal sinus, but they may be carried by the blood stream from distant parts, especially the lung. The meningococcus comes from the cavity of the nose or throat. It is an intracellular organism, usually found inside polymorphonuclear leucocytes. (Fig. 107).

The tubercle bacillus is carried by the blood from some distant tuberculous focus, usually the lung or a lymphatic gland. Meningitis may assume an epidemic form, with many cases developing in one locality or in many places throughout the country. Such epidemic meningitis is always due to the meningococcus. The infection is spread by *carriers*, who harbor the organisms in their throat, but do not themselves develop infection of the meninges. The term *cerebrospinal meningitis* is often applied to the meningococcal type, but the other forms are also cerebrospinal in the sense that the meninges of both the brain and the spinal cord are inflamed.

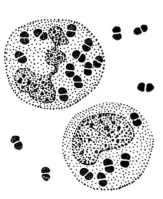

Fig. 107.—Meningococci, mostly intracellular.

Diagnosis.—The diagnosis is made by *lumbar puncture*. When normal cerebrospinal fluid is removed by this means it is as clear as water, and the pressure is so low that it flows out drop by drop. In meningitis due to the pyogenic bacteria the fluid is turbid, because in reality it is thin pus, and the pressure is raised to such a degree that it may spurt from the needle. When the fluid is examined under the microscope it is found to be crowded with polymorphonuclear leucocytes (pus cells), and to contain varying numbers of the bacteria responsible for the infection. In tuberculous meningitis the spinal fluid is only slightly milky or may be almost clear, for, as the inflammation is less acute, the cells are much fewer in number and are for the most part lymphocytes. The pressure is raised, as in the other

forms of meningitis. The finding of tubercle bacilli in the fluid clinches the diagnosis.

At autopsy the subarachnoid space is filled with an acute inflammatory exudate in the meningococcal, streptococcal, and pneumococcal forms, so that the brain and cord are covered with yellow pus. In tuberculous meningitis, however, there is only a thin milky white layer in which tubercles may be distinguished with difficulty. As the subarachnoid space over the brain is continuous with that of the cord, lumbar puncture serves to show what is going on inside the skull in cases of meningitis.

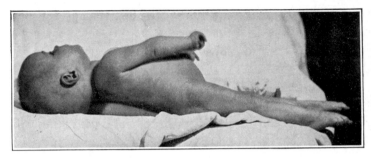

Fig. 108.—Acute meningitis, showing stiffening of the body, retraction of the head, and arching of the back.

The Basis of Symptoms.—The symptoms of meningitis are partly general and partly local. The general symptoms are those of any severe infection, *i.e.*, fever, malaise, and leucocytosis. The *local symptoms* are due to meningeal irritation, both cerebral and spinal, *i.e.*, severe headache, stiffness of the neck, and pains in the back. In severe cases the head is retracted and the back arched, presenting a highly characteristic clinical picture. (Fig. 108). The onset is often very sudden, frequently with vomiting, and the patient is at first restless and irritable, but later becomes drowsy, and finally sinks into a stupor. During the stage of irritability the patient may be very sensitive to bright light (*photophobia*), and to loud noises. The irritation symptoms are due to stimulation of the meninges and the nerves which enter the brain and cord. The drowsiness and stupor of the later stages are due to increasing intracranial pressure with compression of the brain. This is largely due to a condition of acute hydrocephalus which develops, for the inflammatory exudate blocks the small openings through which the cerebrospinal fluid escapes from the ventricles, so that the fluid collects increasingly in these cavities and presses the brain against the skull.

Principles of Treatment.—In the case of meningococcal meningitis, penicillin and sulfonamide drugs have reduced the previous high mortality rate very considerably. Large doses of these drugs are used until the infection is combatted. The use of antiserum is no longer considered necessary. Similarly, in streptococcal and pneumococcal meningitis the antibiotics and sulfonamides have provided a cure in many cases, although the number of recoveries in pneumococcal meningitis is not as high as in other forms.

Tuberculous meningitis was considered uniformly fatal until the introduction of streptomycin. Now prolonged treatment with streptomycin, both intramuscularly and injected into the spinal canal, has resulted in improvement and apparent cure in some cases, but the disease still cannot be completely controlled in all cases.

ACUTE ANTERIOR POLIOMYELITIS

Poliomyelitis or *infantile paralysis* is an acute infectious disease of the spinal cord and brain caused by a filterable virus (the virus of poliomyelitis) and chiefly affecting children. The name signifies an inflammation of the gray matter of the spinal cord or marrow (*polios*, gray; *myelos*, marrow). It is the anterior part of the gray matter of the cord containing the motor nerve cells which is chiefly affected, thus explaining the term anterior in the full title (Fig. 109). The disease may occur in sporadic, *i.e.*, occasional, form, or it may become epidemic. An epidemic usually begins about the end of June and for some unknown reason disappears with the onset of cold weather.

The virus is carried from one person to another in the throat where it can live without producing any symptoms and without invading the nervous system. Such individuals are called carriers. They are immune to the disease, but they can carry the infection. During an epidemic there are far more carriers than patients suffering from the disease, that is to say, there is a much larger carrier epidemic than disease epidemic. The virus has also been found in the feces of patients convalescing from the disease, and even in sewage. This at once suggests the analogy of typhoid fever, and opens the question as to whether the virus of poliomyelitis may gain entrance through the mouth rather than through the nose. It will probably be some time before this question can be answered. The importance of the correct answer in relation to prevention of the disease is self-evident.

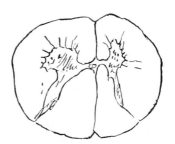

Fig. 109. — Late effects of poliomyelitis: atrophy of right anterior (motor) horn of the spinal cord.

The infection starts in the throat and nose, and spreads up through the floor of the skull to reach the brain. The route which it follows is a remarkable one, quite unlike that by which bacteria spread (lymph stream and blood), but similar to that of a number of other viruses which attack the nervous system. It travels along the nerves, actually inside the nerves, which pass from the brain through the floor of the skull to the nose, *i.e.*, the olfactory nerves or nerves of smell. Having reached the brain, the virus traverses that organ and passes down the nerve fibers of the spinal cord, where it attacks and destroys the motor nerve cells in the anterior part of the gray matter. The motor nerve cells of the lower part of the brain (pons or medulla) may also be attacked, and if death occurs it is due to destruction

of these cells. The meninges are also inflamed, so that the cerebrospinal fluid may be expected to show changes.

The Basis of Symptoms.—The child shows *general symptoms* of infection, such as fever, malaise, irritability, and loss of appetite. After a day or two of these symptoms the *paralysis,* which is so characteristic and tragic a feature of the disease, suddenly makes its appearance. Only one arm or one leg may be paralyzed, or both legs.

Nerve cells differ from most cells of the body in being unable to proliferate, so that no repair or replacement of the injured cells is possible. For this reason the paralysis is permanent. The paralyzed muscles atrophy from disease, so that the limb becomes wasted and shrivelled (Fig. 110).

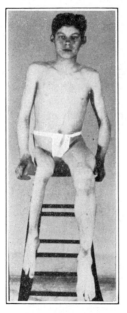

Fig. 110.—End-result of poliomyelitis; marked atrophy of right leg.

If the vital centers in the lower part of the brain are also affected there may be *paralysis of swallowing and respiration,* which may result in death. The symptoms are not purely motor, for there is usually *pain* in the back and the affected limbs. *Stiffness of the neck* and *rigidity of the back* are constant and early symptoms. The explanation of these sensory symptoms is not certain, but they are supposed to be due to irritation of the meninges and the sensory nerves. During an epidemic many children manifest only the sensory disturbances and never develop paralysis, owing probably to their motor nerve cells possessing a certain degree of immunity against the virus.

The *cerebrospinal fluid* shows changes which are useful in making a diagnosis in the early stages before paralysis has developed, but which are not distinctive of the disease. The pressure is raised and there is a moderate increase in the number of lymphocytes. Both of these changes are also present in tuberculous meningitis, but the absence of tubercle bacilli serves to distinguish the two diseases.

Principles of Treatment.—There is no specific treatment for this disease at the present time. So far all attempts to attack this virus infection have resulted in failure. During the acute phase of the disease it is important that the patient have careful nursing care, with protection of paralyzed muscles. Heat in the form of hot packs to the painful muscles will relieve spasm and symptoms of pain. Some cases suffering from paralysis of the respiratory muscles can be saved by the use of the artificial respirator. It is important to utilize all methods of exercise and physiotherapeutic measures during the rehabilitation period which may be many weeks or months. If sufficient recovery of muscle strength does not occur splints may be required to provide the maximum degree of functional usefulness.

RABIES

The popular name of this disease is *hydrophobia*, indicating an aversion or repulsion to water. It is primarily a disease of animals, dogs, cats and wolves, being rarely transmitted from a rabid animal to man. The virus of rabies is found in the saliva of the rabid animal, and gains entrance to man through wounds from bites or scratches. Like poliomyelitis, rabies is a disease of the central nervous system, and the virus passes from the infected wound along the nerves to the spinal cord, in much the same way as the tetanus toxin travels. The time this takes is the incubation period, and fortunately it is long, from forty to sixty days.

The principal *symptoms*, whether in animal or man, are terrific cerebral excitement and rage, spasm of the muscles of the pharynx especially at the sight of water so that the patient is unable to drink, and generalized convulsions. It is one of the most terrible of all diseases, and when symptoms have developed all cases die.

It is remarkable that the modern *treatment* of rabies is that introduced by Pasteur, who knew nothing of filterable viruses. He found that the spinal cord of rabbits infected with the disease was rich in the infective agent (of the nature of which he knew nothing), as shown by the results of animal inoculation. He also found that he could lower the virulence by drying the cord—the longer the drying, the lower the virulence. He then used the material of low virulence as a vaccine, with which he inoculated repeatedly the person bitten by the rabid animal. By this means he built up resistance to the virus, so that by the time it reached the spinal cord some two months later the patient had become immune. If the Pasteur treatment was commenced immediately after the bite, there was complete prevention in every case. Surely a stroke of pure genius in the earliest days of bacteriology!

SYPHILIS OF THE NERVOUS SYSTEM

Among the most tragic manifestations of syphilis are those due to infection of the central nervous system. A peculiarity of these lesions is that they do not develop for many years after the original infection; it may be ten, fifteen, or even twenty years later. The patient may have been without symptoms for years, may have almost forgotten that he ever had syphilis, when suddenly, without warning the sword of Damocles may fall. Various parts of the nervous system may be attacked, so that the symptoms may be very varied, but there are two clearly cut clinical pictures or diseases which alone will be described here. The first and most terrible of these is general paresis or general paralysis of the insane, the second is tabes dorsalis or locomotor ataxia.

General Paresis.—The name is descriptive for it implies not only a weakness of the muscles but a general weakening of all the faculties of the mind. The even more sinister "general paralysis of the insane" describes the final state of the patient. The spirochetes of syphilis are scattered widely throughout the brain, and produce multiple areas of inflammation together with destruction of the nerve cells and nerve fibers. As a result

of this destruction the brain atrophies and wastes away, becoming much smaller than normal. This wasting affects particularly the cerebral cortex in the frontal region, that is to say the part of the brain concerned with the highest functions of the mind. The areas concerned with muscular movements and with sensation are also involved.

The Basis of Symptoms.—The symptoms of the disease are as diverse as the lesions are widely disseminated. The first indication that all is not well is a painful *deterioration in the higher life of the mind* and the soul. The moral sense is impaired, and there is a weakening of the faculties of judgment, reason, and self-control. *Delusions of grandeur* lead to domestic and financial difficulties, for if a man believes that he is worth millions and orders motor cars and grand pianos in corresponding amount, it is not conducive to domestic happiness. The structure of the mind crumbles, and the final stage is one of childishness and *complete dementia*. All of these changes are due to destruction of the nerve cells in the cerebral cortex. *Tremors* are highly characteristic; they involve the face, lips, and tongue so that the speech becomes thick and indistinct, and the hands are tremulous. These tremors are due to lesions in the motor centers. The sensory centers are also involved, so that sensibility is dulled and pain may hardly be felt. The pupil of the eye no longer contracts when exposed to bright light, although it still does so when the eye looks at a near object, a condition known as the *Argyll-Robertson pupil*. *Convulsive seizures* followed by unconsciousness are common. The *weakness of the muscles* implied in the name of the disease becomes extreme. In the end the patient is not only mindless but helpless. To describe his existence as that of an animal is unjust to even the lowest member of the animal kingdom.

The *cerebrospinal fluid* shows changes which are of great importance, because they allow the physician to make an early diagnosis at a time when treatment may arrest the progress of the disease. The cells of the fluid, particularly lymphocytes, are markedly increased, especially at the beginning of the malady, but far more significant is the fact that the Wassermann test on the fluid is positive, showing that the patient is suffering from syphilis of the central nervous system.

Principles of Treatment.—Penicillin treatment has largely replaced all other forms of therapy in the handling of these patients. A course of penicillin injections over a period of three or four weeks is used. In addition to this, in some cases, the use of fever therapy has been of value. Formerly the fever was produced by the introduction of a malarial infection into the patient's blood stream. This has now largely been carried out by the production of artificial fever by means of placing the patient in a chamber which is heated to raise the patient's temperature to 105°.

Tabes Dorsalis.—The word tabes means a wasting away, and as the lesion in this syphilitic disease of the spinal cord is a wasting of the posterior or dorsal part of the cord, the condition is called tabes dorsalis (Fig. 111). In the dorsal columns of the cord run the nerves which carry the sensation of position, what is called muscle sense and joint sense. When these are lost the patient is no longer certain of the position of his legs, so that he becomes unsteady or *ataxic* in his locomotion. For this reason the disease is also known as *locomotor ataxia*. The first name is a pathological term

indicating the lesion, the second is a clinical term indicating one of the principal symptoms.

Anyone wishing to read a description of the onset of the symptoms of tabes by a master of literature should look up Kipling's wonderful little story, "Love o' Women." There is no muscular weakness, for the lesion is confined to the sensory nerves, but the power of muscular coördination is gradually lost, so that the patient is unable to make his legs do what he wants them to. Things are not so bad as long as he has the assistance of sight, but in the dark he is completely at sea. The ordinary person walks by faith (without watching the ground), but the tabetic walks by sight. He walks with his legs wide apart to increase his stability, and is unable to stand with his feet together and his eyes closed without swaying or falling (*Romberg's sign*). To the trained eye the tabetic can be recognized at once as he walks down the street by his peculiar wide-based gait and the way he throws his feet out and brings them down with a stamp (Fig. 112).

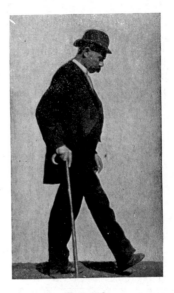

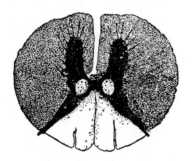

FIG. 111.   FIG. 112.

FIG. 111.—Spinal cord in tabes dorsalis; marked degeneration (white) of posterior columns.

FIG. 112.—A tabetic walking. He watches the ground and throws out his feet. (Church and Peterson; courtesy of W. B. Saunders Company.)

Other sensory disturbances are sudden, severe shooting pains passing down the legs known as *lightning pains*, and occasional attacks of abdominal pain and vomiting, called *gastric crises*, which may be mistaken for acute appendicitis. There is *loss of the knee-jerks*, *i.e.*, lack of response when the tendon below the knee cap is tapped, loss of the normal contraction of the pupil to light (*Argyll-Robertson pupil*) as in general paresis, and gradual wasting of the optic nerve, *optic atrophy*, with corresponding impairment of vision. The disease may last many years, because it involves no vital centers. The *cerebrospinal fluid* shows the same changes as in general paresis so that its examination is of the greatest help in diagnosis.

Treatment.—Again, in this form of central nervous system syphilitic infection, penicillin now is the best method of treatment and may often serve to arrest the progress of the condition and relieve many of the symptoms.

DISSEMINATED SCLEROSIS

This condition, also known as multiple sclerosis, is a chronic disease of the nervous system, characterized by curious remissions and relapses, and by the presence of multiple patches of sclerosis or hardening scattered diffusely throughout the gray and white matter of the brain and spinal cord. The nerve fibers in the white matter degenerate and are replaced by glial (neuroglial) scar tissue. The cause of the condition is unknown.

The *clinical picture* is extremely varied. The patient, usually a young man, suffers from an assortment of sensory and motor symptoms, some of which may be quite fleeting. The sensory disturbances take the form of numbness and tingling in the hands and feet, or definite loss of sensation. Motor disturbances are seen in the gait, which is peculiarly stiff, in fleeting paralyses, in tremor of the hands when they are used (intention tremor), a jerky movement of the eyes (nystagmus), and a characteristic staccato speech.

There is no satisfactory treatment, but on account of the remissions the patient may live for many years.

BRAIN TUMORS

We have already seen that the brain is composed of two types of cells, the nerve cells and the neuroglial cells. Tumors of the brain only arise from and are composed of neuroglial cells so that they are called *gliomas*. Not uncommonly a tumor grows from the meninges which cover the brain, and is therefore called a *meningioma*. There is a fundamental difference between these two types of tumor, for the meningioma is an innocent tumor which is encapsulated and merely presses upon the brain (Fig. 113), whereas the glioma is a malignant tumor which infiltrates the brain and is not demarcated from it in any way. It follows that it is very much easier to remove a meningioma than a glioma. Although gliomas are malignant by virtue of their infiltrative power, they vary greatly in their degree of malignancy, and whilst some are rapidly growing and kill the patient in a few months, others grow very slowly and the patient may live for many years, especially if he receives skillful surgical treatment. Moreover, gliomas do not form metastases or secondary growths in other parts of the body like most malignant tumors do.

There are many different kinds of glioma, but only four of these will be described. Of these four, two occur principally in the adult, namely, glioblastoma multiforme and astrocytoma; two occur in children, namely, medulloblastoma and ependymoma. The *glioblastoma multiforme* is a highly malignant tumor occurring in middle life and is usually found in one or other of the cerebral hemispheres. The margin is ill-defined so that the surgeon may have great difficulty in knowing where the tumor ends

and the normal brain begins. It is highly invasive and is likely to kill the patient in the course of a few months. The *astrocytoma* is much less malignant, and the average time of survival after operation is six years. It may occur in any part of the brain, and in children the common site is the cerebellum. This tumor in children is usually completely innocent. The *medulloblastoma* is a highly malignant and rapidly growing tumor. The prognosis of this tumor of children is therefore the very opposite to that of astrocytoma. The *ependymoma* is the rarest of the four. It usually occurs in children and in the same location as the medulloblastoma. It is, however, much less malignant than that tumor.

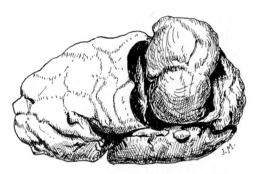

FIG. 113.—Meningioma lifted out of cavity in brain which it has produced by pressure.

Another intracranial tumor which is much more closely related to meningioma than to the gliomas is the *acoustic nerve tumor*. It grows from the eighth cranial nerve at the angle between the pons and the cerebellum and forms a firm, round, well-encapsulated tumor. It presses upon the nerve supplying the muscles of the face as well as upon the acoustic or auditory nerve. The principal symptoms are therefore facial paralysis and deafness on one side. It is important to realize that the tumor is perfectly benign, so that when removed surgically there is no chance of its return.

The Basis of Symptoms.—The symptoms of a brain tumor may be divided into two groups, the first general and the second localizing. The *general symptoms* are due to the increased intracranial pressure produced by the mass of new tissue inside the skull, and are more or less the same in whichever part of the brain the tumor is situated. The chief of these is *headache*, which may become excruciating in intensity. The *cerebrospinal fluid pressure* is greatly increased, as shown by lumbar puncture. *Vomiting* may be marked in the later stages, but is often absent. The pressure on the optic nerves produces swelling of the termination of these nerves in the eye, a condition called *optic neuritis* which can be recognized when the retina of the eye is viewed with the ophthalmoscope. Roentgen-ray examination may show *thinning of the skull*.

The *localizing symptoms* are naturally very varied, because they depend on the site of the tumor in the brain. If the motor centers are involved there will be weakness of the muscles of the face, arm or leg. If the sensory centers are affected there will be corresponding disturbance of sensation.

Involvement of the special senses, such as sight or hearing, will point to the areas concerned with these functions. It is for this reason that these symptoms are known as localizing, because by a careful analysis of these disturbances the physician is able to arrive at a conclusion as to the exact location of the tumor, and the surgeon is then able to open the skull at the correct spot where he will have access to the lesion. Unfortunately, there are fairly extensive regions of the brain known as *silent areas*, so-called because lesions of these areas do not give rise to any localizing symptoms. If the tumor is situated in one of the silent areas, it may be impossible to determine its exact location, impossible even to decide on which side of the brain to operate.

If the reader would like to get a vivid idea of what it is like to be a patient with a brain tumor, he should read "A Journey Round My Skull," by the distinguished Hungarian novelist, Frigyes Karinthy, who himself was the patient. The rather terrifying description of the operation under a local anesthetic is perhaps somewhat highly colored.

Treatment.—The treatment of brain tumors is discouraging but by no means hopeless. If the tumor can be located, much or the whole of it may be removed. In the case of a meningioma a complete cure may be expected. With the gliomas it is very much more difficult for the surgeon to know if he has removed all the tumor, so that there is great danger that some of it may be left behind and that the growth will recur. But even if a cure cannot be assured, several years of comfort and comparative health may be added to the patient's life. Perhaps the most important point for the patient with a brain tumor to decide is to choose the right surgeon.

THE CEREBROSPINAL FLUID

The normal spinal fluid is as clear as water, contains sugar and chlorides, no protein, less than 5 lymphocytes per c.mm., and no polymorphonuclears. In acute meningitis the vessels in the inflamed meninges allow the constituents of the blood to pour into the fluid, so that it contains much protein and great numbers of polymorphonuclears (pus cells). The fluid is therefore purulent and turbid. The bacteria feed on and destroy the sugar, so that this substance is reduced in amount or disappears entirely. Bacteria are found in smears of the pus and in culture. Tuberculous meningitis, which is much less acute, gives rather different spinal fluid findings. The fluid is clear or only slightly milky, as it usually contains less than 100 cells per c.mm., most of which are lymphocytes. The protein (globulin) is only moderately increased, and the sugar correspondingly diminished. The most characteristic findings are a marked diminution in the chlorides and the presence of tubercle bacilli in the smears. In poliomyelitis the picture is identical with that of tuberculous meningitis, except that the chlorides are normal and there are, of course, no tubercle bacilli.

Chapter

21

DISEASES OF THE BONES AND JOINTS

Structure and Function.—It is rational as well as convenient to consider diseases of the bones and joints together, because a joint is merely a movable union between two bones, so that disease of a bone may involve the joint and disease of a joint may spread to the adjoining bones.

A bone is not a dead thing. It is true that it is impregnated with a nonliving material which gives it its rigidity, but the bone itself is just as much alive as the heart or the brain. It consists of bone cells surrounded by a modified fibrous tissue saturated with salts of calcium, in which there are spaces or interstices which are particularly numerous at the ends of the bone. In the center of the shaft of the bone there is a cavity, the *medullary cavity*, filled with the *bone-marrow* which manufactures the red blood cells and the leucocytes (Fig. 114). The marrow also extends into the interstices of the bone, and is therefore particularly abundant at the ends of the bone. Lining the medullary cavity and the interstices are primitive bone cells called *osteoblasts*, which are the precursors of the adult bone cells, and whose function it is to form new bone. It is from these cells that the commonest form of malignant bone tumor, the osteogenic sarcoma, is formed. In the same situations there are much larger cells, giant cells containing several nuclei, called *osteoclasts*. They are concerned with removal instead of formation of bone, and from them also a tumor, the giant-cell tumor, may arise, but unlike the osteogenic sarcoma it is essentially benign.

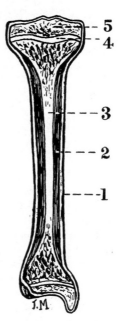

Fig. 114.—Long bone. 1, Periosteum; 2, shaft; 3, medullary cavity; 4, epiphyseal cartilage; 5, epiphysis.

It is a mistake to imagine that bone is the stable and enduring structure which it appears to be. The bones of the skeleton form a great storehouse for calcium, which is combined with phosphorus in the form of calcium phosphate. When the body needs more calcium it is taken from the bones, where it is later replaced. During pregnancy there is a great demand for calcium to form the bones of the growing baby, and if the food does not contain a sufficient amount it is taken from the bones of the mother. The

(273)

movement of calcium to and from the bones is governed largely by the parathyroid glands, those minute structures in the neck situated behind the thyroid. When the parathyroids become overactive, as in parathyroid tumor, the bones become so decalcified that they are softened and bend under any strain, giving rise to marked deformities.

During childhood and adolescence the bones grow in length. This they do entirely by virtue of a layer of cartilage at each end of the bone known as the *epiphyseal cartilage.* When the child grows up this cartilage becomes calcified and converted into bone, after which no more growth is possible. The growth of the cartilage is under the control of the pituitary gland. When this gland becomes overactive in early life as the result of a pituitary tumor, the growth of the epiphyseal cartilage is speeded up and the individual becomes a giant. It is evident that gigantism is not possible once the cartilage has become converted into bone. Conversely, if the pituitary is insufficiently active, growth ceases and the person remains a dwarf. But whilst there is only one cause of gigantism, there are many causes of dwarfism. Indeed the study of dwarfism is a subject in itself, a subject so extensive that to discuss it here is out of the question.

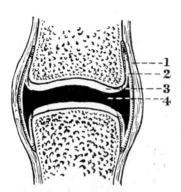

FIG. 115.—Normal joint. 1, Capsule; 2, synovial membrane; 3, articular cartilage; 4, joint cavity.

A bone must grow in thickness as well as in length. This increase of thickness is brought about by the *periosteum,* a fibrous membrane which closely covers the bone and which contains osteoblasts on its deep surface. It is through the periosteum that the superficial part of the bone receives its blood supply, so that anything which injures or removes the periosteum will threaten the health and even the life of the bone.

We have said that the epiphyseal cartilage is at the end of the bone, but this is not strictly true. It is separated from the actual end of the bone, *i.e.,* the joint surface, by a small piece of bone known as the *epiphysis.* The epiphyseal cartilage therefore intervenes between the shaft of the bone and the epiphysis. Many of the most important diseases of bone (inflammation, tuberculosis, sarcoma) commence in this region of the bone on one or other side of the epiphyseal cartilage.

It now becomes evident that it is the epiphyses which enter into the formation of a joint. The surface of each epiphysis is covered by a hard layer of cartilage, the *articular cartilage,* which provides an exquisitely smooth surface for the movements of the joint, a surface just as smooth as the piston and cylinder of an automobile. If anything interferes with the smoothness of this surface there will be a corresponding interference with the function of the joint. Each epiphysis is therefore bounded by two layers of cartilage, the articular cartilage on the side next the joint, the epiphyseal cartilage (in the growing bone) on the side next the shaft.

A *joint* or articulation consists of two *articular surfaces*, a *capsule* or strong fibrous structure which joins the two ends of the bone together, and a *synovial membrane*, which lines the capsule and produces an oily fluid that lubricates the articular surfaces and ensures the smooth working of the mechanism (Fig. 115). Any or all of these structures may be damaged by disease.

ACUTE OSTEOMYELITIS

The word osteomyelitis means inflammation of the bone (osteitis) and of the bone-marrow (myelitis). The inflammation actually involves only the soft parts of the bone, *i.e.*, the marrow in the medullary cavity and the interstices of the bone, but the calcium is dissolved away from the hard structures as the result of the inflammation, so that the bone becomes softened.

The inflammation is nearly always caused by staphylococci, which generally gain access to the body through the skin causing a boil, and are then carried to the bone by the blood stream. The disease is essentially one of children and adolescents in whom the bone is still growing. As growth takes place only in the region of the epiphyseal cartilage, and as this is therefore the part most abundantly supplied with bloodvessels, it follows that the disease affects the end of the bone, usually on the side of the epiphyseal cartilage next to the shaft. Injury to the bone is a common accessory factor, because this is apt to cause rupture of a small vessel, and the circulating staphylococci are enabled to settle down in the blood clot and grow rapidly. The injury may be a twist or a direct blow. I once saw a boy develop acute osteomyelitis twelve hours after he had been struck on the knee by a golf ball. The bones most frequently affected are the femur, tibia, and humerus.

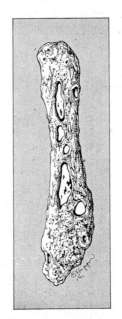

FIG. 116. — Extensive osteomyelitis showing the rough new bone, cloacæ, and sequestra (white.)

The lesion begins as an *abscess of the bone*. As the result of acute inflammation pus is produced, and this tends to spread down the medullary cavity and outward to the surface. When it reaches the surface it raises the periosteum from the bone, and may spread along the surface for a considerable distance. As it is from the periosteum that the bone receives a considerable proportion of its blood supply, it follows that a considerable area of the shaft may become devitalized and die. Such a piece of dead bone is called a *sequestrum*, and in the course of time this becomes separated from the living bone by the action of the osteoclasts. The inflamed periosteum is stimulated to form a thick layer of new bone, called the *new case*, which surrounds the sequestrum. In the new case there are a number of openings,

cloacæ, through which purulent discharge escapes from the interior (Fig. 116). The infection may also spread through the epiphyseal cartilage into the epiphysis, and may finally destroy the articular cartilage and infect the adjacent joint. One of the most serious results of the inflammation is thrombosis of the vessels in the marrow. The thrombi become heavily infected with staphylococci, and they may break down and be carried by the blood to the lungs and other organs, where they set up multiple abscesses, a condition of *pyemia*. Great numbers of bacteria enter the blood stream from the suppurative area in the bone, so that the patient suffers from *septicemia*.

The Basis of Symptoms.—From what has been said it is apparent that osteomyelitis tends to be both a local and a general infection, and the symptoms are therefore both local and general. The *local symptoms* are *pain* and *tenderness* at the end of one of the long bones, usually in the region of the knee, together with *heat, redness*, and *swelling:* the classical signs, in short, of acute inflammation. As the lesions are so close to a joint the serious mistake may be made of confusing the condition with acute rheumatism. The pain and tenderness are very severe, because the inflammation is going on in dense unyielding bone, so that the tension becomes extreme with accompanying pressure on the sensory nerves. All acute inflammation of bone causes severe pain and tenderness, whether it be in the long bones, mastoid or jaw (from toothache), and always for the same reason.

The *general symptoms* are those of any severe acute infection, *i.e.*, high fever, chills, rapid pulse, marked leucocytosis, and the presence of staphylococci in blood culture. Although it is the local lesions which cause the patient the pain that is his chief complaint, it is the general infection which threatens his life.

Principles of Treatment.—The entire picture of osteomyelitis has been changed since the introduction of antibiotic therapy. The disease used to be a surgical one, the only treatment being opening up the bone so as to allow the pus and the infecting organisms to escape. The condition is now treated by medical means and if the diagnosis is made early and correct treatment started at once, the widespread bacterial infection described in the preceding paragraphs will be prevented. It is evident also that if the case is properly treated there will be no development of a sequestrum nor sinuses.

BONE AND JOINT TUBERCULOSIS

Tuberculosis of bone is like osteomyelitis except that it is a chronic disease from the beginning. Like the acute disease, it affects the ends of the bones, but begins in the epiphysis much more frequently than does osteomyelitis. The bones most often attacked are the long bones of the arms and legs, the bones of the wrist and ankle, and the vertebræ. The disease may commence in the bone and spread to the joint, or commence in the synovial membrane of the joint and spread to the bone. In the late stages, both structures are usually affected. The tubercle bacilli are carried to the bone or joint by the blood stream from some other focus in the body, usually the lung or a lymphatic gland. In about one-fifth of the cases the infection is

due to the bovine type of tubercle bacillus, having been derived from infected milk. Growing bones are particularly susceptible to the infection, so that the disease is commoner in youth, but the age incidence is not so marked as in osteomyelitis.

The lesion consists of a slow destruction of the end of the bone, not a wholesale destruction but a nibbling here and there, giving the bone a worm-eaten appearance known as *caries*, a word which means dry rot. If the disease begins in the shaft, the epiphyseal cartilage is gradually eaten away and the epiphysis is invaded. From the epiphysis, whether it is infected primarily or secondarily, the disease spreads to the articular cartilage, which is eroded bit by bit until the articular surface comes to be formed by the diseased and roughened bone (Fig. 117). A similar destruction of the smooth articular surface occurs when the disease begins in the joint, because the infection extends from the synovial membrane to the articular cartilage, which is again eaten away bit by bit.

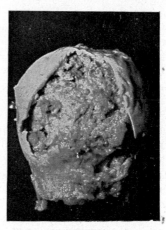

Fig. 117.—Tuberculosis of head of femur. Only a small part of smooth articular cartilage remains at the left. (Boyd, Surgical Pathology; courtesy of W. B. Saunders Company.)

Tuberculosis of the spine, also known as *Pott's disease*, is of frequent occurrence in children, although it may also occur in the adult. The disease affects one or more vertebræ, which it slowly destroys, just as the ends of the long bones are destroyed. The pressure from above causes the softened vertebræ to collapse, with resulting deformity of the spine, so that the child develops a "hump-back" (Fig. 118). A more serious result is pressure on the spinal cord, with the gradual production of paralysis of the legs (Fig. 119). A tuberculous or *cold abscess* may develop, the peculiarity of which is that it tends to spread along the psoas muscle which passes from the lumbar part of the spine to the upper end of the femur. This *psoas abscess*, as it is called, will therefore tend to appear in the groin as a soft swelling which may easily be mistaken for a hernia.

The Basis of Symptoms.—Whichever joint is affected, be it the wrist, the knee, or the joints of the spine, the first symptom will be *limitation of movement*. This is natural, because no one will move a diseased joint more than is absolutely necessary. If the disease starts in the bone, symptoms will not appear until the joint also is involved. The joint will be *swollen* owing to tuberculous swelling of the synovial membrane. The *affected limb* tends to be *shorter* than the normal one, partly because of the bone destruction, but mainly because the epiphyseal cartilage which is responsible for the growth in the length of the bone is killed. When the articular cartilage is destroyed and the roughened ends of the bones come in contact,

18

pain will develop. There may be no pain during the day, because the muscles around the joint contract and prevent movement from occurring. But
when the child falls asleep the muscle watch dogs are no longer on guard,
and the joint may be moved, causing intense pain, the child waking up with
a start and a cry, so that these pains are known as "starting pains" or
"night pains." For a long time the patient may show none of the general
symptoms of tuberculosis such as fever or loss of weight.

Principles of Treatment.—The treatment of bone and joint tuberculosis
is general and local. The general treatment is fresh air, good food, plenty
of sunshine, etc. The local treatment is rest to the joint. This is brought
about by means of splints or a plaster cast. If these fail to arrest the progress of the disease, or if the damage
is already too great, the diseased ends
of the bones may have to be removed
surgically. After such an operation
the two bones fuse in the same way
as a fracture unites, and the joint
becomes permanently stiff; indeed, it
ceases to be a joint at all.

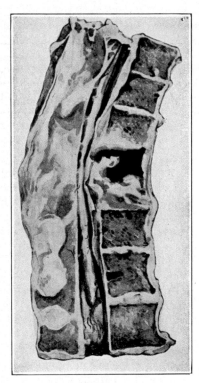

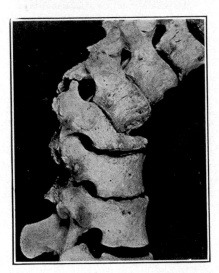

FIG. 118   FIG. 119

FIG. 118.—Pott's disease, showing destruction of the middle vertebra.

FIG. 119.—Pott's disease of spine. A vertebra is destroyed (right) and the spinal
cord is compressed.

ACUTE RHEUMATISM

A general description of acute rheumatic fever has already been given in
Chapter ,6 p. 69, but reference may be made here to the condition of the
joints. It is an acute inflammation, an acute arthritis, but without suppuration. Several joints are affected, one after the other. The affected
joint is swollen, and is so acutely tender that even jarring of the bed will

cause the patient severe anguish. Fortunately the inflammation is short-lived, but as one joint clears up another may become affected.

Treatment.—Treatment consists of keeping the joint carefully wrapped up, and in the administration of salicylates which produce a remarkable relief in the pain and swelling.

RHEUMATOID ARTHRITIS

This very common, tragic, and crippling disease, known also as chronic arthritis, is a chronic inflammatory condition affecting particularly the small joints of the hands and feet, although the larger joints may be affected later. It is the oldest of all known diseases, having been observed in many of the Egyptian mummies. Rheumatoid arthritis is one of the greatest causes of disability, and it has been estimated that it is responsible for

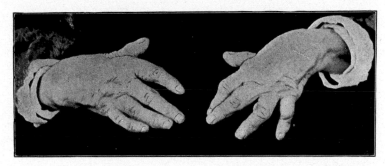

FIG. 120.—Chronic arthritis causing marked deformity of the fingers.

an annual loss of $200,000,000 in the United States. It is undoubtedly due to an infection, but the exact organism responsible has not so far been determined with certainty, although suspicion is centered chiefly on the streptococcus group. Many patients have some chronic focus of infection in the teeth, tonsils or elsewhere, and removal of this focus may be followed by arrest of the disease. It is most common in women between twenty and forty years of age, but men are also frequently affected.

The pathological changes resemble in certain respects those of joint tuberculosis, although it attacks many joints instead of a single one, and does not lead to destruction of the bone. There is the same swelling of the synovial membrane which causes the joints to be enlarged, the same gradual destruction of the articular cartilage, the same interference with the function of the joint resulting finally in complete disability and fusion of the joint surfaces. The course of the disease is marked by curious remissions and exacerbations, and at any stage the progress may be arrested, but as in tuberculosis the injury to the joint is permanent, and the hands and feet are twisted, gnarled, and crippled for life (Fig. 120). On this account and because of its commonness, the disease is of great industrial importance.

Symptoms.—The symptoms are *pain* and *swelling* of the joints, together with increasing *stiffness* and *disability*. In the later stages the joints

become distorted and deformed. During the exacerbations the patient often suffers from mild fever, malaise, anemia, and sweating, all pointing to a chronic infection.

Treatment. During the acute phase of the rheumatoid disease rest is of great importance together with methods of physiotherapy which help to restore function and particularly to prevent crippling deformities. The maintenance of correct posture of the joints involved provides for the maximum of function when the acute process subsides. Relief of pain with heat and mild analgesics is necessary in most cases. The use of cortisone and ACTH in rheumatoid arthritis has provided marked benefit in many cases. This treatment is accompanied by relief of pain, decrease in swelling and increase in movement of affected joints. Unfortunately in many instances this improvement is not maintained after the drug is stopped. However, this form of treatment represents the first specific method of combatting this condition and offers to many patients the hope of relief and improvement.

Gonorrheal Arthritis.—This is an occasional complication of acute gonorrhea, fortunately occurring in only 3 to 5 per cent of cases. The arthritis varies greatly in severity, often being merely a mild synovitis, but sometimes a purulent inflammation. As a rule the joint condition appears four or five weeks after the acute inflammation of the urethra, but occasionally it occurs many months later. The true nature of such cases is often completely missed.

Several joints are usually attacked, especially the knee, ankle, shoulder, and the small joints of the hand or foot. Pain, especially on movement, is the chief symptom. At a later stage stiffness due to adhesions between the joint surfaces may cause great disability.

This complication of gonorrhea has largely disappeared as the result of the present adequate treatment of the infection with penicillin in the acute stage of the disease. If arthritis develops, the use of penicillin and sulfonamides will shorten the course of the arthritis.

TUMORS OF BONE

We have already seen that bone is a complex structure into the composition of which a number of tissues enter, e.g., bone cells, marrow, periosteum, and cartilage. Tumors of various kinds may arise from any of these elements. For the purpose of this brief outline, however, bone tumors may be divided into primary and secondary, whilst the primary tumors may again be divided into innocent and malignant.

Primary Tumors.—Primary tumors of bone may be innocent or malignant. The three chief *innocent* tumors are osteoma, chondroma, and giant-cell tumor. The *osteoma* and *chondroma* are very similar tumors, the former consisting of bone cells and the latter of cartilage. Both of these are hard tumors which usually arise at the end of a long bone, although they may occur in practically any bone in the body. Being benign they are localized and usually remain small, but occasionally they grow to a great size. When removed they show no tendency to recur. The *giant-cell*

tumor develops in children and young adults, usually before the age of thirty. It occurs principally at the ends of long bones, and the common location is the knee. It is highly destructive locally, but does not cause metastases nor kill the patient. It consists of a soft red hemorrhagic mass which greatly distends the bone and almost completely destroys it. This gives the highly characteristic picture in the *x*-ray film of large bubbles separated by thin strips of bone. The tumor gets its name from the large number of giant cells which are seen in the microscopic section.

The three chief primary malignant tumors of bone are osteogenic sarcoma, Ewing's tumor, and multiple myeloma. *Osteogenic sarcoma* is the commonest of the three. It is a disease of young persons between the ages of ten and thirty and is very rarely seen after the age of fifty. The location is similar to that of giant-cell tumor, namely, at the ends of the long bones, usually in the region of the knee joint. The tumor expands the end of the bone, so as to give it a "leg of mutton" appearance. Spread takes place by the blood stream, and secondary growths are formed first in the lungs. *Ewing's tumor* occurs at an earlier age period than osteogenic sarcoma, usually between the ages of five and fifteen. It is rarely seen over the age of thirty. It involves the bone much more diffusely than does osteogenic sarcoma, giving rise to a uniform thickening. The tumor does not begin at the end of a bone. One of the more striking features of the disease is that as the tumor progresses other growths become apparent in many widely distant bones, particularly those bones known as the flat bones, such as the scapula, sternum, vertebræ, and skull. The tumor is highly sensitive to radiation, but in spite of this the prognosis is extremely bad. *Multiple myeloma* is also characterized by multiplicity, and it is really a tumor of bone-marrow rather than of the bone itself. By the time the patient comes to the doctor a large number of the flat bones may be involved. In about half the cases the urine shows what is called Bence-Jones protein, a protein which appears as a cloud when the urine is heated to 55° C., disappears at 85° C., but reappears on cooling. The tumor is highly malignant and invariably fatal. The age incidence is entirely different from that of the other two primary bone tumors, for multiple myeloma is never seen before the age of forty.

Treatment.—Treatment of malignant bone tumors consists in amputation at the earliest possible moment, in the hope that metastases may not yet have been set up. Roentgen-ray examination of the lungs must first be made, because if secondary growths are found in these organs no treatment is of any avail. Some forms of sarcoma respond well to roentgen-ray treatment, and the tumor may disappear for a time, but the relief is only temporary, and sooner or later the tumor will recur.

Secondary Tumors.—Secondary tumors of bone are carcinomas, the tumor cells coming from a cancer in some other organ. The most common forms of cancer which are likely to metastasize to bone are cancer of the breast, lung, prostate, and kidney. The metastatic tumor destroys the bone, and the first indication of its presence may be the occurrence of a fracture from a very trivial injury. It is evident from the nature of the condition that nothing in the way of treatment is of any avail.

RICKETS

Rickets is a disease in which a deficiency in certain elements of the food interferes with the proper calcification of the bones. In order to understand it, a brief consideration of the process of calcification is therefore necessary. The chief mineral constituents which impart rigidity to the bones are *calcium* and *phosphorus*, combined in the form of *calcium phosphate*. These substances are absorbed from the food and deposited in the bones. If they are not present in the food in sufficient amount, the bones remain soft and are easily bent. A deficiency in phosphorus is much more serious than a deficiency in calcium.

But there is another factor in deficiency which is even more fatal to proper calcification. This factor is *vitamin D*. The ordinary food of a child usually contains a reasonable amount of calcium and phosphorus, but may be gravely lacking in vitamin D. This vitamin is necessary for the proper absorption of calcium and phosphorus from the food, and in its absence, no matter how abundant the minerals may be in the food, the body is unable to utilize them and rickets will result. Vitamin D is a fat-soluble vitamin, in contrast with some of the other vitamins which are water-soluble. It is therefore contained principally in fatty foods, although also found in certain vegetables.

A third factor is *light* (ultra-violet light). The relation between ultra-violet light and vitamin D has already been discussed on page 33.

The *cause* of rickets is therefore a deficiency in some of the factors necessary for the proper calcification of bone. The most important of these is vitamin D. A marked deficiency in phosphorus and to a lesser degree in calcium is a predisposing factor. The fault lies in the quality not the quantity of the food. A child may be starved and emaciated but show no sign of rickets, whilst a plump baby may show marked rickets. The disease is much commoner in artificially-fed infants than in those which are breast-fed. Owing to the absence of light it is commoner in large smoky cities and during the winter months. Negro children are especially susceptible, as their dark skin prevents the light from acting on the ergosterol. All the factors are included in the statement that rickets is a disease of the slums of large cities in countries which get little sunshine.

Symptoms.—The symptoms are partly connected with bones, partly constitutional. The disease is one of infancy and early childhood (six months to two years), and a period at which there is the greatest demand for calcium and phosphorus by the rapidly growing bones. The softened bones become deformed, especially those which bear the weight of the body (Fig. 121), and curvature of the spine develops. The head is large and square. The sternum is pushed forward (pigeon-breast), and a series of nodules develop at the anterior ends of the ribs called the rickety rosary. Nodular swellings are formed at the wrists, knees, and ankles. The most serious deformity is a narrowing of the inlet of the pelvis, which in the female may make normal delivery impossible in later life. Among the constitutional disturbances are sweating, restlessness, flabbiness of the muscles giving the child a "pot belly," and enlargement of the spleen. The blood phosphorus is markedly decreased.

Principles of Treatment.—Treatment consists in making good the deficiencies which may have been present. Cod-liver oil is an old and well-proved remedy. Halibut (haliver) oil is also rich in vitamin D, and is more palatable than cod-liver oil. The most potent form of vitamin D is viosterol, *i.e.*, ergosterol which has been irradiated by ultra-violet light. An

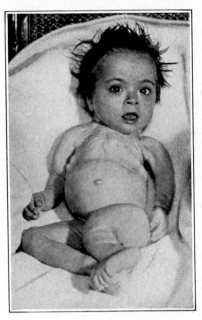

FIG. 121.—Rickets, showing large forehead, deformed chest, curvature of arms and legs, and pot belly.

abundance of sunlight is desirable. Sunlight loses its ultra-violet rays when passed through window glass, for the short-wave rays are screened out by the lead in the glass. Special lead-free glass may be used in the nursery, or the child may be exposed to the light of a lamp capable of producing ultra-violet rays, such as the mercury vapor lamp or the carbon arc lamp.

Chapter

22

DISEASES OF THE TEETH

Structure.—A tooth is composed of four structures: (1) enamel, (2) dentine, (3) pulp, and (4) cementum (Fig. 122). The *enamel* is the outer covering or crown of the tooth. It is calcified and extremely hard, so that it can stand the wear and tear of a long life and can enable a dog to crunch bones without itself becoming worn away. It forms a perfect covering for the dentine, but unfortunately it is brittle and easily cracked. Moreover, fissures may form in the course of development, especially if the food at that period is lacking in vitamins, and through these fissures infection may reach the underlying dentine. The *dentine* forms the main bulk of the tooth. Like the enamel it is calcified. It is traversed by large numbers of minute channels, the dentinal tubules, which pass from the enamel down to the pulp. It is along these channels that infection may find its way once it has reached the dentine. The *pulp* consists of soft connective tissue filled with bloodvessels and nerves. From our knowledge of inflammation it is evident that this is the part of the tooth which alone is capable of showing the usual inflammatory changes, because the dentine contains no vessels, and the enamel is really a dead tissue. The *cementum* covers the dentine in the root portion of the tooth. It resembles bone in its structure, and joins with the enamel at the line of the gum. The *peridental membrane* is the periosteum of the tooth and joins the cementum to the bone of the jaw, so that it is responsible for holding the tooth in position.

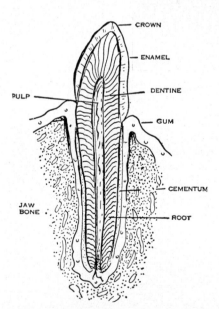

FIG. 122.—Section through a tooth to show its structure. (Best and Taylor, The Human Body and Its Functions; courtesy of Henry Holt & Co.)

The two important diseases of the teeth are caries and pyorrhea.

(284)

CARIES

Caries or dental caries is one of the most widespread of diseases. It is found in the teeth of Egyptian mummies, so that it is no new affliction of mankind, and it is world-wide in its distribution, although certain races such as the Eskimos and African natives are remarkably exempt. It is principally a disease of childhood and adolescence; when that period is past the threat of caries becomes very much less. Both the milk teeth and the permanent teeth are liable to the disease, but it is most likely to attack the permanent teeth at the time of their eruption. The molars are most frequently affected.

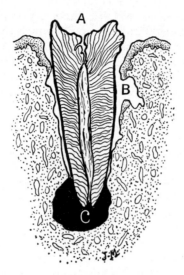

Fig. 123.—Dental disease. *A*, Caries affecting crown of tooth and penetrating down to the pulp. *B*, Pyorrhea; shrinking of bone and gum away from tooth. *C*, Root abscess.

There is no single *cause* of caries, for various factors may play a part. Anything which endangers the integrity of the enamel covering is liable to lead to caries. *Heredity* is a potent factor. Just as some persons inherit weak arteries which are certain to develop arteriosclerosis, so some families appear to be unable to produce good enamel and are certain to suffer from caries. *Lack of vitamins* in the early period of life interferes with the development of the enamel. Once the teeth have fully developed, it is doubtful if vitamins have any effect on their health. An *excess of cereals* appears definitely to interfere with the proper calcification of the teeth and therefore exposes them to caries. These are predisposing factors. The exciting factor is the presence of *bacteria* that break up the carbohydrates of the food débris and form acids which attack the teeth. Proper care of the mouth by removing the material from which these acids are formed is a valuable means of prevention. And yet the Eskimos and African natives manage to avoid caries without the assistance of a toothbrush.

Lesions.—The lesions of caries can only be appreciated when the structure of the tooth is understood. Like the caries of bone tuberculosis, it is a gradual eating away of the tooth. All the elements of the tooth may be affected. The acids produced by the bacteria enter the enamel through cracks and defects, and gradually dissolve away the calcium of this hard substance. In time they reach the dentine, which is now exposed by the erosion of the enamel not only to the acids but to the bacteria themselves. Destruction of the dentine occurs much more rapidly and widely, so that a large cavity may be formed in the dentine although there is only a small defect in the overlying enamel. The bacteria readily pass along the dentinal tubules and thus reach the pulp where they set up a true and often a violent inflammation. It is this inflammatory reaction in the pulp which is responsible for the pain of caries. The infection may pass down through the opening in the root of the tooth through which the dental nerve enters the pulp, and may give rise to a *root abscess* (Fig. 123). Such an abscess may become chronic, and is apt to be a source of *focal infection* from which bacteria pass into the blood in small quantities, causing chronic arthritis and other forms of chronic infection.

PYORRHEA

The full name of this disease is pyorrhea alveolaris, that is to say, a discharge of pus from the alveolus or margin of the jaw. It is a very common disease, but it has nothing to do with caries, for caries is a disease of the tooth, whilst pyorrhea is a disease of the surroundings of the tooth which itself may be perfectly sound. Caries is a disease of youth, whilst pyorrhea is a disease of middle age.

The exact nature of the first step in the process is uncertain, but there is a falling away of the bony surroundings of the tooth, so that a gap is formed between the root of the tooth and the bone (Fig. 123). In this gap food collects and decomposes so that there is a chronic inflammation with copious discharge of pus and bleeding of the gums as shown by pink staining of the toothbrush. In the course of time the root of the tooth will become loosened and the tooth, often quite healthy, will fall out. As soon as this occurs the pus is free to escape, the infection subsides, and the pyorrhea clears up. The usual explanation of the first step is that an atrophy of the bone around the tooth occurs, as a result of which the above-mentioned gap is formed. It appears more probable than an accumulation of food occurs in the crevice which normally exists between the gum and tooth, that this gives rise to infection, and that the infection leads to softening of the bone and the formation of a gap between tooth and bone, a gap in which food continues to accumulate and the infection becomes increasingly severe.

The S
medical p
ment of i
streptoco
microörg
group of
Bacillus
dysenter
this are
thiazol a
A rem
directly a
bacteria.
of bacter
fences of
the invac
The di
the blood
ineffectiv
acts on
urine, so
free part
All me
to a smal
drugs, or
result of
evident t
who mer
be given
to the p
toxic effe
be low-gr
and twell
velop dru
may invc
fall rapid
be a corr
clears, a
complicat
the urine
being dep
dangerou
tubules.
The nu
(1) She n
must keep
the intak
twenty-fc

PART III. PRACTICAL APPLICATIONS

Chapter

23

THE PRINCIPLES OF TREATMENT

TREATMENT, therapy or therapeutics is still more of an art than a science, despite the resounding advances which have been made in recent years in the management of bacterial infections. One still treats a man or a woman, not a disease. In this respect the position of the nurse remains supreme. For the doctor also, his duty cannot be confined to prescribing drugs or wielding a scalpel. He must assume benevolent command of the situation, with the nurse acting as his trusted lieutenant. The human relationship between the patient and his attendants remains as fundamental as ever.

The infinite variety of things which can be done for the sick person may be divided into a number of main groups. It is seldom, however, that any one form of therapy can be used alone.

GENERAL MEASURES

Rest.—This is perhaps the most important single therapeutic measure in combating disease. Rest in bed is the oldest and still the best household remedy. It is difficult to explain on scientific grounds the exact manner in which rest helps the sick person. All infections are benefited by rest, which may be general or local. An example of the value of local rest is afforded by immobilization of an infected hand by a splint or a sling. By this means upward spread of the invading organisms, particularly streptococci, along the lymphatics as a result of muscular movements is reduced to a minimum.

It is important, however, to remember that rest is not simply a state of inactivity, of freedom from toil. There must be rest of the mind as well as rest of the body, relaxation, and freedom from unnecessary worry. Mental fatigue is often more harmful than physical fatigue and more difficult to relieve. Sometimes the best way of resting a tired person is by changing from mental work to recreation through physical activity. The patient who lies in bed with his mind occupied with worries is far from resting. Rest is a state of tranquillity, of quiet and repose, a freedom from all that harasses and disturbs. The nurse may play a most important part in enabling the patient to attain this state of tranquillity. A simple example is her function of protecting a very sick patient from importunate visitors, who are certain to exhaust him both physically and mentally. As improvement sets in one visitor at a time may be allowed, and when two are present they

288

sho
tier
con

I
in t
are
Suc
dis
hig
hav
die
cip:
wel
im
iod
bee

A
me
gra
res
rep
im
wh
Co
the

1
is i
the
Th
co
sor
it i

alv
ca
ch
th

a s
bo
pa
an
in
ac
of

Antibiotics.—Many microörganisms such as moulds and soil bacteria secrete metabolic products which inhibit or prevent the growth of other microörganisms. These chemical substances of microbial origin are known as antibiotics, because they inhibit growth and even destroy bacteria in dilute solution.

The first antibiotic to be discovered was penicillin. In 1928 a British bacteriologist, Alexander Fleming, noticed that a culture of staphylococci accidentally contaminated with green mould ceased to grow and was destroyed. This mould is the common green mould Penicillium notatum, which grows on moist bread, old cheese and jams. Fleming, therefore, gave the name of penicillin to the active substance in the culture fluid. In 1940 Florey and his associates at Oxford worked out methods for its isolation and purification, and applied it to the treatment of human infections. So incredibly powerful is the substance thus obtained that it inhibits the growth of staphylococci in a dilution of one in eighty million. Streptomycin was discovered by Waksman in 1944, being obtained from a soil organism.

Penicillin acts against Gram-positive bacteria, particularly the staphylococcus, hemolytic streptococcus and pneumococcus, but also inhibits the growth of a few Gram-negative organisms, especially the gonococcus and meningococcus, as well as spirochetes, so that it is invaluable in the treatment of syphilis. *Streptomycin*, on the other hand, is effective only against Gram-negative bacteria, but also has some inhibitory action on the tubercle bacillus. Neither has any effect on viruses. Both of these agents have a narrow range of activity. From these facts it will be apparent that an accurate bacteriological diagnosis is of the greatest importance in determining the choice between penicillin and streptomycin. An important distinction between the two is that individual strains of organisms within penicillin's relatively narrow spectrum of activity are fairly uniform in their sensitivity to the antibiotic (although some strains of staphylococci are now beginning to develop resistance), whereas the strains within species sensitive to streptomycin vary considerably in their degree of sensitivity to that antibiotic. There is thus often an effect of apparently acquired resistance to streptomycin; less resistant strains succumb, and the more resistent strains multiply and predominate. The three newer antibiotics *chloromycetin* (chloramphenicol), *aureomycin* and *terramycin*, are active against a wide variety of organisms, not only Gram-positive and Gram-negative bacteria, but spirochetes and viruses as well. They are, therefore, spoken of as "wide spectrum antibiotics."

Penicillin and streptomycin tend to be destroyed by the gastric juice and the bacteria of the large intestine, so that they are given by intramuscular injection, penicillin in the form of procaine penicillin. Oral tablets of penicillin can be used, but a higher dosage is required and there is some danger of poor absorption. Aureomycin, chloramphenicol and terramycin are given orally every four to six hours, because success depends on maintaining a high antibiotic level in the infected area. Where there are collections of pus separated by some distance from bloodvessels, local injections of penicillin or streptomycin are made into the pus cavity. Topical applications of the antibiotics are used in the form of ointment in skin infections or as drops in infections of the eye.

PART III. PRACTICAL APPLICATIONS

Chapter

23

THE PRINCIPLES OF TREATMENT

TREATMENT, therapy or therapeutics is still more of an art than a science, despite the resounding advances which have been made in recent years in the management of bacterial infections. One still treats a man or a woman, not a disease. In this respect the position of the nurse remains supreme. For the doctor also, his duty cannot be confined to prescribing drugs or wielding a scalpel. He must assume benevolent command of the situation, with the nurse acting as his trusted lieutenant. The human relationship between the patient and his attendants remains as fundamental as ever.

The infinite variety of things which can be done for the sick person may be divided into a number of main groups. It is seldom, however, that any one form of therapy can be used alone.

GENERAL MEASURES

Rest.—This is perhaps the most important single therapeutic measure in combating disease. Rest in bed is the oldest and still the best household remedy. It is difficult to explain on scientific grounds the exact manner in which rest helps the sick person. All infections are benefited by rest, which may be general or local. An example of the value of local rest is afforded by immobilization of an infected hand by a splint or a sling. By this means upward spread of the invading organisms, particularly streptococci, along the lymphatics as a result of muscular movements is reduced to a minimum.

It is important, however, to remember that rest is not simply a state of inactivity, of freedom from toil. There must be rest of the mind as well as rest of the body, relaxation, and freedom from unnecessary worry. Mental fatigue is often more harmful than physical fatigue and more difficult to relieve. Sometimes the best way of resting a tired person is by changing from mental work to recreation through physical activity. The patient who lies in bed with his mind occupied with worries is far from resting. Rest is a state of tranquillity, of quiet and repose, a freedom from all that harasses and disturbs. The nurse may play a most important part in enabling the patient to attain this state of tranquillity. A simple example is her function of protecting a very sick patient from importunate visitors, who are certain to exhaust him both physically and mentally. As improvement sets in one visitor at a time may be allowed, and when two are present they

should both be at the same side of the bed. A good nurse can keep a patient's mind off his troubles much better than can the doctor, and thus contribute to his state of rest.

Diet.—Correct food is assuming a position of ever-increasing importance in the treatment of disease as well as in the preservation of health. Proteins are the sole source of material for the maintenance and repair of tissues. Such maintenance and repair may be specially needed in febrile and other diseases where there is marked breakdown of tissue. The proteins of the highest biological value are contained in meat, fish, milk and eggs, as they have the most essential amino acids. This is of special importance when the diet is restricted, as in conditions associated with albuminuria. The principal rôle of fats and carbohydrates is to furnish energy, a requisite of the well rather than the sick person. It is only necessary to mention the all-important rôle of food, and particularly of vitamins and minerals such as iodine, calcium and iron, in the dietary deficiency diseases. These have been fully discussed in Chapter 3.

As a rough guide it may be said that a diet containing liberal amounts of meat, milk and dairy products, eggs, fruit and vegetables, and some whole grain cereal may be depended on to be adequate. On the nurse rests the responsibility of seeing that the patient eats the prescribed diet; she must report to the doctor if he does not do so. The regulation of fluids may be as important as the regulation of food. Thus when there is much fluid loss, which may be due to vomiting, diarrhea, etc., that loss must be made up. Conversely, when the tissues are water-logged, as in myocardial failure, the intake of fluid must be diminished.

Nursing.—This needs no more than mention in a book of this type. This is not because the subject is not of supreme importance, but rather because the author is much less qualified to speak on the subject than is the reader. There are endless services by which the nurse not only ministers to the comfort of the patient but contributes to his eventual recovery. There are some diseases, of which typhoid fever is perhaps the best example, in which it is better to have a good nurse than a good doctor.

DRUGS

It has been said of drugs that they sometimes cure, often relieve, and always console. Only a limited number of drugs are very useful. These can be divided into the two great groups of specific agents and the new chemotherapeutic agents exemplified by the sulfonamide drugs and the antibiotics.

Specific Drugs.—These are usually understood to be those which have a selective action on one particular infective agent or on one organ of the body. Examples of the former are the action of quinine on the malarial parasite and arsenical preparations on the spirochæta pallida of syphilis; an excellent example of the latter group is the action of digitalis on the heart in certain forms of heart failure. Opium and its derivatives have a specific action in relieving pain, and are on that account amongst the most valuable of all drugs.

The Sulfonamides.—The sulfonamide drugs were first introduced into medical practice in 1936, and their advent marked a revolution in the treatment of infections caused by such common bacteria as the staphylococcus, streptococcus, pneumococcus and gonococcus, as well as by many other microörganisms. A notable exception was the Gram-negative bacilli, a group of bacteria not stained by Gram's method of staining, and including Bacillus coli and the bacilli causing typhoid and paratyphoid fever and dysentery. The first member of the sulfonamides was sulfanilamide. From this are derived all the others in common use, such as sulfapyridine, sulfathiazol and sulfadiazine.

A remarkable feature of their action is that they do not kill bacteria directly as do antiseptics, but merely delay or inhibit multiplication of the bacteria. This inhibiting process is known as *bacteriostasis*. As a result of bacteriostasis spread of the infection is prevented, and the natural defences of the body such as leucocytes and antibodies have time to overcome the invading organisms and neutralize their toxins.

The drug is absorbed from the stomach and enters the blood stream. In the blood, part of it becomes combined or "conjugated"; this part is quite ineffective. The rest remains "free" or active, and it is this part which acts on the bacteria. Unfortunately the drug is rapidly excreted in the urine, so that repeated administration is necessary if the blood level of the free part is to remain sufficiently high to be effective.

All members of the group are potentially dangerous. The danger is only to a small number of people who are either naturally unduly sensitive to the drugs, or, as more commonly happens, have acquired sensitivity as the result of previous sulfonamide treatment. With this in mind it becomes evident that it is a dangerous mistake to administer sulfa drugs to anyone who merely happens to have developed a little fever. They should only be given when there is real need for them, because a grave disservice is done to the patient if he is needlessly made sulfa-hypersensitive. The chief toxic effects are fever, blood changes, and renal complications. *Fever* may be low-grade or high and sustained. It usually begins between the fifth and twelfth days, but if the patient has had a previous course he may develop drug fever a few hours after receiving it a second time. *Blood changes* may involve the red cells or the leucocytes. The number of red cells may fall rapidly, a condition known as acute hemolytic anemia. Or there may be a corresponding fall in the leucocytes, particularly the polymorphonuclears, a condition of leucopenia. Both of these may prove fatal. *Renal complications* may be either hematuria or suppression of urine. Blood in the urine is caused by crystals of the drugs, particularly sulfanilamide, being deposited in the kidney. Suppression of urine, which is much more dangerous and may readily prove fatal, is due to damage to the renal tubules.

The nurse has important duties in all cases receiving sulfonamide drugs. (1) She must report at once any unusual fever or skin eruption. (2) She must keep an accurate record of the output of urine. (3) She must see that the intake of fluid is sufficient to provide a total volume of 1000 cc. in twenty-four hours.

Antibiotics.—Many microörganisms such as moulds and soil bacteria secrete metabolic products which inhibit or prevent the growth of other microörganisms. These chemical substances of microbial origin are known as antibiotics, because they inhibit growth and even destroy bacteria in dilute solution.

The first antibiotic to be discovered was penicillin. In 1928 a British bacteriologist, Alexander Fleming, noticed that a culture of staphylococci accidentally contaminated with green mould ceased to grow and was destroyed. This mould is the common green mould Penicillium notatum, which grows on moist bread, old cheese and jams. Fleming, therefore, gave the name of penicillin to the active substance in the culture fluid. In 1940 Florey and his associates at Oxford worked out methods for its isolation and purification, and applied it to the treatment of human infections. So incredibly powerful is the substance thus obtained that it inhibits the growth of staphylococci in a dilution of one in eighty million. Streptomycin was discovered by Waksman in 1944, being obtained from a soil organism.

Penicillin acts against Gram-positive bacteria, particularly the staphylococcus, hemolytic streptococcus and pneumococcus, but also inhibits the growth of a few Gram-negative organisms, especially the gonococcus and meningococcus, as well as spirochetes, so that it is invaluable in the treatment of syphilis. *Streptomycin*, on the other hand, is effective only against Gram-negative bacteria, but also has some inhibitory action on the tubercle bacillus. Neither has any effect on viruses. Both of these agents have a narrow range of activity. From these facts it will be apparent that an accurate bacteriological diagnosis is of the greatest importance in determining the choice between penicillin and streptomycin. An important distinction between the two is that individual strains of organisms within penicillin's relatively narrow spectrum of activity are fairly uniform in their sensitivity to the antibiotic (although some strains of staphylococci are now beginning to develop resistance), whereas the strains within species sensitive to streptomycin vary considerably in their degree of sensitivity to that antibiotic. There is thus often an effect of apparently acquired resistance to streptomycin; less resistant strains succumb, and the more resistent strains multiply and predominate. The three newer antibiotics *chloromycetin* (chloramphenicol), *aureomycin* and *terramycin*, are active against a wide variety of organisms, not only Gram-positive and Gram-negative bacteria, but spirochetes and viruses as well. They are, therefore, spoken of as "wide spectrum antibiotics."

Penicillin and streptomycin tend to be destroyed by the gastric juice and the bacteria of the large intestine, so that they are given by intramuscular injection, penicillin in the form of procaine penicillin. Oral tablets of penicillin can be used, but a higher dosage is required and there is some danger of poor absorption. Aureomycin, chloramphenicol and terramycin are given orally every four to six hours, because success depends on maintaining a high antibiotic level in the infected area. Where there are collections of pus separated by some distance from bloodvessels, local injections of penicillin or streptomycin are made into the pus cavity. Topical applications of the antibiotics are used in the form of ointment in skin infections or as drops in infections of the eye.

IMMUNOTHERAPY

The natural means by which the body defends itself against infection is by immunity reactions, in which antibodies and leucocytes play a leading part. It is possible to assist these reactions by immunotherapy. There are two ways in which this can be done.

1. The production of antibodies may be stimulated by the injection of vaccines, which consist of the dead bodies of bacteria. In this way an *active immunity* is built up. It will be evident that the great field for active immunity is in the *prevention* of infection. Outstanding success in prevention has been attained in connection with typhoid fever, smallpox and diphtheria. It should be noted that the technique differs in each of these three examples. In the case of typhoid the vaccine consists of the dead bodies of typhoid bacilli. Smallpox vaccine contains a greatly attenuated living virus. The agent used in immunization against diphtheria is not really a vaccine, but is neutralized diphtheria toxin, known as toxoid. The result, however, is the same in all three, namely, active immunity.

2. An animal may be used for the production of the antibodies by means of inoculation; the blood serum containing these antibodies is then injected into the patient. The patient is given a *passive immunity*, so called because the patient himself takes no active part in producing the immune state. The serums or sera used in the treatment of disease are usually antitoxins, which are prepared by injecting gradually increasing doses of toxin into an animal. If bacteria instead of toxins are employed, the serum is an antibacterial one. One of the oldest and still the most efficient of the antitoxic sera is that used against diphtheria. The antibacterial sera on the whole have been disappointing.

ORGANOTHERAPY

This form of treatment may be employed in two ways. The first is also known as substitution therapy, because it consists in the administration of the extract of an organ which has become deficient in activity. This deficiency is likely to be permanent, so that the organotherapy must be continued for the duration of the patient's life. In spite of this drawback organotherapy has achieved some of the most brilliant results in the entire field of therapeutics. Examples of substitution therapy are provided by insulin in diabetes, liver extract in pernicious anemia, and thyroid extract in myxedema. A breath-taking illustration of what may be achieved by this method of treatment is shown in Figure 124. Organotherapy may also be used to produce a temporary physiological effect rather than prolonged replacement therapy.

PHYSIOTHERAPY

This form of therapy, also known as physical therapy, is probably the most ancient of all forms of treatment, and within recent years it has assumed increasing importance, particularly in the treatment of injuries.

Physiotherapy may take the form of massage, heat therapy, electrotherapy and radiation therapy.

Massage.—Massage is essentially manipulation of the tissues. It may be either stimulating or sedative. While in theory it can be applied by anyone, it must be realized that it demands skill and training, just as do other forms of treatment, and in the hands of an inexperienced person it may be responsible for much harm. The movements must be carried out rhythmically and smoothly. Not all persons can become masters of the art, for they may lack the necessary rhythm, or the strength of hand which is needed to manipulate the great muscles of the back. A thorough knowledge of anatomy is necessary, and also a knowledge of the physiological

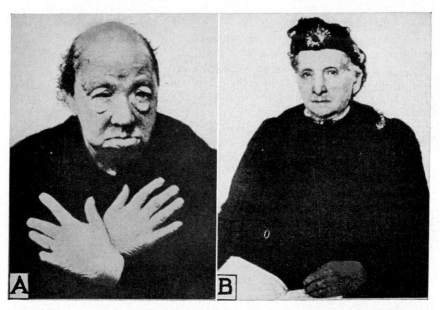

FIG. 124.—*A*, Myxedema of twenty years duration; patient bed-ridden and imbecile. *B*, After treatment with thyroid extract; the same patient thirty years later, aged ninety-four years. (Harington: The Thyroid Gland—Its Chemistry and Physiology, courtesy of Oxford University Press.)

effects which it is desired to produce. The principal types or techniques of massage are stroking (superficial or deep), kneading and friction. These techniques are used for different purposes. Massage is employed both for local and general conditions. Examples of local conditions in which it may prove useful are organic nervous diseases associated with paralysis and wasting of the muscles, *e.g.*, poliomyelitis, chronic arthritis, fractures, sprains and strains, and atonic conditions of the alimentary canal. Amongst general conditions are debilitating diseases with loss of muscular tone, and neurasthenia (for its soothing effect). Massage is also valuable in patients who are inactive or bedridden, although not necessarily seriously ill.

It is not easy to state with certainty the exact mechanism by means of which massage produces its valuable effects. It appears to be partly mechanical and partly reflex. The flow of venous blood and lymph is mechanically assisted by stroking in the direction of that flow. The lightest touch will serve to empty the superficial veins and lymphatics. Some reflex mechanism must be presumed as the basis of the remarkable relief of muscular spasm which follows massage in cases of fracture. Skillful massage may cause rapid disappearance of the swelling after a fracture, and in such cases the mechanism is probably as much reflex as mechanical. Massage does not produce lactic acid in the muscles, but it serves to remove the lactic acid produced by violent muscular exertion. It appears to stimulate the interchange between the blood and the tissues. Finally it soothes the nervous system in a remarkable manner, as can be demonstrated in many cases of neurasthenia.

Heat.—Heat may be applied to the body in a variety of forms. *Radiant heat* utilizes the infra-red rays, which produce heat within the body. The source of these rays is not in contact with the body. The usual source is the ordinary electric light bulb, but an infra-red baker may be used, which gives out no light but much heat. In *conducted heat* therapy the source of heat is in direct contact with the body. The source may be: (1) hot packs or a hot bath; (2) electric or other dry forms of heat; (3) *diathermy*, in which heat is generated in the tissues as the result of the passage through them of an electric current.

Heat acts in various ways, but particularly by dilating the small blood-vessels and increasing the capillary circulation in the part. This leads to muscular relaxation and reduction in the amount of pain. Radiant heat acts principally on the skin, but diathermy goes much deeper into the muscles. The commonest of all physiotherapeutic prescriptions is baking followed by massage. The baking produces dilatation of the superficial vessels, whilst massage helps to eliminate waste products from the part. This combination frequently provides great relief and comfort.

Cold plays a much less important part in therapy than does heat, but it has its place. It is of particular value in stopping hemorrhage after a sprain, in which a ligament is torn, together with the surrounding vessels.

Electrotherapy.—This may be applied in the form of the sinusoidal current or diathermy. The *sinusoidal current* is a galvanic current which increases from zero to a maximum in voltage, then returning to zero and to a negative voltage equal to the positive maximum. It is thus an electric current which oscillates between a given positive and negative voltage. A slow rate of oscillation is valuable for producing painless contractions of muscles which have been weakened from long disuse. *Diathermy* creates heat as the result of the passage of a high frequency alternating current. A very high rate of frequency of alternation is employed, between 500,000 and 3,000,000 cycles per second. The advantage of the high frequency is that the passage of the current is harmless and painless. The tissues act as a high resistance to the current, and heat is generated as a result. The special field of diathermy is in the application of heat to a limited, deep-seated, inaccessible part of the body. It is of no value for heating a large area of body surface; for this purpose radiant heat should be used.

19

Radiation Therapy.—Various forms of radiation have been used in the treatment of disease. *Infra-red radiation, i.e.*, the long waves beyond the red end of the visible spectrum, has already been considered. These long waves are produced by any heated body.

Ultra-violet Radiation.—Ultra-violet radiation represents the short waves beyond the violet end of the visible spectrum. The common sources are the carbon arc lamp and the mercury-vapor quartz lamp; in the latter an electric current is passed through a quartz tube containing mercury which becomes vaporized by the heat of the current. The reason that the tube is made of quartz instead of glass is that ultra-violet rays do not penetrate ordinary glass because of the lead which it contains. Ultra-violet radiation is of particular value in the treatment of rickets, because it activates the ergosterol which lies in the subcutaneous tissues and converts it into vitamin D. It is also believed to be of value in tuberculosis.

Radiotherapy.—This is a special form of radiation treatment in which *x*-rays and radium are employed. The gamma rays of radium produce the same effects on the tissues as do *x*-rays. The chief field of usefulness of radiotherapy is in the treatment of malignant tumors and allied conditions. Radiation arrests the reproduction of cancer cells, and at the same time leads to degeneration and destruction of these cells. Not all malignant tumors are equally suitable for this form of therapy. Some are very radio-sensitive and melt away under the influence of radiation almost under the eye of the observer. Others are equally radioresistant. Rapid disappearance of the tumor does not necessarily indicate a good prognosis, for unless all the tumor cells are killed it will inevitably reappear. The question as to whether *x*-rays or radium should be used depends a good deal on the location of the tumor. A small superficial growth, such as carcinoma of the lip, is better treated with radium. In a widespread condition such as lympho-sarcoma *x*-rays would be employed. Experience has shown that radiation is of particular value in carcinoma of the mouth, cervix, skin, and in lympho-sarcoma. It may be used alone or in conjunction with surgery. In the latter case it may be used preoperatively or postoperatively. Radiation is used as a palliative measure in leukemia and in Hodgkin's disease, but cure of these conditions cannot be expected. In conclusion it may be pointed out that the safe use of *x*-rays and radium demands as great skill and as extensive a training as does the safe use of a knife by the surgeon. Indeed, much more irreparable damage may be done by radiotherapeutic agents than by the surgeon's knife.

Psychotherapy.—A pathologist who spends his life studying the organic manifestations of disease is manifestly completely unfitted to discuss the subject of psychotherapy. Such a one is the present writer. It will therefore be merely alluded to in this place. The physician conducting a busy practice soon discovers that more than half the patients who walk into his office fail to show evidence of organic disease; there is apparently nothing really wrong with any one organ. And yet they are sick and need to be treated with skill, consideration, and sympathy. When a person is out of mental harmony with his environment, when he finds the stresses of life too hard to be borne, he may feel as ill as if an organ was seriously diseased, and the symptoms complained of may be similar to those of an organic

disease. These symptoms are real and not imaginary. Moreover, much of the state of distress induced by organic disease is due to the emotional and mental disturbances resulting from a realization that disease exists. It is inherent in human nature to magnify the unknown. The manner in which the patient reacts to the disease may be more important than the disease itself. The object of these remarks is to emphasize that from the patient's point of view the pathological lesions are by no means the sum total of the disease. The relief of mental distress and the promotion of contentment are just as vital as the alleviation of the physical suffering. In bringing about this relief the skilled, wise and understanding nurse may play an even more important part than the doctor who pays the patient an occasional and often too brief visit. In the wise words of a great physician: "the secret of the care of the patient is in caring for the patient."

Chapter

24

THE COLLECTION OF MATERIAL
FOR THE LABORATORY

In the diagnosis of disease by modern methods the laboratory plays an important part. Some of the material for laboratory tests which is taken from the patient is obtained by trained laboratory technicians, but much of it must be collected by the nurse. Especially is this the case in the smaller hospitals, which are not plentifully supplied with technicians. Upon the care and exactness with which she carries out this work depends much of the success of the test performed in the laboratory. The strength of a chain is its weakest link. Carelessness on the part of the nurse in collecting the specimen and labelling it with the name of the right patient will render the most accurate test completely worthless. Many of the points have already been touched on in the preceding pages, but some others will be referred to in this place.

Swabs.—A swab of infected material is taken in order that a culture may be made of any bacteria present. Bacteria die when removed from their source of nourishment, especially when the material which contains them is allowed to dry up. It is evident, therefore, that a swab should be sent to the laboratory as soon after it has been taken as may be convenient. In taking a throat swab it is important that the swab be taken from the throat itself, and not from the tongue, palate, or uvula. Any patch of exudate or membrane must be specially swabbed. The tongue is held down by a tongue depressor so that a full view of the back of the throat may be obtained. After douching or gargling with an antiseptic solution it is advisable to allow two hours to elapse before obtaining a specimen which will be used to make a culture.

Smears.—Some bacteria are examined more conveniently in a smear on a glass slide than by culture. This is true particularly of the gonococcus, so that a gonorrheal discharge must always be smeared instead of swabbed. In examining *genital smears* for gonorrhea in the adult female, a smear is taken from the cervix, not from the vagina; a vaginal smear is useless for this purpose. A clear view of the cervix must be obtained by means of a vaginal speculum, the cervix is wiped dry of vaginal secretion, and a wooden applicator or metal probe (not a swab) is passed into the cervical canal. In children, on the other hand, in whom vaginal infection may be caused by the fingers (gonorrheal vaginitis), a vaginal smear is made with a probe or applicator. *Eye smears* are made in addition to cultures, as it is desirable to know if the discharge from an eye contains pus cells. The lower lid is pulled down, and the smear and culture made by means of a platinum

(296)

wire loop. Two smears must always be made, because an ordinary methylene blue stain is used on the one and a Gram stain on the other. The two slides must never be placed face to face, lest they stick together. They should be separated by a rubber band round each end of one slide; the second slide is then bound to the first (face inward) by another rubber band. In this way there is neither danger of spread of infection, nor can the smears become spoiled.

Syphilitic Material.—When material has to be collected from a primary syphilitic sore for examination for the Spirochæta pallida by the dark-field method, a special technique is employed. The discharge from the ulcer is drawn into a fine capillary tube by means of a rubber nipple, and the apparatus is placed in a test-tube which is then plugged with cotton wool. As the motility on which recognition of the spirochetes depends is of short duration, the specimen must be dispatched at once to the laboratory. It must be remembered that this material is extremely infective and therefore highly dangerous.

When vaginal secretion has to be examined for Trichomonas vaginalis, a pathogenic protozoön parasite causing an irritating purulent vaginitis, the material is usually collected with a swab which is returned to a sterile tube containing a small amount of sterile isotonic saline.

Sputum.—When sputum is examined it is for the purpose of determining the presence of bacteria in the bronchi or lungs, not the mouth. The mouth is well rinsed and the patient then asked to cough up the discharge directly from the bronchi. If possible, send the first morning specimen. A specimen of sputum to be examined for tubercle bacilli may be collected in a bottle containing a little phenol, but if the sputum is to be *cultured* for other bacteria this antiseptic must be omitted from the container.

Stomach Contents.—Reference has already been made to the collection of stomach contents. The composition of the various test-meals will be found in the books on laboratory medicine.

Duodenal Contents.—Examination is usually for bile, pus, crystals, etc. In this case no special precautions need be taken. Occasionally, however, a bacteriological examination has to be made for typhoid bacilli, because these bacilli are discharged from the gallbladder into the duodenum both in the active disease and in typhoid carriers. In such a case it is necessary to use a sterile tube.

Stools.—As the specimen may have to be examined bacteriologically, the receptacle in which it is placed must contain no antiseptic. Only a very small quantity need be placed by means of a spatula in a wide-mouthed bottle. Do not put in enough to spill over. When a tapeworm has to be looked for, the whole specimen must be sent to the laboratory. Examination for the ameba of dysentery is only possible on the fresh warm specimen, so that the sample of stool must be sent down immediately it is passed.

Urine.—A urinalysis may be either a general examination (reaction, specific gravity, and chemical tests for albumin and sugar) or a microscopic examination. The requisition sent with the specimen should be marked either "general" or "microscopic" or both. A specimen for microscopic examination should be fresh, as red blood cells and casts disappear when the urine is allowed to stand for some time. If the total output of sugar, etc.,

in the twenty-four hours is to be measured, a twenty-four-hour specimen is obtained in a Winchester bottle, mixed well, and a sample taken and sent to the laboratory with a note of the twenty-four-hour output, which is charted at the same time. From this information the total amount excreted in the twenty-four hours can readily be calculated. The measurement must be in cubic centimeters, not in ounces. The addition of a small amount of toluol prevents decomposition which might otherwise make the estimation quite valueless. This is done most conveniently by placing 25 cc. of toluol in a Winchester bottle and adding each specimen as it is passed, shaking each time so as to mix the new specimen with the toluol. A catheterized specimen of urine taken from the two ureters should be collected in sterile tubes or bottles, as a bacteriological examination is frequently required. The vital importance of the correct labelling of such specimens has already been referred to.

Wassermann Reaction.—There is no test in which proper collection of the material is more important than in the case of the Wassermann reaction because of the significance attached to a positive result. A gummed label should be filled in before the specimen is collected, and attached at once to the tube before a specimen from another patient is taken. The blood can be taken from a vein in a Keidel vacuum tube (with needle attached), or a large syringe and needle can be used, the blood being expelled into a clean test-tube. It is of vital importance that the syringe, needle, and test-tube be absolutely dry and contain no trace of antiseptic, otherwise the test, which is a most delicate one, may be completely spoiled.

Blood Chemistry.—The chemical substances present in the blood are not all evenly distributed between the blood cells and the plasma. Therefore, some estimations are performed on whole blood, others on plasma, and others on serum, so the laboratory should be consulted when there is doubt about the type of specimen required. If whole blood or plasma is needed for an estimation, it is necessary to prevent the blood from clotting after it has been withdrawn from a vein and so an anticoagulant is added to the specimen tube. Several different anticoagulants are available, but the one most commonly used for chemical estimations is neutral potassium oxalate. It is important that blood is not collected into a tube containing Wintrobe's oxalate mixture (the anticoagulant commonly used for hematological estimations) as this mixture contains ammonia, which will interfere with some chemical estimations. If the test is to be performed on serum, then the specimen is collected in the same manner as for a Wassermann reaction. It is important to avoid hemolysis in the collection of the blood. Remove any alcohol with which the skin has been rubbed. The syringe and needle may be washed with sterile normal saline but not with water before venipuncture. Remove the needle from the syringe before transferring the blood to the container, so as to prevent the red cells being broken up. The oxalate bottle is to be gently inverted several times, not vigorously shaken. If the test for blood sugar cannot be done for some hours, and especially in the case of specimens sent by mail, much of the sugar disappears (glycolysis). In order to obviate this fallacy, sodium fluoride (a mass of the dry powder the size of a pea) is added to the blood. This prevents both clotting and glycolysis, and will preserve the sugar in the blood for a week.

Basal Metabolic Rate (B.M.R.).—The only details which the nurse needs to know about this test are that the patient must be given no breakfast on the morning of the test, and that a "preliminary test" is done on the preceding day. The sole object of the latter is to accustom the patient to the procedure, which may otherwise excite him unduly and thus send up the basal metabolic rate. No breakfast is given, because the biochemical activity needed to digest a meal is sufficient to raise the B.M.R.

Cerebrospinal Fluid.—Examination of the spinal fluid is most commonly done for suspected meningitis. The tube in which the fluid is collected must therefore be sterile. There is always a danger that the tube may be broken or upset, the fluid running into the cotton-wool plug; in either case the patient has to undergo the discomfort and pain of a second lumbar puncture. It is therefore better to collect the fluid in a small, strong, flat-bottomed sterile bottle. A similar precaution may well be observed in the collection of urine from both ureters, a procedure which requires the passage of a cystoscope into the bladder and is attended by great discomfort to the patient.

Surgical Tissues.—All tissues removed in the operating room are placed in a 10 per cent solution of formalin, which acts as a "fixative" and prevents decomposition. In the case of some tissues, such as tonsils, a bacteriological examination is required. When this is ordered, the specimen must on no account be put into formalin, otherwise all the bacteria will be killed. The specimen is merely placed in a sterile tube or bottle, and sent as soon as possible to the laboratory.

Collection of Drinking Water for Bacteriological Examination.—A nurse doing public health work in the country may be called upon to collect water for this purpose. Obtain glass sample bottles sterilized in an autoclave by the laboratory doing the bacteriological examination. Fill one with a representative sample from the well, spring, reservoir, or lake used for drinking purposes. The sample should be labelled with the location of the source and the date and hour taken. It should reach the laboratory within six hours and should be kept at refrigeration temperature during transit. All samples containing more than 500 bacteria per cc. of water are undrinkable, but much depends on the type of bacteria. Bacillus coli suggest contamination with feces which may contain typhoid or dysentery bacilli.

Bacteriological Examination of Milk.—The unopened milk bottle should be handed over to the laboratory as soon as possible after it is received and packed in ice during the interval, which should not be more than four hours. If a longer time is required, record it.

Milk having less than 50,000 bacteria per cc. is graded as good. Poor grades of milk may have 500,000 bacteria per cc. and be drunk without apparent harm. All depends on whether the bacteria are Bacillus coli from uncleanliness, tubercle bacilli, typhoid, virulent streptococci, diphtheria, or Brucella abortus. The same type of examination can be applied to ice-cream.

In cases of food poisoning, samples of all suspected food should be wrapped in sterile sheets or if these are not available use fresh clean wrapping paper. Then pack in ice and dispatch immediately to the laboratory.

INDEX

A

ABSCESS, 59
  cold, 277
  of bone, 275
  of brain, 262
  of lung, 133
  psoas, 277
Acetone in urine, 184, 203
Acidosis, 183, 184
Acoustic nerve tumor, 271
Acromegaly, 237
ACTH, 234
Actinomycosis, 90
Acute anterior poliomyelitis, 265
  hemorrhagic pancreatitis, 181
  ulcerative endocarditis, 118
Addison's disease, 234
Adenocarcinoma, 109
Adenoma, 107
  of pituitary, 239
Adhesions, 57, 165
Adrenalin, 234
Adrenals, 233
  cortical tumors of, 235
  structure of, 233
Adrenogenital syndrome, 235
Agranulocytic angina, 254
Agranulocytosis, 254
Albuminuria, 191, 297
Allergy, 65
  food, 66
Amenorrhea, 208
Amœba histolytica, 173
Amœbic dysentery, 160, 173
  treatment of, 161
Anaerobic bacteria, 86
Anemia, 30, 151, 246
  hyperchromic, 248
  macrocytic, 248
  pernicious, 246
  primary hypochromic, 250
  secondary, 250
Aneurism, aortic, 121
Angina pectoris, 119
Angioma, 108
Animal parasites, 26, 95
Anisocytosis, 248
Ankylostoma duodenale, 98
Anthracosis, 139
Anthrax, 84
Antibiotics, 290
Antigens, 80, 244
Antitoxins, 57, 64
Aortic aneurism, 121
  incompetence, 116
Aphasia, 260
Apoplexy, 260
Appendicitis, 162

Argyll-Robertson pupil, 269
Arterial hypertension, 120
Arteries, diseases of, 125
  arteritis, 126
Arteriosclerosis, 41, 47, 125, 191
Arthritis, gonorrheal, 280
  rheumatoid, 279
Asbestosis, 139
Ascaris lumbricoides, 98, 172
Aschheim-Zondek test, 215, 232
Ascites, 176
Asthma, 66
Atelectasis, 142
  congenital, 142
Atheroma, 47, 125
Athlete's foot, 90
Auricular fibrillation, 117, 122
Avitaminosis, 31

B

BACILLARY dysentery, 161
Bacilli, 67
  anaerobic, 86
  botulinus, 88
  coli, 155
  diphtheria, 71
  dysenteriæ, 160
  pestis, 84
  tetani, 87
  tubercle, 73
  typhosus, 155
  welchii, 86
Bacteria, 29, 67
Basal metabolic rate, 299
Beri-beri, 32
Biliary calculi, 178
Bladder, 188
  carcinoma of, 199
Blastomycosis, 90
Blood, 241
  chemistry, 298
  grouping, 244
  in urine, 204
  matching, 244
  transfusion, 243
Boil, 59
Bone, abscess of, 273
  giant cell tumor, 280
  sarcoma of, 281
  secondary tumors, 281
  tuberculosis of, 276
  tumors of, 280
Botulism, 88
Brain, abscess of, 262
  tumors of, 279
Breast, cancer of, 220
  fibroadenoma of, 220
  lobular hyperplasia, 219

(300)